MRI of the Knee

Editor

KIRKLAND W. DAVIS

MAGNETIC RESONANCE IMAGING CLINICS OF NORTH AMERICA

www.mri.theclinics.com

Consulting Editors
SURESH K. MUKHERJI
LYNNE S. STEINBACH

November 2014 • Volume 22 • Number 4

ELSEVIER

1600 John F. Kennedy Boulevard • Suite 1800 • Philadelphia, Pennsylvania, 19103-2899

http://www.mri.theclinics.com

MRI CLINICS OF NORTH AMERICA Volume 22, Number 4
November 2014 ISSN 1064-9689, ISBN 13: 978-0-323-32379-6

Editor: John Vassallo (j.vassallo@elsevier.com)
Developmental Editor: Yonah Korngold

Magnetic Resonance Imaging Clinics of North America (ISSN 1064-9689) is published quarterly by Elsevier Inc., 360 Park Avenue South, New York, NY 10010-1710. Months of issue are February, May, August, and November. Business and Editorial Offices: 1600 John F. Kennedy Blvd., Ste. 1800, Philadelphia, PA 19103-2899. Customer Service Office: 3251 Riverport Lane, Maryland Heights, MO 63043. Periodicals postage paid at New York, NY and additional mailing offices. Subscription prices are $375.00 per year (domestic individuals), $581.00 per year (domestic institutions), $190.00 per year (domestic students/residents), $420.00 per year (Canadian individuals), $755.00 per year (Canadian institutions), $545.00 per year (international individuals), $755.00 per year (international institutions), and $275.00 per year (international and Canadian students/residents). International air speed delivery is included in all *Clinics* subscription prices. All prices are subject to change without notice. **POSTMASTER:** Send address changes to *Magnetic Resonance Imaging Clinics*, Elsevier Health Sciences Division, Subscription Customer Service, 3251 Riverport Lane, Maryland Heights, MO 63043. Customer Service (orders, claims, online, change of address): Elsevier Health Sciences Division, Subscription Customer Service, 3251 Riverport Lane, Maryland Heights, MO 63043. Tel:1-800-654-2452 (U.S. and Canada); 314-447-8871 (outside U.S. and Canada). Fax: 314-447-8029. E-mail: journalscustomerservice-usa@elsevier.com (for print support); journalsonlinesupport-usa@elsevier.com (for online support).

Reprints. For copies of 100 or more of articles in this publication, please contact the Commercial Reprints Department, Elsevier Inc., 360 Park Avenue South, New York, NY 10010-1710. Tel.: 212-633-3874; Fax: 212-633-3820; E-mail: reprints@elsevier.com.

Magnetic Resonance Imaging Clinics of North America is covered in the *RSNA Index of Imaging Literature, MEDLINE/PubMed (Index Medicus),* and *EMBASE/Excerpta Medica.*

Printed in the United States of America.

Contributors

CONSULTING EDITORS

SURESH K. MUKHERJI, MD, MBA, FACR
Professor and Chairman; W.F. Patenge
Endowed Chair, Department of Radiology,
Michigan State University, East Lansing,
Michigan

LYNNE S. STEINBACH, MD, FACR
Professor of Clinical Radiology and
Orthopaedic Surgery, Department of
Radiology and Biomedical Imaging, University
of California San Francisco, San Francisco,
California

EDITOR

KIRKLAND W. DAVIS, MD
Professor of Radiology; Section Chief,
Musculoskeletal Imaging and Intervention,
Department of Musculoskeletal Radiology,
University of Wisconsin School of Medicine
and Public Health, Madison, Wisconsin

AUTHORS

WON C. BAE, PhD
Assistant Professor, Department of Radiology,
University of California San Diego Medical
Center, San Diego, California

STEPHANIE A. BERNARD, MD
Associate Professor, Department of Radiology,
Penn State Milton S. Hershey Medical Center,
Hershey, Pennsylvania

ROBERT DOWNEY BOUTIN, MD
Clinical Professor, Department of Radiology,
School of Medicine, University of California,
Davis, Sacramento, California

PAMELA S. BRIAN, MD
Assistant Professor, Department of Radiology,
Penn State Milton S. Hershey Medical Center,
Hershey, Pennsylvania

ERIC Y. CHANG, MD
Assistant Clinical Professor, Radiology
Service, VA San Diego Healthcare System;
Department of Radiology, University of
California San Diego Medical Center, San
Diego, California

RAJEEV CHAUDHARY, BS
Graduate Student Research Assistant,
Department of Radiology, University of
Wisconsin School of Medicine and Public
Health, Madison, Wisconsin

KAREN C. CHEN, MD
Department of Radiology, VA San Diego
Healthcare System; Department of Radiology,
University of California San Diego Medical
Center, San Diego, California

CHRISTINE B. CHUNG, MD
Professor, Radiology Service, VA San Diego
Healthcare System; Department of Radiology,
University of California San Diego Medical
Center, San Diego, California

KIRKLAND W. DAVIS, MD
Professor of Radiology; Section Chief,
Musculoskeletal Imaging and Intervention,
Department of Musculoskeletal Radiology,
University of Wisconsin School of Medicine
and Public Health, Madison, Wisconsin

QIAN DONG, MD
Associate Professor, Department of Radiology,
University of Michigan, Ann Arbor, Michigan

DONALD J. FLEMMING, MD
Professor of Radiology and Orthopedics,
Department of Radiology, Penn State Milton
S. Hershey Medical Center, Hershey,
Pennsylvania

MICHAEL C. FORNEY, MD
Section of Musculoskeletal Imaging, Imaging
Institute, Cleveland Clinic, Cleveland, Ohio

RUSSELL C. FRITZ, MD
Medical Director, National Orthopedic Imaging
Associates, Greenbrae, California

GLENN GAVIOLA, MD
Musculoskeletal Radiologist, Department
of Musculoskeletal Radiology, Brigham and
Women's Hospital, Boston, Massachusetts

DANIEL GEIGER, MD
Radiologist, Department of Radiological,
Oncological and Pathological Sciences,
Sapienza University of Rome, Rome, Italy

KARA G. GILL, MD
Assistant Professor, Division of Pediatric
Radiology, Department of Radiology,
University of Wisconsin School of Medicine
and Public Health, Madison, Wisconsin

HIGOR GRANDO, MD
Department of Radiology, University of
California San Diego Medical Center,
San Diego, California; Department of
Radiology, Hospital do Coração (HCor) and
Teleimagem, São Paulo, Brazil

AMIT GUPTA, MD
Section of Musculoskeletal Imaging, Imaging
Institute, Cleveland Clinic, Cleveland, Ohio

THOMAS W. HASH II, MD
Assistant Professor, Department of Radiology,
Duke University Hospital, Durham, North
Carolina

JON A. JACOBSON, MD
Professor, Department of Radiology, University
of Michigan, Ann Arbor, Michigan

BHARTI KHURANA, MD
Emergency Radiologist, Department of
Emergency Radiology, Brigham and
Women's Hospital, Boston,
Massachusetts

RICHARD KIJOWSKI, MD
Professor, Department of Radiology, University
of Wisconsin School of Medicine and Public
Health, Madison, Wisconsin

RICHARD A. MARDER, MD
Chair and Professor of Orthopaedic Surgery;
Chief, Sports Medicine, Department of
Orthopaedics, University of California,
Davis, Sacramento, California

TOM MINAS, MD
Department of Orthopedic Surgery,
Cartilage Repair Center, Brigham and
Women's Hospital, Chestnut Hill,
Massachusetts

ALI NARAGHI, MD
Joint Department of Medical Imaging,
University Health Network, Mount Sinai
Hospital and Women's College Hospital,
University of Toronto; Department of Medical
Imaging, Toronto Western Hospital, Toronto,
Ontario, Canada

BLAISE A. NEMETH, MD, MS
Associate Professor, Department of
Orthopedics and Rehabilitation, University of
Wisconsin School of Medicine and Public
Health, Madison, Wisconsin

DEEPA PAI, MD
Assistant Professor, Department of
Radiology, University of Michigan,
Ann Arbor, Michigan

MINI N. PATHRIA, MD
Professor, Department of Radiology,
University of California-San Diego, San Diego,
California

HUMBERTO G. ROSAS, MD
Associate Professor, Department of Radiology,
University of Wisconsin School of Medicine
and Public Health, Madison, Wisconsin

SCOTT E. SHEEHAN, MD, MS
Musculoskeletal Radiologist, Department of
Musculoskeletal Radiology, University of
Wisconsin School of Medicine and Public
Health, Madison, Wisconsin

LAWRENCE M. WHITE, MD
Joint Department of Medical Imaging,
University Health Network, Mount Sinai
Hospital and Women's College Hospital,
University of Toronto; Department of Medical

Imaging, Toronto General Hospital, Toronto,
Ontario, Canada

CARL S. WINALSKI, MD
Section of Musculoskeletal Imaging, Imaging
Institute, Cleveland Clinic; Department of
Biomedical Engineering, Lerner Research
Institute, Cleveland Clinic, Cleveland, Ohio

CORRIE M. YABLON, MD
Assistant Professor, Department of Radiology,
University of Michigan, Ann Arbor, Michigan

Contents

> The treatment of meniscal tears has evolved secondary to a better understanding of the essential roles that the menisci play in the normal function of the knee, including load transmission, stress distribution, shock absorption, joint lubrication, resistance to capsular and synovial impingement, and maintenance of joint congruity. Imaging evaluation of the menisci requires an understanding of the normal anatomy, the imaging criteria necessary to accurately diagnose a meniscal tear, meniscal tear patterns, and awareness of common diagnostic pitfalls.

> Meniscus surgery is common, and surgical indications and techniques continue to evolve. After highlighting relevant anatomy and emerging magnetic resonance (MR) imaging techniques, this article reviews the current indications and techniques used for meniscus surgery, evaluates the use of MR imaging protocols with and without arthrography, and focuses on MR imaging interpretation of the postoperative meniscus, with particular attention to clinical outcomes and diagnostic criteria.

> Cruciate ligament injuries, and in particular injuries of the anterior cruciate ligament (ACL), are the most commonly reconstructed ligamentous injuries of the knee. As such, accurate preoperative diagnosis is essential in optimal management of patients with cruciate ligament injuries. This article reviews the anatomy and biomechanics of the ACL and posterior cruciate ligament (PCL) and describes the magnetic resonance (MR) imaging appearances of complete and partial tears. Normal postoperative appearances of ACL and PCL reconstructions as well as MR imaging features of postoperative complications will also be reviewed.

> Posterolateral (PLC) and posteromedial (PMC) corners of the knee represent complex anatomic regions because of intricate soft tissue and osseous relationships in small areas. Concise knowledge of these relationships is necessary before approaching their evaluation at imaging. Magnetic resonance imaging offers an

provides the radiologist with an overview of the surgical strategies for repairing cartilage lesions in the knee followed by a discussion of their postoperative appearance on MR imaging in normal and abnormal cases. Guidelines for adequate reporting of the MR imaging findings after cartilage repair in the knee are also included.

MAGNETIC RESONANCE IMAGING CLINICS OF NORTH AMERICA

FORTHCOMING ISSUES

February 2015
Updates in Cardiac MRI
Karen G. Ordovas, *Editor*

May 2015
Chest MRI
Prachi P. Agarwal, *Editor*

August 2015
MRI of the Elbow and Wrist
Kimberly K. Amrami, *Editor*

RECENT ISSUES

August 2014
Hepatobiliary Imaging
Peter S. Liu and Richard G. Abramson, *Editors*

May 2014
The Male Pelvis
Mukesh G. Harisinghani, *Editor*

February 2014
Bowel Imaging
Jordi Rimola, *Editor*

RELATED INTEREST

Radiologic Clinics of North America, May 2013 (Vol. 51, No. 3)
Imaging of the Lower Extremity
Kathryn J. Stevens, *Editor*

PROGRAM OBJECTIVE

The goal of *Magnetic Resonance Imaging Clinics of North America* is to keep practicing physicians up to date with current clinical practice by providing timely articles reviewing the state of the art in patient care.

TARGET AUDIENCE

All practicing physicians and healthcare professionals who provide patient care utilizing findings from Magnetic Resonance Imaging.

LEARNING OBJECTIVES

Upon completion of this activity, participants will be able to:
1. Review magnetic resonance imaging of the pediatric knee.
2. Discuss a biomechanical approach to interpreting MRI of knee injuries.
3. Review considerations in imaging the knee in the setting of metal hardware.

ACCREDITATION

The Elsevier Office of Continuing Medical Education (EOCME) is accredited by the Accreditation Council for Continuing Medical Education (ACCME) to provide continuing medical education for physicians.

The EOCME designates this enduring material for a maximum of 15 *AMA PRA Category 1 Credit*(s)™. Physicians should claim only the credit commensurate with the extent of their participation in the activity.

All other health care professionals requesting continuing education credit for this enduring material will be issued a certificate of participation.

DISCLOSURE OF CONFLICTS OF INTEREST

The EOCME assesses conflict of interest with its instructors, faculty, planners, and other individuals who are in a position to control the content of CME activities. All relevant conflicts of interest that are identified are thoroughly vetted by EOCME for fair balance, scientific objectivity, and patient care recommendations. EOCME is committed to providing its learners with CME activities that promote improvements or quality in healthcare and not a specific proprietary business or a commercial interest.

The planning committee, staff, authors and editors listed below have identified no financial relationships or relationships to products or devices they or their spouse/life partner have with commercial interest related to the content of this CME activity:

Won C. Bae, PhD; Stephanie A. Bernard, MD; Robert Downey Boutin, MD; Pamela S. Brian, MD; Eric Y. Chang, MD; Rajeev Chaudhary, BS; Karen C. Chen, MD; Christine B. Chung, MD; Kirkland W. Davis, MD; Qian Dong, MD; Michael C. Forney, MD; Russell C. Fritz, MD; Glenn Gaviola, MD; Daniel Geiger, MD; Kara G. Gill, MD; Higor Grando, MD; Amit Gupta, MD; Thomas W. Hash, II, MD; Kristen Helm; Brynne Hunter; Jon A. Jacobson, MD; Bharti Khurana, MD; Richard Kijowski, MD; Sandy Lavery; Richard A. Marder, MD; Jill McNair; Suresh K. Mukherji, MD; Ali Naraghi, MD; Blaise A. Nemeth, MD, MS; Deepa Pai, MD; Mini N. Pathria, MD; Humberto G. Rosas, MD; Scott E. Sheehan, MD, MS; Lynne S. Steinbach, MD, FACR; Karthikeyan Subramaniam; John Vassallo; Lawrence M. White, MD; Carl S. Winalski, MD; Corrie M. Yablon, MD.

The planning committee, staff, authors and editors listed below have identified financial relationships or relationships to products or devices they or their spouse/life partner have with commercial interest related to the content of this CME activity:

Donald J. Flemming, MD has royalties/patents with Elsevier BV.

Tom Minas, MD is on Speakers Bureau and is a consultant for The Sanofi Group; has stock ownership in ConforMIS, Inc.; has royalties, patents with Elsevier BV and ConforMIS, Inc.

Carl S. Winalski, MD both he and his spouse/partner have stock ownership with Pfizer, Inc.; and his spouse/partner has stock ownership with General Electric.

UNAPPROVED/OFF-LABEL USE DISCLOSURE

The EOCME requires CME faculty to disclose to the participants:
1. When products or procedures being discussed are off-label, unlabelled, experimental, and/or investigational (not US Food and Drug Administration (FDA) approved); and
2. Any limitations on the information presented, such as data that are preliminary or that represent ongoing research, interim analyses, and/or unsupported opinions. Faculty may discuss information about pharmaceutical agents that is outside of FDA-approved labelling. This information is intended solely for CME and is not intended to promote off-label use of these medications. If you have any questions, contact the medical affairs department of the manufacturer for the most recent prescribing information.

TO ENROLL

To enroll in the *Magnetic Resonance Imaging Clinics of North* Continuing Medical Education program, call customer service at 1-800-654-2452 or sign up online at http://www.theclinics.com/home/cme. The CME program is available to subscribers for an additional annual fee of $250 USD.

METHOD OF PARTICIPATION

In order to claim credit, participants must complete the following:

1. Complete enrolment as indicated above.
2. Read the activity.
3. Complete the CME Test and Evaluation. Participants must achieve a score of 70% on the test. All CME Tests and Evaluations must be completed online.

CME INQUIRIES/SPECIAL NEEDS

For all CME inquiries or special needs, please contact elsevierCME@elsevier.com.

Foreword
MRI of the Knee

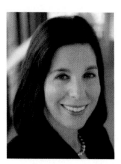

Lynne S. Steinbach, MD, FACR
Consulting Editor

This issue of *Magnetic Resonance Imaging Clinics of North America* focuses on the knee. Kirkland Davis, a Professor of Radiology and Section Chief in Musculoskeletal Imaging at the University of Wisconsin, has done a fantastic job of assembling some of the most accomplished North American musculoskeletal radiologists for this project. The esteemed authors are from highly regarded institutions that specialize in musculoskeletal MRI. State-of-the-art material is presented on important subjects with excellent figures, diagrams, and up-to-date references enhancing learning for even the most experienced radiologist. Although many of us feel comfortable reading knee MRIs, it is helpful to keep up with all of the new information regarding anatomy and pathology. The menisci, ligaments, and tendons along with the patellofemoral joint can be challenging to assess. When radiologists understand biomechanics, they become more adept at knowing what abnormalities to look for in the study. More and more we are imaging postoperative knees, and it is important to know about the surgery and what to expect after surgery along with the best way to image when there is metal in the mix. The cartilage is a very important structure to evaluate, and there are many different sequences that we can use for this assessment. We need to be accurate in our descriptions of cartilage abnormalities and postoperative cartilage assessment because cartilage repair is frequently performed. A volume such as this makes us more able to master this subject during our readouts. Bravo for a job well done!

Lynne S. Steinbach, MD, FACR
Department of Radiology and Biomedical Imaging
University of California San Francisco
505 Parnassus
San Francisco, CA 94143-0628, USA

E-mail address:
lynne.steinbach@ucsf.edu

Magn Reson Imaging Clin N Am 22 (2014) xiii
http://dx.doi.org/10.1016/j.mric.2014.08.003
1064-9689/14/$ – see front matter © 2014 Elsevier Inc. All rights reserved.

Preface
MR Imaging of the Knee

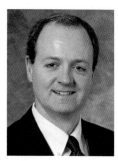

Kirkland W. Davis, MD
Editor

MR imaging has become an indispensable tool in the diagnosis of a wide range of knee pathology. Knee scans are among the most frequently performed in most MR suites, and the knee often is the first joint that residents feel comfortable interpreting. However, the knee mirrors the broader musculoskeletal system in that it is deceptively complex. It continues to present new challenges as our technology advances, our understanding of anatomy and biomechanics evolves, and our desire to investigate pathology in finer detail and in more challenging circumstances only increases.

This issue on MR Imaging of the Knee takes a fresh look at the basics of imaging the menisci, ligaments, and tendons; affords a comprehensive look at MR imaging in the pediatric knee; provides new perspectives on the biomechanics of knee injuries and assessment of knee arthritis and regional inflammatory conditions; summarizes the current thinking on MR imaging after surgery on the menisci and on articular cartilage; and addresses the latest and ongoing developments in assessing cartilage degradation as well as MR imaging in the setting of knee hardware. This all-star team of authors has produced a wonderful set of works, and I offer them my heartfelt thanks and gratitude. It is my hope and expectation that this issue will be a useful tool for the radiologist and nonradiologist alike and will provide new, helpful, and exciting information for all those interested in the knee, from trainee to expert. Moreover, I hope that all find this to be enjoyable reading.

Kirkland W. Davis, MD
Professor of Radiology
Section Chief, Musculoskeletal Imaging and
Intervention
University of Wisconsin School of Medicine
and Public Health
Madison, WI 53792, USA

E-mail address:
kdavis@uwhealth.org

Magn Reson Imaging Clin N Am 22 (2014) xv
http://dx.doi.org/10.1016/j.mric.2014.08.002
1064-9689/14/$ – see front matter © 2014 Elsevier Inc. All rights reserved.

CrossMark

Magnetic Resonance Imaging of the Meniscus

Humberto G. Rosas, MD

KEYWORDS

- Meniscus • Knee • Tear • Magnetic resonance imaging • MRI
- ISAKOS (International Society of Arthroscopy, Knee Surgery and Orthopaedic Sports Medicine)

KEY POINTS

- The magnetic resonance (MR) criteria for diagnosing a meniscal tear include either increased signal unequivocally contacting the articular surface or abnormal meniscal morphology in the absence of previous surgery.
- Accurate description of tear patterns is vital in guiding treatment options. The ISAKOS (International Society of Arthroscopy, Knee Surgery and Orthopaedic Sports Medicine) arthroscopic tear classification system includes longitudinal-vertical, horizontal, radial, vertical flap, horizontal flap, and complex.
- Displaced tears may be overlooked on MR imaging and should be sought in the recesses, the posterior intercondylar notch, and popliteal hiatus in the setting of a blunted meniscus.
- Secondary signs may accompany meniscal tears and increase diagnostic confidence. The indirect signs with the highest positive predictive value include parameniscal cysts, linear subchondral edema, and meniscal extrusion.

INTRODUCTION

Arthroscopic partial meniscectomy is the most common orthopedic surgery performed in the United States.[1] Perspectives on the function of the menisci, biomechanical effects after meniscectomy, and treatment algorithms continue to evolve, placing a greater emphasis on meniscal preservation and outcome measures. The potential deleterious effects of surgery have been known for some time: the landmark study in 1948 by Fairbank[2] recognized that "meniscectomy is not wholly innocuous…" in the sentinel article recognizing the chronic maladaptive changes after a meniscectomy. More recently, studies[1] have shown no difference in long-term improvement between patients undergoing partial meniscectomies and a sham procedure in the treatment of degenerative meniscal tears. In addition, symptomatic patients with meniscal tears and underlying chondrosis showed no difference in functional status when comparing surgery versus physical therapy alone.[3]

Since its inception into clinical practice in the 1980s, magnetic resonance (MR) has become the preferred imaging method for evaluating the meniscus, with reported accuracies, sensitivities, and specificities ranging between 85% and 95% in detecting meniscal tears.[4] Given the evolving treatment strategies, one must not only identify a tear but describe the location, extent, tear pattern, and any associated chondrosis to guide treatment options. The International Society of Arthroscopy, Knee Surgery and Orthopaedic Sports Medicine (ISAKOS) Knee Committee formed a Meniscal Documentation Subcommittee in 2006, with the objective of developing a reliable classification system in the evaluation of the meniscus to

Disclosure: none.
Department of Radiology, University of Wisconsin School of Medicine and Public Health, 600 Highland Avenue, Madison, WI 53792-3252, USA
E-mail address: hrosas@uwhealth.org

Magn Reson Imaging Clin N Am 22 (2014) 493–516
http://dx.doi.org/10.1016/j.mric.2014.07.002
1064-9689/14/$ – see front matter © 2014 Elsevier Inc. All rights reserved.

facilitate outcome assessment. The tear patterns in this classification system include longitudinal-vertical, horizontal, radial, vertical flap, horizontal flap, and complex.[5]

Therefore, the role of MR imaging has expanded to be not only a simple diagnostic study but a critical decision-making tool providing information that may not only alter the surgical technique but also provide information that would obviate surgery. This review focuses on normal anatomy, technical factors involved when imaging the meniscus, the imaging criteria for diagnosing meniscal tears, the imaging appearance of the various patterns of meniscal tears, secondary signs of meniscal injury, and common diagnostic pitfalls.

ANATOMY

The shape and composition of the menisci confer an ability to absorb shock, distribute axial load, assist in joint lubrication, and maintain joint congruity in extremes of flexion and extension.[6] The semilunar, triangular, fibrocartilaginous menisci are C-shaped, with a concave surface tapered centrally, conforming to the morphology of the femoral condyle, and a flat base attached to the condylar surface of the tibia via the anterior and posterior root ligaments (**Fig. 1**). The intimate

anatomic relationship and contiguous fibers between the anterior root ligament of the lateral meniscus and anterior cruciate ligament (ACL) insertion site result in a striated or comblike appearance, which can be mistaken for a meniscal tear (**Fig. 2**).[7] Although rarely identified on MR, a similar connection between the ACL and medial meniscus through the meniscocruciate ligament has been noted in several anatomic studies.[8] A common variant of the anterior root of the medial meniscus is an insertion along the far anterior margin of the tibia, giving the false impression of extrusion or pathologic subluxation (**Fig. 3**).[9] The typical meniscal tibial attachment sites and their relationship with the cruciate ligaments are shown in **Figs. 1** and **2**.

The configuration of 3 distinct layers of collagen within the meniscus and formation of collagen bundles oriented along both the long and short axes of the menisci allow for efficient load transmission and shock absorption. The longitudinal fibers are circumferentially oriented, resulting in the ability of the meniscus to distribute axial loads and provide what is commonly referred to as hoop strength. The more loosely organized radial fibers help form a lattice and act to tie the longitudinal bundles together and resist forces that would lead to longitudinal splitting of the meniscus (**Fig. 4**).[10]

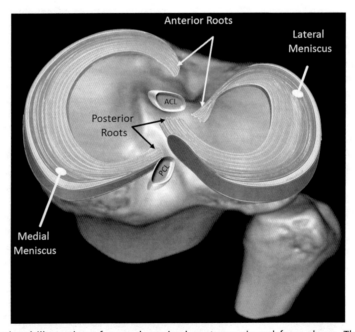

Fig. 1. Three-dimensional illustration of normal meniscal anatomy, viewed from above. The concave superior surface conforms to the morphology of the femoral condyles and results in increased contact area. The root ligaments attach centrally close to the cruciate ligaments. Although larger, the medial meniscus covers a smaller percentage of the articular surface of the tibia (50% compared with 70% for the lateral meniscus). ACL, anterior cruciate ligament; PCL, posterior cruciate ligament.

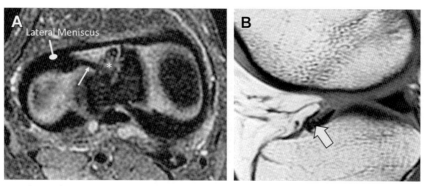

Fig. 2. (*A*) Axial MRI reconstruction showing contiguous fibers (*arrow*) between the lateral meniscus and the ACL (*asterisk*). (*B*) This anatomic relationship results in the striated appearance typically seen in this region on sagittal images (*block arrow*).

Each meniscus can be divided into thirds: an anterior horn, body, and posterior horn. The shape of the meniscus can be described best as an elongated semilunar triangle, with a concave hypotenuse and tapered ends. The result is a cross-sectional appearance, resembling either a slab or triangle, based on the orientation of the imaging plane in respect to the axis of the meniscus. The menisci resembles a triangle when imaged perpendicular to the free edge or long axis of the meniscus, such as sagittal images through the horns or coronal images through the body. The menisci takes on a more slab or bow tie configuration if the imaging plane parallels the long axis of the meniscus (eg, sagittal images through the body or coronal images through the horns).

Despite the similarities, the medial and lateral menisci are distinctly different. The larger, more open C-shaped medial meniscus increases in width from anterior to posterior, resulting in a larger posterior horn compared with the anterior horn

when viewed in cross section. The more circular lateral meniscus maintains a relatively constant width, resulting in the anterior and posterior horns being nearly equal in size in cross section (**Fig. 5**). Peripherally, the menisci are anchored to the fibrous capsule, with the medial meniscus firmly attached to the deep fibers of the medial collateral ligament, limiting its mobility and presumably leading to an increased susceptibility to injury compared with the more mobile lateral meniscus.[6,11] The popliteomeniscal fascicles arise from the periphery of the posterior horn of the lateral meniscus and form a posterolateral meniscocapsular extension, which creates the popliteus hiatus. The fascicles not only form the hiatus, which allows the popliteus tendon an avenue to course intra-articularly and maintain the integrity of the joint, but stabilize and control the motion of the posterior horn.[12] On MR imaging, the anteroinferior and posterosuperior fascicles are visualized in approximately 90% of knee examinations and best

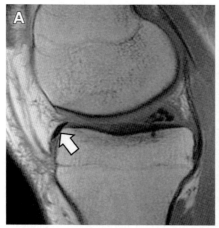
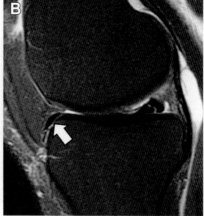

Fig. 3. Sagittal proton density (*A*) and fat-suppressed T2 (*B*) images showing a far anterior attachment of the anterior root of the medial meniscus (*arrow*), giving the false impression of extrusion or pathologic subluxation.

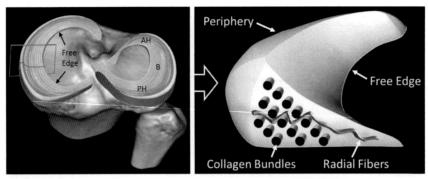

Fig. 4. Three-dimensional illustrations of normal meniscal anatomy. The meniscus typically is divided into thirds: the anterior horn (AH), body (B), and posterior horn (PH). The circumferential collagen fibers connect the anterior and posterior portions of the menisci and provide hoop strength, resulting in the ability to distribute axial loads. These fibers are more concentrated along the periphery of the menisci. Radial fibers form a lattice and act to tie the longitudinal fibers together, coursing and connecting the peripheral portion of the meniscus to the free edge.

visualized on the sagittal fluid-sensitive sequences (**Fig. 6**).[13] Tearing of the posterosuperior fascicle is highly associated with tears of the posterior horn of the lateral meniscus, with a sensitivity, specificity, and positive predictive value of 89%, 96%, and 79% respectively.[14,15]

Other normal anatomic structures and anatomic variants that can mimic a tear if not recognized include the meniscofemoral ligaments, oblique meniscomeniscal ligament, and the transverse meniscal ligament. The most commonly described meniscofemoral ligaments originate from the posterior horn of the lateral meniscus and insert onto the lateral aspect of the posterior medial femoral condyle, with the ligament of Humphry (**Fig. 7**) coursing anterior to the genu of the posterior cruciate ligament (PCL) and the ligament of Wrisberg traveling behind the genu of the PCL.[16,17] One potential pitfall occurs when a peripheral longitudinal tear is confused for a far lateral insertion of the meniscofemoral ligament. As a general rule, the attachment of the meniscofemoral ligaments to the posterior horn of the lateral meniscus should not extend greater than 14 mm beyond the lateral border of the PCL.[18] Therefore, if the meniscofemoral ligament is identified on 4 or more sequential sagittal MR images beyond the PCL, a peripheral longitudinal tear should be suspected and reported as such. The lesser known and extremely uncommon anterior meniscofemoral ligament connects the anterior horn of the medial meniscus to the roof of the intercondylar notch and lies parallel and posterior to the ligamentum mucosum (**Fig. 8**).[19] This variant should not be confused for a displaced meniscal fragment.

The oblique meniscomeniscal ligament attaches the anterior horn of 1 meniscus to the posterior horn of the contralateral meniscus, coursing through the intercondylar notch between the cruciate ligaments. Present in 1% to 4% of knees, this structure should not be mistaken for a bucket handle meniscal tear.[20]

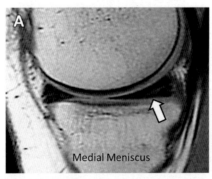

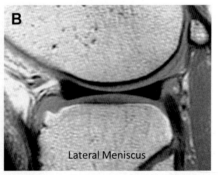

Fig. 5. Sagittal proton density images through the menisci (A, B) show the normal anatomy of the meniscal horns, with the posterior horn of the medial meniscus (A, arrow) being larger than the anterior horn. Laterally (B), the horns are nearly equal in size in cross section, because the lateral meniscus maintains a relatively constant width.

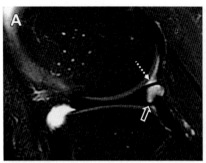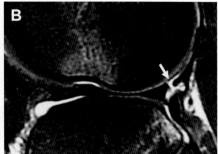

Fig. 6. Popliteomeniscal fascicles. (*A*) The posterosuperior popliteomeniscal fascicle (*dashed arrow*) forms the roof of the popliteus hiatus, extending from the posterosuperior margin of the lateral meniscus to the posterior capsule. The anteroinferior popliteomeniscal fascicle (*block arrow*) is a coronary ligament, which forms the floor of the popliteus hiatus. (*B*) Tear of the posterosuperior fascicle (*arrow*) is highly associated with tears involving the posterior horn of the lateral meniscus, as was confirmed surgically in this case.

The anterior transverse meniscal (geniculate) ligament typically connects the anterior horns of the menisci, although variations in its attachment exist. This structure is identified in 90% of dissections and 83% of MR examinations and can simulate an anterior root tear (**Fig. 9**).[21,22]

Recognizing and localizing each of these normal anatomic structures on serial images prevent inadvertently reporting a tear.

MR APPEARANCE OF MENISCAL TEARS: CRITERIA, DISTRIBUTION, AND TECHNICAL FACTORS

MR is an established imaging method for the diagnosis of meniscal injuries, showing high diagnostic accuracy. A 2003 meta-analysis of 29 publications between 1991 and 2000[4] reported a pooled sensitivity and specificity of 93.3% and 88.4% for medial meniscal tears and 79.3% and 95.7% for lateral meniscal tears.

Normally, the menisci show low signal intensity on all imaging sequences. In certain circumstances, increased intrameniscal signal can be observed either secondary to increased vascularity in children, mucoid degeneration in adults, or after trauma resulting in a meniscal contusion, all of which lack the characteristic imaging features of a tear. The MR criteria for diagnosing meniscal tears in the absence of previous surgery include either increased intrasubstance signal unequivocally contacting the articular surface or meniscal distortion, such as alterations in the shape or size of the meniscus.[23,24] If these criteria are present on 2 or more images, thereby fulfilling the 2-touch slice rule, the specificity increases, with reported positive predictive values of 94% and 96%, respectively, for medial and lateral meniscal tears, and should be reported as a torn

meniscus.[25] A common misconception is that the findings must be identified on contiguous slices when if either meniscal distortion or intrameniscal signal contacting the articular surface is seen in the same region on any 2 MR images, including consecutive slices, or alternatively on 1 coronal and 1 sagittal image, the criteria have been met. If the findings are seen solely on a single image, the positive predictive value decreases to 43% and 18% for medial and lateral meniscal tears, respectively, and should be described as a possible tear. Signal confined to the substance of the meniscus without definitive extension to the articular surface, even signal characterized as possibly contacting the surface, has been shown to be no more likely to represent a tear than a meniscus with no internal signal.[26]

Most tears involve the posterior horn of the meniscus, more frequently occurring in the more constrained medial meniscus. This distribution accounts for the fact that most tears are best visualized on sagittal sequences. However, the coronal sequences not only act as a supplement and cross-reference but have been shown to be superior to the sagittal images in depicting certain tears, including root tears, most displaced/bucket handle tears, and tears involving the meniscal body.[9,27] More recently, studies have advocated for the use of thin axial sequences through the meniscus to improve accuracy, description, and detection of small radial tears, displaced tears, and peripheral tears of the lateral meniscus.[28]

Tears isolated to the anterior horn of the meniscus are uncommon and should be diagnosed with caution, because they comprise 2% all medial meniscal and 16% of all lateral meniscal tears.[25] In the setting of an ACL tear, there is an increased incidence of peripheral longitudinal-vertical tears, with diminished sensitivities for the

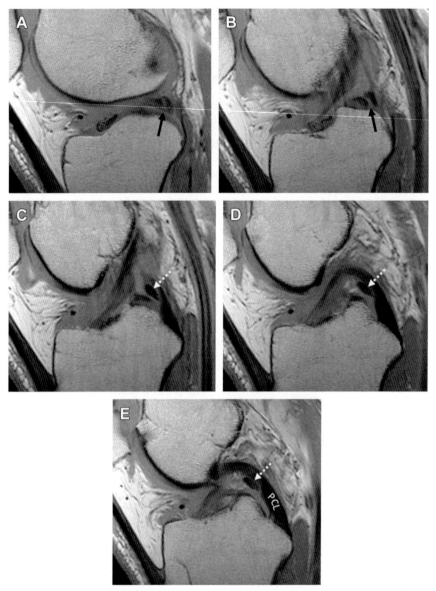

Fig. 7. Serial sagittal proton density images (*A–E*) from lateral to medial showing the course of the ligament of Humphry (*C–E, dashed arrow*) from the posterior horn of the lateral meniscus traveling anterior to the genu of the posterior cruciate ligament (PCL) en route to the femoral condyle. The meniscofemoral ligaments may mimic a peripheral vertical longitudinal tear (*A, B, black arrow*), but can be differentiated by following these structures on serial images (*A–E*).

detection of tears on both clinical examination and imaging interpretation, particularly tears involving the posterior horn of the lateral meniscus.[29] One must be cognizant of the typical distribution of meniscal tears and association with ligamentous injuries.

Although optimization of scanning parameters and protocols is beyond the scope of this review, the ability to detect meniscal tears is improved with high spatial resolution. Measures such as maximizing matrix size and maintaining a small field of view and slice thickness increase spatial resolution. Typical parameters required to achieve adequate resolution include a field of view 16 cm or less, a matrix size of at least 192 (phase-encoding direction) x 256 (frequency-encoding direction), and a slice thickness no greater than 3 to 4 mm.[30,31] These modifications come at a cost to signal-to-noise ratio, which can be preserved by using high field strength magnets ($\geq$1.5 T),

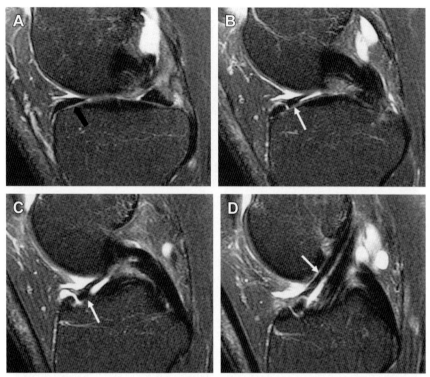

Fig. 8. Rare anterior meniscofemoral ligament (*B–D, white arrow*) connecting the anterior horn of the medial meniscus (*A, black arrow*) to the roof of the intercondylar notch as seen on serial sagittal T2-weighted sequences (*A–D*).

increasing the number of acquisitions, and using dedicated high-performance extremity gradient coils.[32,33]

As a general rule, meniscal tears are typically best delineated on short echo time sequences, such as T1-weighted or proton density sequences.[34,35] This factor is postulated to be a result of shorter T2 relaxation time from bound hydrogen nuclei to macromolecules within the tear.[36] As with any rule, there are exceptions, one of which includes evaluation of the meniscal roots, in which fluid-sensitive sequences have been shown to result in higher diagnostic accuracies. Therefore, when assessing for a meniscal tear, it is imperative to evaluate all imaging sequences.

As our understanding of both the function of the menisci and deleterious long-term biomechanical effects after meniscetomy increases, both surgical and nonsurgical treatments continue to evolve, placing a greater emphasis on meniscal preservation to maintain normal knee physiology and reduce the potential for accelerated degenerative changes. This situation places an even greater role on the imaging assessment of internal derangement and the necessity for a standardized classification system.

MENISCAL TEAR CLASSIFICATION

Treatment options and surgical techniques vary considerably based on several factors, including meniscal tear pattern. Longitudinal tears are often amenable to repair, whereas horizontal tears and partial radial tears typically require debridement.[37] Therefore, it is critical to not only diagnose a meniscal tear but to provide an accurate morphologic description to guide treatment options and assess long-term outcome measures. The ISAKOS arthroscopic meniscal tear classification system includes longitudinal-vertical, horizontal, radial, vertical flap, horizontal flap, and complex. This system can be adapted for use when interpreting imaging studies, as detailed later.

Longitudinal-Vertical Tears

A longitudinal-vertical tear courses parallel to the long axis of the meniscus and perpendicular to the tibial plateau and can involve a single articular surface or both articular surfaces, separating the meniscus into inner and outer segments (**Figs. 10–12**). Peripheral longitudinal-vertical tears involving the posterior horn of the lateral meniscus are often difficult to identify because of the

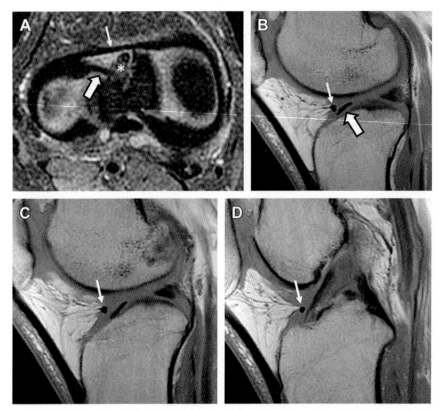

Fig. 9. Axial reconstructed MR image (*A*) and sagittal proton density images (*B–D*) show the anterior transverse meniscal ligament (*white arrow*) connecting the anterior horns of the medial and lateral meniscus coursing anterior to the ACL (*asterisk*). Because the ligament branches from the anterior root (*black outlined arrow*) of the lateral meniscus (best seen in *A* and *B*), one could mistake this structure for a meniscal tear or meniscal fragment if not followed on serial images.

complex anatomy and posterior attachments of the meniscus. As discussed in the anatomy section, disruption of the posterosuperior popliteomeniscal fascicle has a high positive predictive value for arthroscopically confirmed tears of the posterior horn of the lateral meniscus, and a far lateral meniscofemoral ligament attachment exceeding 14 mm beyond the lateral border of the PCL likely represents a tear. In our experience, this type of tear can be more conspicuous on sagittal T2-weighted images. Unlike horizontal or radial tears, pure longitudinal-vertical tears do not involve the free edge of the meniscus. Several normal anatomic structures may mimic a longitudinal-vertical tear, including the popliteus tendon as it courses intra-articularly; the attachment sites of the popliteomeniscal fascicles, transverse ligament, and meniscofemoral ligaments; and the normal striated appearance of the anterior root ligament of the lateral meniscus formed from fibers originating from the ACL.[25,38–40]

Longitudinal-vertical tears are typically seen in younger patients after trauma and are highly associated with tears of the ACL.[41] This relationship is so strong that 90% of medial and 83% of lateral peripheral longitudinal-vertical tears occur in the setting of an ACL injury. The propensity of these types of tears to heal or be amenable to repair is related to the more robust vascular supply from the capillary plexus to the outer 10% to 25% of the meniscus, the most common location of a longitudinal-vertical tear.[42] A recent study[43] confirmed that peripheral longitudinal-vertical tears closer to the meniscocapsular junction were more likely to heal, and that the presence of low T2 signal intensity strands coursing across the tear and lack of visualization of the tear on fluid-sensitive sequences were highly predictive of tears that would go on to heal. The study also showed that tears wider than 2 mm with central fluid signal were unlikely to heal.

A bucket handle tear represents a longitudinal-vertical tear with central migration of the inner handle segment and is the most frequent type of displaced tear (**Fig. 13**). Several imaging findings have been described with this type of meniscal

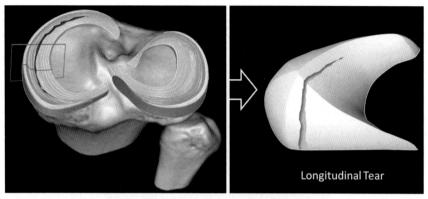

Fig. 10. Three-dimensional and cross-sectional illustrations of a longitudinal-vertical tear extending to both articular surfaces, coursing parallel to the long axis of the meniscus and separating the meniscus into central and peripheral segments. This type of tear characteristically remains equidistant from the inner and outer margins and therefore should not involve the free edge.

injury, including the absent bow tie sign, double PCL sign, double anterior horn or flipped meniscus sign, and fragment within the intercondylar notch sign (**Fig. 14**).[44–46]

The absent bow tie sign is based on the typical appearance of the meniscal body resembling a slab or bow tie on at least 2 successive sagittal images. If a portion of the meniscal body is displaced

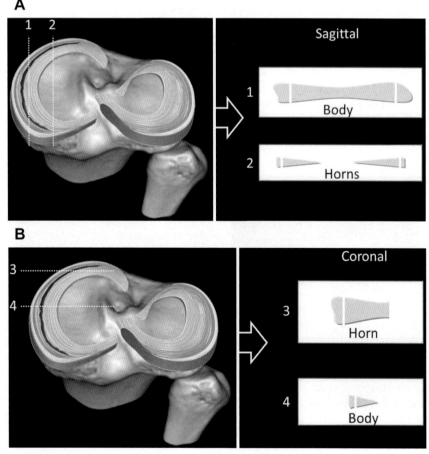

Fig. 11. Three-dimensional renderings of longitudinal-vertical tears, with the insets showing the typical MR imaging appearance in cross section in the sagittal (*A*) and coronal (*B*) planes.

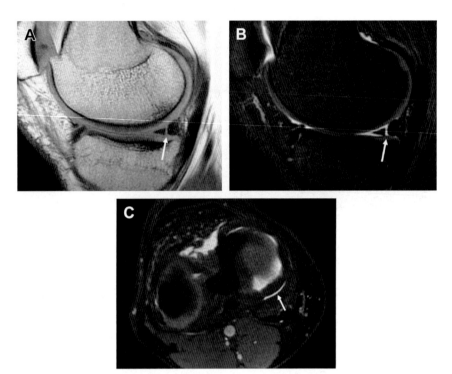

Fig. 12. Sagittal proton density (*A*) and T2 fat-suppressed (*B*) MR images showing vertically oriented increased signal intensity contacting both articular surfaces of the posterior horn of the medial meniscus (*arrrows*) consistent with a complete longitudinal-vertical tear. The axial reconstructed image (*C*) shows how this type of injury parallels the long axis of the meniscus (*arrow*), maintaining the same distance from the periphery.

and therefore blunted, the result is either lack of visualization of the body or visualization reduced to a single slice on the sagittal sequences. However, this finding is not reserved solely to bucket

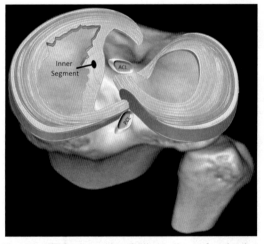

Fig. 13. Three-dimensional illustration of a bucket handle tear. Typically beginning as a longitudinal-vertical tear, the inner segment migrates and displaces centrally. Patients may present with mechanical symptoms, such as locking and catching.

handle tears and can be seen with radial tears of the body of the meniscus, previous partial meniscectomy, a macerated meniscus secondary to severe underlying degenerative changes, or younger patients with naturally smaller menisci. The double PCL sign refers to the migration of the central fragment into the intercondylar notch anterior to and paralleling the PCL. The double anterior horn sign describes the scenario in which a meniscal fragment is located immediately posterior to the native anterior horn with a truncated appearing posterior horn. Although these signs are sensitive, they are not specific and should be used to increase confidence in the diagnosis when considering a bucket handle tear.

Horizontal Tears

A horizontal tear classically involves either the free edge or one of the articular surfaces and propagates peripherally, thereby separating the meniscus into upper and lower halves (**Figs. 15–17**). Meniscal cyst formation is associated with tears that extend to the peripheral rim, presumably secondary to joint fluid permeating through the leaves of the tear (**Fig. 18**). If identified on MR imaging, this indirect sign has a positive predictive value of greater than 90% for arthroscopically confirmed meniscal

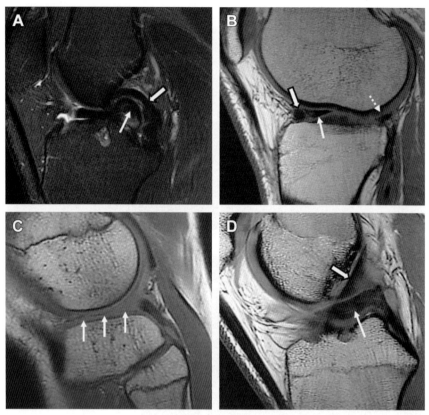

Fig. 14. Bucket handle tears. (*A*) Sagittal fat-suppressed T2 image shows the double PCL sign, with a centrally displaced meniscal fragment (*arrow*) from the medial meniscal located anterior and parallel to the PCL (*block arrow*). (*B*) Sagittal proton density image depicts the double anterior horn sign with a flipped meniscal fragment (*arrow*) posterior to and deforming the native anterior horn of the lateral meniscus (*block arrow*) associated with a truncated posterior horn (*dashed arrow*). (*C*) On this far lateral sagittal proton density image, the absent bow tie sign describes lack of visualization of the meniscal body (*arrows*). (*D*) Fragment within the intercondylar notch (*arrow*) eccentric to the PCL as the intact ACL (*block arrow*) impedes further central migration of the fragment to the level of the PCL on this midsagittal proton density image.

tear, except alongside the anterior horn of the lateral meniscus.[47] Parameniscal cysts located alongside the anterior horn of the lateral meniscus have been shown to have underlying tears in only 64% of cases. Unlike longitudinal tears, horizontal tears are usually degenerative, without an inciting traumatic event and typically are seen in patients older than 40 years.[34] Treatment often requires

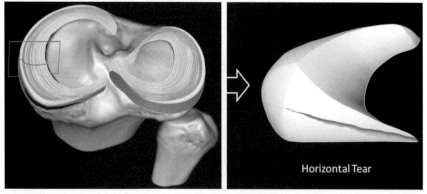

Fig. 15. Three-dimensional and cross-sectional illustrations of a horizontal tear involving the free edge and dividing the meniscus into upper and lower halves. The circumferential longitudinal fibers are typically spared with this type of injury, because the tear courses between the bundles.

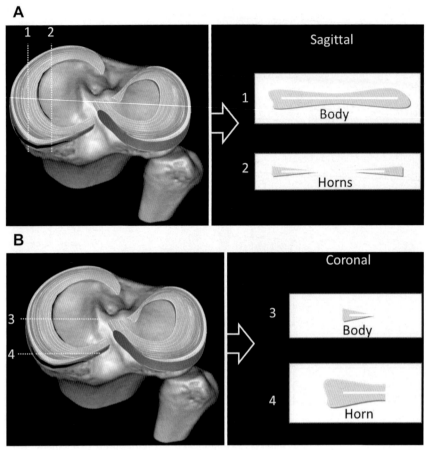

Fig. 16. Three-dimensional illustrations of horizontal tears, with the insets showing the typical MR imaging appearance in cross section in the sagittal (*A*) and coronal (*B*) planes.

debridement of the unstable leaflet of the torn meniscus and, potentially, decompression of an associated parameniscal cyst.

Radial Tears

A radial tear involves the free edge of the meniscus but, in contrast to a horizontal tear, follows a path perpendicular to the tibial plateau and long axis of the meniscus, dividing the meniscus into anterior and posterior portions (**Figs. 19** and **20**). These injuries degrade the ability of the meniscus to resist hoop stress, because the circumferential collagen fibers are sequentially disrupted. These injuries are infrequently amenable to repair, given the low likelihood of regaining function and typical

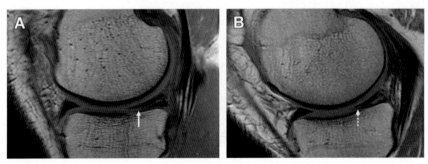

Fig. 17. Sagittal proton density images of horizontal tears extending to the inferior articular surface (*A, arrow*) and the free edge (*B, dashed arrow*) of the meniscus in 2 different patients.

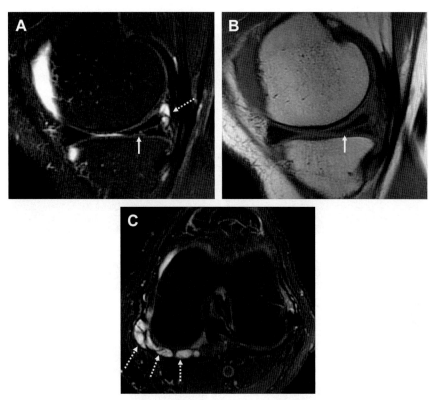

Fig. 18. Sagittal T2-weighted fat-suppressed (*A*) and proton density (*B*) images of a horizontal tear (*white arrow*) with an associated parameniscal cyst (*dashed arrow*). Axial T2-weighted fat-suppressed image (*C*) shows the extent of the multiloculated parameniscal cyst (*dashed arrows*) dissecting into the adjacent soft tissues.

central location, where blood supply to aid healing is nonexistent.[48] The depth of the tear should be described as partial or complete. The deeper the tear, the more devastating are the consequences to the biomechanical function of the meniscus.

Four imaging signs of radial tears have been described: the truncated triangle sign, the cleft sign, the marching cleft sign, and the ghost meniscus (**Figs. 21** and **22**).[37] The variable appearance is dependent on the location of the tear relative to the imaging plane and depth of the tear. As an example, a radial tear involving the posterior horn of the medial meniscus appears truncated or absent (based on the depth of the tear) when

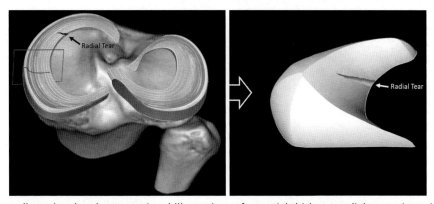

Fig. 19. Three-dimensional and cross-sectional illustrations of a partial-thickness radial tear oriented perpendicular to the long axis of the meniscus and involving the free edge. The circumferential collagen fibers responsible for providing hoop strength are sequentially torn with this type of injury. The deeper the extent of the tear, the more severe are the consequences to the biomechanical function of the menisci.

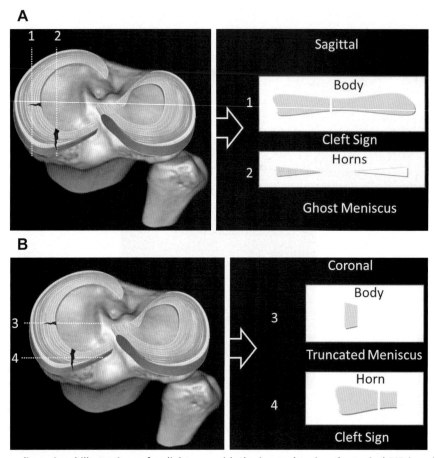

Fig. 20. Three-dimensional illustrations of radial tears, with the insets showing the typical MR imaging appearance in cross section in the sagittal (*A*) and coronal (*B*) planes.

imaged in-plane (sagittal sequence). The same tear typically resembles a cleft when imaged perpendicular to the axis of the tear, in this case on a coronal sequence. Tears that occur at the junction of the anterior horn and body are typically oriented obliquely relative to the imaging planes and therefore take on the appearance of a marching cleft, because the location of the tear appears to migrate on sequential sequences. Radial tears most commonly involve either the posterior horn of the medial meniscus or junction of the anterior horn and body of the lateral meniscus.

Flap Tears

Horizontal and vertical flap tears are unstable injuries in which a portion of the torn segment of the meniscus becomes displaced. Clinical manifestations include mechanical obstruction in the form of locking or catching in addition to pain. Preoperative identification is imperative, because displaced fragments may be difficult to visualize

arthroscopically and require the use of a probe or hook to localize and reduce.

A vertical flap tear, otherwise known as a parrot beak tear, comprises both radial and longitudinal components (**Figs. 23** and **24**).[48] Classically, the injury begins as a radial tear centrally but assumes a longitudinal orientation as it propagates peripherally. This configuration allows the torn portion of the meniscus to displace centrally and take on an appearance likened to a parrot's beak.

Horizontal flap tears involve a short segment of the meniscus with displacement of a meniscal leaf.[49] In most cases, the displaced meniscal fragment can be localized either within the posterior intercondylar notch or the gutters (**Fig. 25**). The medial meniscus is involved 6 to 7 times more frequently than the lateral meniscus, with the fragment displaced in two-thirds of the cases posteriorly toward the posterior intercondylar notch near or posterior to the PCL. The remaining one-third of cases show the fragment coursing into one of the recesses of the medial gutter,

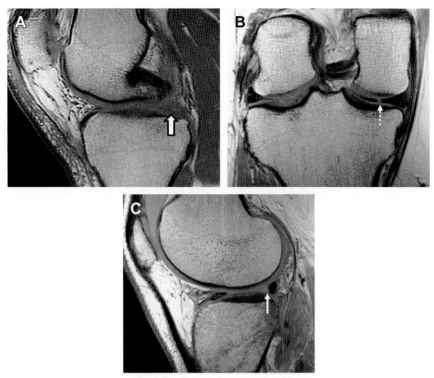

Fig. 21. MR appearance of radial tears. Sagittal proton density–weighted images showing a ghost meniscus (*black outlined arrow*) (*A*) caused by a full-thickness radial tear and absence of normal meniscal tissue, the cleft sign (*dashed white arrow*) (*B*), and the truncated triangle sign (*white arrow*) (*C*) seen with partial-thickness radial tears. All of these tears involve the free edge of the meniscus.

with a preference for the superior recess. Flipped meniscal fragments are identified with equal frequencies along the posterior joint line and lateral recess in the setting of a horizontal flap tear of the lateral meniscus.[50] As a rule, in the absence of previous surgery, if a meniscus appears blunted, a careful search for a displaced fragment should be performed, focusing particular attention on the intercondylar notch and recesses.

Root Tears

Although root tears typically represent radial type tears, a small subset represents a more complex injury. The ISAKOS classification system can be used to describe tears in this location; however, the unique anatomy of the posterior root ligaments and their undulating course along the tibial slope predispose to diagnostic dilemmas as a result of MR magic angle effect compounded by pulsation artifacts (**Figs. 26** and **27**). If recognized preoperatively, this situation can alter the surgical technique, because the posterior roots are not easily accessible at the time of arthroscopy and require placement of additional portals for adequate visualization and treatment.[51]

Underdiagnosis of root tears on both MR imaging and arthroscopy has led to increased attention in the surgical and radiologic literature recently and alterations in the imaging evaluation of this region. For example, by reporting all probable tears as torn, the sensitivity and specificity of detecting lateral posterior root tears improved to 94% and 89%, respectively, when using arthroscopy as the gold standard.[52] Unlike the situation for most tear types, coronal and fluid-sensitive sequences result in better delineation of the roots and partially compensate for the artifacts mentioned earlier.

On coronal sequences, the roots should be identified draping over the tibial plateau on at least a single image. On sagittal sequences, if the posterior root of the medial meniscus is not clearly visualized on the image immediately medial to the PCL, one should suspect a tear.[48]

The increased awareness of root tears in concert with improved in-plane resolution and thinner slice thickness has resulted in the detection of areas of fraying and synovitis surrounding the roots. The diagnostic challenge is determining which cases represent fraying versus a shallow partial-thickness radial tear, although

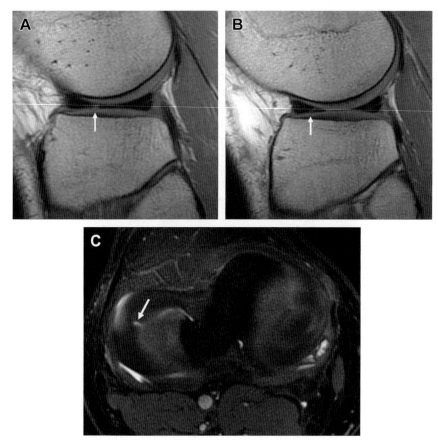

Fig. 22. Marching cleft sign. Typically seen with obliquely oriented radial tears centered at the junction of 1 of the horns and body of the meniscus, the appearance on sagittal images (*A, B*) is that of a vertically oriented cleft (*white arrows*) marching peripherally from the free edge into the substance of the meniscus. The example shown is that of a radial tear involving the junction of the anterior horn and body of the lateral meniscus best characterized on the axial MR reconstruction (*white arrow*) (*C*).

this distinction cannot always be made with imaging. In patients younger than 30 years, particularly patients with concomitant ACL injuries, any abnormal signal within the posterior root of the lateral meniscus indicates a tear. The situation is more ambiguous in patients older than 40 years without

an acute inciting event. In these cases, a differential of synovitis, partial radial tear, and fraying is warranted.[9]

The posterior roots should be scrutinized, especially in the setting of an ACL tear or meniscal extrusion. One series[51] reported an incidence of

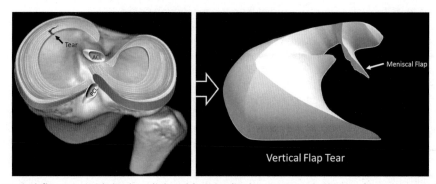

Fig. 23. A vertical flap tear with both radial and longitudinal components. This configuration predisposes the torn portion of the meniscus to displace centrally and assume an appearance likened to a parrot's beak.

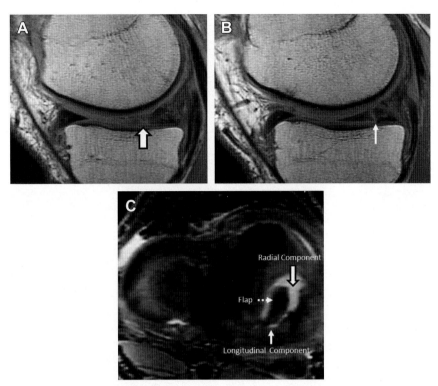

Fig. 24. Imaging appearance of a vertical flap tear. Contiguous sagittal proton density–weighted sequences show both the radial component (*black outlined arrow*) of this type of tear with a truncated posterior horn (*A*) and a longitudinal component (*white arrow*) as the tear propagates centrally (*B*). Axial reconstruction delineates these 2 components in addition to the displaced meniscal flap (*C*).

9.8% and 3.0% for lateral and medial meniscal posterior root tears in patients with ACL tears. Although not exclusively seen with root tears, extrusion can be seen in up to 76% of all medial posterior root tears (**Fig. 28**).[53]

Complex Tears

A tear that cannot be classified into a single category and shows components extending into multiple planes should be described as complex (**Fig. 29**). Typically comprising a combination of radial, horizontal, or longitudinal tears, the meniscus appears fragmented on imaging. The collagen fibers are typically injured, disabling the ability of the meniscus to resist hoop stress.

SECONDARY SIGNS

Indirect signs of an underlying meniscal tear can be helpful in equivocal cases and increase diagnostic confidence and diagnostic accuracy. Several imaging findings associated with meniscal tears were discussed earlier, including meniscal extrusion, injuries to the popliteomeniscal fascicles, and parameniscal cysts. Two additional signs

include linear subchondral edema and bone contusions (**Fig. 30**).

Linear subchondral bone marrow edema adjacent to the meniscal attachment sites, particularly the posterior root ligaments, can be seen in greater than 60% of medial and greater than 90% of lateral meniscal tears. Reported sensitivities and specificities for this finding range between 64% and 70% and 94% and 100%, respectively, for the medial meniscus and 88% and 89% and 98% and 100% for the lateral meniscus.[54]

A more diffuse bone contusion underlying the meniscus is also highly suggestive of a meniscal injury in the setting of trauma. Twenty-four of 25 patients with ACL injuries and bone contusions involving the posterior tibia showed MR imaging findings of either a meniscocapsular separation or a peripheral posterior meniscal tear in 1 study.[55]

DIAGNOSTIC ERRORS AND ANATOMIC VARIANTS

De Smet and colleagues[56] evaluated the sources of diagnostic errors, subdividing them into

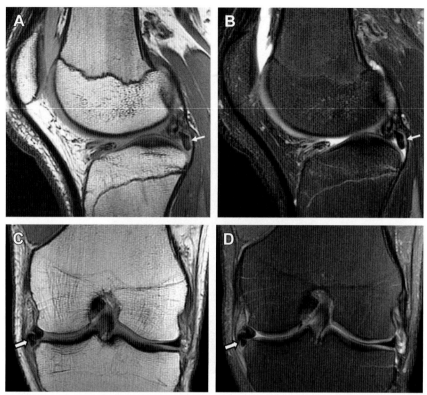

Fig. 25. Horizontal flap tears. Sagittal proton density and fat-suppressed T2-weighted sequences (*A*,*B*) of a horizontal flap tear (*arrow*) flipped posteriorly into the popliteus hiatus. Coronal proton density (*C*) and coronal proton density fat-suppressed (*D*) images of a horizontal flap tear, with a large meniscal fragment seen coursing into the inferior recess of the medial gutter (*arrow*).

unavoidable errors, interpretation errors, and errors secondary to equivocal findings. The study showed the inherent limitations of MR imaging, because many of the arthroscopically confirmed tears were undetectable even in retrospect. The investigators calculated a theoretic maximal sensitivity of 96% from medial meniscal tears and 94% for lateral meniscal tears.

Twenty-two percent of errors were attributed to misinterpretation of the imaging findings. False-positive results were primarily caused by mistaking normal structures or anatomic variants for tears. As alluded to in the anatomy section, the menisco-femoral ligaments, popliteomeniscal fascicles, popliteus tendon, transverse ligament, and striated appearance of the anterior root ligament of the lateral meniscus may all mimic a meniscal tear. Awareness and identification of each of these normal anatomic structures on serial images help avoid inadvertently mistaking them for a tear.

Two anatomic variants distort the meniscal shape, potentially leading to a false diagnosis of a tear: a discoid meniscus and a meniscal flounce. A discoid meniscus represents an enlarged meniscus diagnosed on MR imaging when the meniscal body measures 15 mm or wider on a midcoronal image (**Fig. 31**).[57,58] Watanabe and Takeda[59] described 3 subgroups: (1) the complete variant resembling a block or slab, which covers most of the tibial plateau; (2) the partial variant, which maintains a triangular morphology and covers 80% or less of the tibial plateau; and (3) the Wrisberg variant, which has altered or absent posterior attachments, with the meniscofemoral ligament acting as the sole posterior stabilizer, resulting in a hypermobile meniscus, often presenting clinically with the sensation of a snapping knee. A discoid meniscus is more commonly seen laterally and in men, with a reported frequency ranging between 0.4% and 3.0%.

Although tears are common in the setting of a discoid meniscus, the diagnosis can be challenging secondary to increased vascularity and often normal diffuse intrameniscal signal. Diffuse intrasubstance signal contacting the articular surface in discoid menisci has a positive predictive value of between 57% and 78%. Therefore, our practice reports this finding as a possible

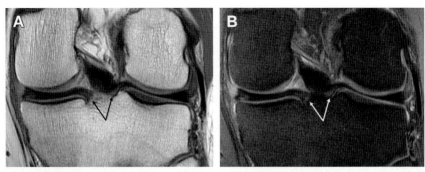

Fig. 26. On coronal images, the roots (*arrows*) should be identified draping over the tibial plateau on at least a single image. (*A*) Often the roots (*arrows*) are best visualized on fluid-sensitive sequences (*B*), which partially compensate for pulsation artifact and magic angle effects.

tear with a likelihood of 60% to 80%. However, linear signal unequivocally contacting the articular surface typically represents a true meniscal tear.[60,61]

A meniscal flounce is a rippled appearance of the free, nonanchored inner edge of the medial meniscus (**Fig. 32**). Typically, this finding is a result of flexion at the knee joint and redundancy of the

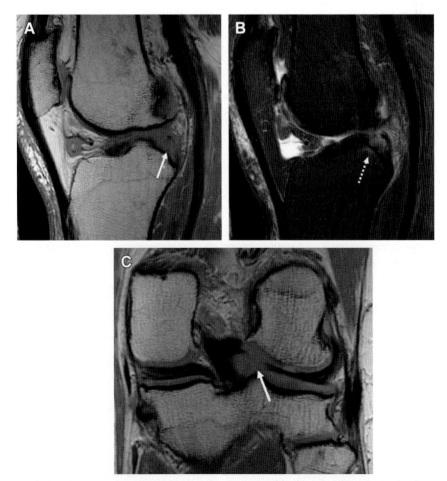

Fig. 27. Root tear. (*A*) The posterior root of the lateral meniscus is not visualized on the sagittal proton density–weighted image (*A, arrow*), with subjacent subchondral bone marrow edema seen on the sagittal T2-weighted sequence (*B, dashed arrow*). The coronal proton density image (*C*) better delineates the gap (*arrow*) from this full-thickness radial tear involving the posterior root ligament.

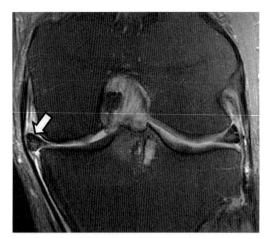

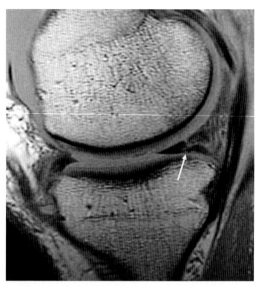

Fig. 28. Meniscal extrusion. On this midcoronal fat-suppressed proton density image in which the medial collateral ligament is visualized, the meniscal body (*arrow*) extends greater than 3 mm beyond the edge of the tibial plateau consistent with extrusion. The patient had a full-thickness radial tear of the posterior root ligament (*not shown*).

Fig. 29. Complex tear. The tear (*arrow*) in this sagittal proton density image is composed of both vertical and horizontal components, resulting in a fragmented appearance.

free edge of the meniscus. This finding is routinely seen at the time of arthroscopy, given the positioning of the knee, and has a high positive predictive value for an intact meniscus. If the meniscus otherwise appears normal, a meniscal flounce should be recognized as a normal variant.[62]

Meniscal ossicles (**Fig. 33**) or calcific deposits such as chondrocalcinosis within the menisci from metabolic disorders such as calcium pyrophosphate dihydrate deposition disease may result in abnormal intrasubstance signal, thereby decreasing the sensitivity and specificity for the detection of meniscal tears.[63,64] Correlation with radiographs is an essential habit when interpreting MR studies, particularly in identifying calcifications or ossification, which could confound one's interpretation and result in misdiagnosis.

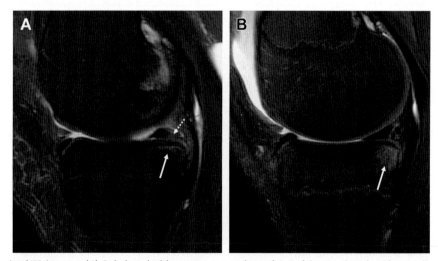

Fig. 30. Sagittal T2 images. (*A*) Subchondral bone marrow edema (*arrow*) is associated with an adjacent tear of the posterior root ligament (*dashed arrow*). (*B*) A more diffuse bone contusion (*arrow*) is seen subjacent to a peripheral longitudinal tear.

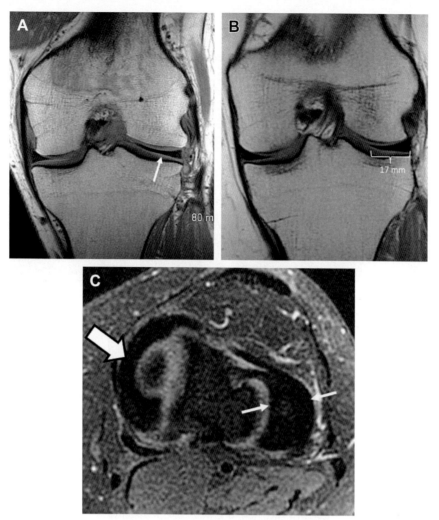

Fig. 31. Discoid meniscus. (*A*) Coronal proton density image showing a complete variant with an enlarged lateral meniscus (*arrow*), resembling a slab measuring 19 mm (normal <15 mm). (*B*) Coronal proton density image of a partial variant, which maintains the normal triangular morphology but is enlarged. (*C*) Axial MR image of the patient in (*B*) showing the enlarged lunar shaped lateral meniscus (*arrows*), covering more of the tibial articular surface. Compare the morphology to the normal C-shaped medial meniscus (*white block arrow*).

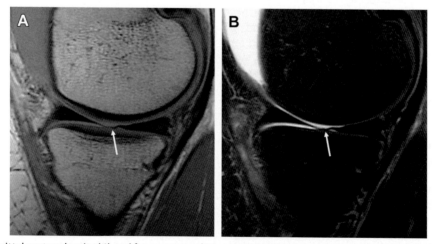

Fig. 32. Sagittal proton density (*A*) and fat-suppressed T2-weighted (*B*) images show the typical rippled appearance of a meniscal flounce (*arrow*) involving the free, nonanchored free edge of the body of the medial meniscus.

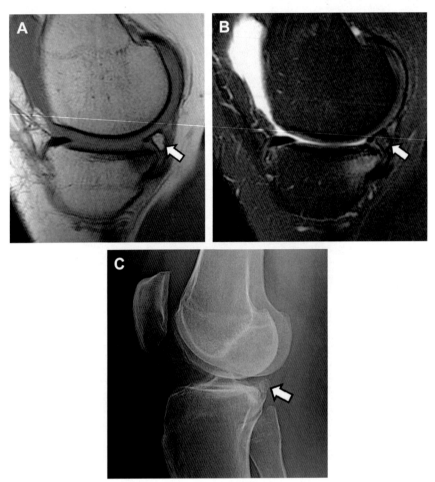

Fig. 33. Sagittal proton density (*A*) and fat-suppressed T2 (*B*) MR images and a lateral radiograph (*C*) of the knee showing the characteristic imaging findings of a meniscal ossicle (*arrows*).

SUMMARY

As treatment options for meniscal injuries continue to evolve, the interpretation of imaging studies becomes more complex. A thorough understanding of technical factors, normal anatomy, causes for misinterpretation, subtypes of meniscal tears, surgical techniques, as well as adhering strictly to established imaging criteria for the diagnosis of meniscal tear are required not only for high diagnostic accuracies but have implications on patient management.

In my opinion, a quality assurance program can lead to improved diagnostic accuracy as well. Standardizing terminology between radiologist and referring physicians in addition to correlating imaging findings with arthroscopic reports allows a practice to not only track the effects of changes in protocol or equipment but to perform outcome measures. Understanding the relevant imaging features to report, including pertinent positive and negative findings, can be achieved only through collaborative efforts.

REFERENCES

1. Sihvonen R, Paavola M, Malmivaara A, et al. Arthroscopic partial meniscectomy versus sham surgery for a degenerative meniscal tear. N Engl J Med 2013;369:2515–24.
2. Fairbank TJ. Knee joint changes after meniscectomy. J Bone Joint Surg Br 1948;30B:664–70.
3. Katz JN, Brophy RH, Chaisson CE, et al. Surgery versus physical therapy for a meniscal tear and osteoarthritis. N Engl J Med 2013;368:1675–84.
4. Oei EH, Nikken JJ, Verstijnen AC, et al. MR imaging of the menisci and cruciate ligaments: a systematic review. Radiology 2003;226:837–48.
5. Anderson AF, Irrgang JJ, Dunn W, et al. Interobserver reliability of the International Society of Arthroscopy, Knee Surgery and Orthopaedic Sports

Medicine (ISAKOS) classification of meniscal tears. Am J Sports Med 2011;39:926–32.

6. Renstrom P, Johnson RJ. Anatomy and biomechanics of the menisci. Clin Sports Med 1990;9:523–38.

7. Shankman S, Beltran J, Melamed E, et al. Anterior horn of the lateral meniscus: another potential pitfall in MR imaging of the knee. Radiology 1997;204:181–4.

8. Berlet GC, Fowler PJ. The anterior horn of the medial meniscus. An anatomic study of its insertion. Am J Sports Med 1998;26:540–3.

9. De Smet AA. How I diagnose meniscal tears on knee MRI. AJR Am J Roentgenol 2012;199:481–99.

10. Petersen W, Tillmann B. Collagenous fibril texture of the human knee joint menisci. Anat Embryol (Berl) 1998;197:317–24.

11. Rath E, Richmond JC. The menisci: basic science and advances in treatment. Br J Sports Med 2000;34:252–7.

12. Simonian PT, Sussmann PS, van Trommel M, et al. Popliteomeniscal fasciculi and lateral meniscal stability. Am J Sports Med 1997;25:849–53.

13. Sakai H, Sasho T, Wada Y, et al. MRI of the popliteomeniscal fasciculi. AJR Am J Roentgenol 2006;186:460–6.

14. De Smet AA, Asinger DA, Johnson RL. Abnormal superior popliteomeniscal fascicle and posterior pericapsular edema: indirect MR imaging signs of a lateral meniscal tear. AJR Am J Roentgenol 2001;176:63–6.

15. Blankenbaker DG, De Smet AA, Smith JD. Usefulness of two indirect MR imaging signs to diagnose lateral meniscal tears. AJR Am J Roentgenol 2002;178:579–82.

16. Cho JM, Suh JS, Na JB, et al. Variations in meniscofemoral ligaments at anatomical study and MR imaging. Skeletal Radiol 1999;28:189–95.

17. Lee BY, Jee WH, Kim JM, et al. Incidence and significance of demonstrating the meniscofemoral ligament on MRI. Br J Radiol 2000;73:271–4.

18. Park LS, Jacobson JA, Jamadar DA, et al. Posterior horn lateral meniscal tears simulating meniscofemoral ligament attachment in the setting of ACL tear: MRI findings. Skeletal Radiol 2007;36:399–403.

19. Anderson AF, Awh MH, Anderson CN. The anterior meniscofemoral ligament of the medial meniscus: case series. Am J Sports Med 2004;32:1035–40.

20. Sanders TG, Linares RC, Lawhorn KW, et al. Oblique meniscomeniscal ligament: another potential pitfall for a meniscal tear–anatomic description and appearance at MR imaging in three cases. Radiology 1999;213:213–6.

21. Marcheix PS, Marcheix B, Siegler J, et al. The anterior intermeniscal ligament of the knee: an anatomic and MR study. Surg Radiol Anat 2009;31:331–4.

22. Nelson EW, LaPrade RF. The anterior intermeniscal ligament of the knee. An anatomic study. Am J Sports Med 2000;28:74–6.

23. Crues JV 3rd, Mink J, Levy TL, et al. Meniscal tears of the knee: accuracy of MR imaging. Radiology 1987;164:445–8.

24. Rubin DA, Paletta GA Jr. Current concepts and controversies in meniscal imaging. Magn Reson Imaging Clin N Am 2000;8:243–70.

25. De Smet AA, Norris MA, Yandow DR, et al. MR diagnosis of meniscal tears of the knee: importance of high signal in the meniscus that extends to the surface. AJR Am J Roentgenol 1993;161:101–7.

26. Kaplan PA, Nelson NL, Garvin KL, et al. MR of the knee: the significance of high signal in the meniscus that does not clearly extend to the surface. AJR Am J Roentgenol 1991;156:333–6.

27. Magee T, Williams D. Detection of meniscal tears and marrow lesions using coronal MRI. AJR Am J Roentgenol 2004;183:1469–73.

28. Gokalp G, Nas OF, Demirag B, et al. Contribution of thin-slice (1 mm) axial proton density MR images for identification and classification of meniscal tears: correlative study with arthroscopy. Br J Radiol 2012;85:e871–8.

29. De Smet AA, Graf BK. Meniscal tears missed on MR imaging: relationship to meniscal tear patterns and anterior cruciate ligament tears. AJR Am J Roentgenol 1994;162:905–11.

30. Burstein DB, Fritts HM, Fischer DA. Diagnosis of meniscal and cruciate ligament tears using MRI. Evaluation of two scanning techniques. Minn Med 1991;74:29–32.

31. Stabler A, Glaser C, Reiser M. Musculoskeletal MR: knee. Eur Radiol 2000;10:230–41.

32. Kneeland JB, Hyde JS. High-resolution MR imaging with local coils. Radiology 1989;171:1–7.

33. Welsch GH, Juras V, Szomolanyi P, et al. Magnetic resonance imaging of the knee at 3 and 7 tesla: a comparison using dedicated multi-channel coils and optimised 2D and 3D protocols. Eur Radiol 2012;22:1852–9.

34. Rubin DA. MR imaging of the knee menisci. Radiol Clin North Am 1997;35:21–44.

35. Mink JH, Levy T, Crues JV 3rd. Tears of the anterior cruciate ligament and menisci of the knee: MR imaging evaluation. Radiology 1988;167:769–74.

36. Crues JV 3rd, Ryu R, Morgan FW. Meniscal pathology. The expanding role of magnetic resonance imaging. Clin Orthop Relat Res 1990;(252):80–7.

37. Harper KW, Helms CA, Lambert HS 3rd, et al. Radial meniscal tears: significance, incidence, and MR appearance. AJR Am J Roentgenol 2005;185:1429–34.

38. Vahey TN, Bennett HT, Arrington LE, et al. MR imaging of the knee: pseudotear of the lateral

meniscus caused by the meniscofemoral ligament. AJR Am J Roentgenol 1990;154:1237–9.

39. Herman LJ, Beltran J. Pitfalls in MR imaging of the knee. Radiology 1988;167:775–81.

40. Watanabe AT, Carter BC, Teitelbaum GP, et al. Normal variations in MR imaging of the knee: appearance and frequency. AJR Am J Roentgenol 1989;153:341–4.

41. Rosas HG, De Smet AA. Magnetic resonance imaging of the meniscus. Top Magn Reson Imaging 2009;20:151–73.

42. Arnoczky SP, Warren RF. The microvasculature of the meniscus and its response to injury. An experimental study in the dog. Am J Sports Med 1983; 11:131–41.

43. Kijowski R, Rosas HG. MRI characteristics of healed and unhealed peripheral vertical meniscal tears. Am J Roentgenol 2014;202(3):585–92.

44. Magee TH, Hinson GW. MRI of meniscal bucket-handle tears. Skeletal Radiol 1998;27:495–9.

45. Dorsay TA, Helms CA. Bucket-handle meniscal tears of the knee: sensitivity and specificity of MRI signs. Skeletal Radiol 2003;32:266–72.

46. Wright DH, De Smet AA, Norris M. Bucket-handle tears of the medial and lateral menisci of the knee: value of MR imaging in detecting displaced fragments. AJR Am J Roentgenol 1995;165:621–5.

47. De Smet AA, Graf BK, del Rio AM. Association of parameniscal cysts with underlying meniscal tears as identified on MRI and arthroscopy. AJR Am J Roentgenol 2011;196:W180–6.

48. Tuckman GA, Miller WJ, Remo JW, et al. Radial tears of the menisci: MR findings. AJR Am J Roentgenol 1994;163:395–400.

49. Ruff C, Weingardt JP, Russ PD, et al. MR imaging patterns of displaced meniscus injuries of the knee. AJR Am J Roentgenol 1998;170:63–7.

50. McKnight A, Southgate J, Price A, et al. Meniscal tears with displaced fragments: common patterns on magnetic resonance imaging. Skeletal Radiol 2010;39:279–83.

51. Lee SY, Jee WH, Kim JM. Radial tear of the medial meniscal root: reliability and accuracy of MRI for diagnosis. AJR Am J Roentgenol 2008;191:81–5.

52. De Smet AA, Blankenbaker DG, Kijowski R, et al. MR diagnosis of posterior root tears of the lateral meniscus using arthroscopy as the reference standard. AJR Am J Roentgenol 2009;192:480–6.

53. Choi CJ, Choi YJ, Lee JJ, et al. Magnetic resonance imaging evidence of meniscal extrusion in medial meniscus posterior root tear. Arthroscopy 2010;26:1602–6.

54. Bergin D, Hochberg H, Zoga AC, et al. Indirect soft-tissue and osseous signs on knee MRI of surgically proven meniscal tears. AJR Am J Roentgenol 2008;191:86–92.

55. Kaplan PA, Gehl RH, Dussault RG, et al. Bone contusions of the posterior lip of the medial tibial plateau (contrecoup injury) and associated internal derangements of the knee at MR imaging. Radiology 1999;211:747–53.

56. De Smet AA, Tuite MJ, Norris MA, et al. MR diagnosis of meniscal tears: analysis of causes of errors. AJR Am J Roentgenol 1994;163:1419–23.

57. Araki Y, Yamamoto H, Nakamura H, et al. MR diagnosis of discoid lateral menisci of the knee. Eur J Radiol 1994;18:92–5.

58. Silverman JM, Mink JH, Deutsch AL. Discoid menisci of the knee: MR imaging appearance. Radiology 1989;173:351–4.

59. Watanabe AT, Takeda S. Arthroscopy of the knee joint. In: Helfet AJ, editor. Disorders of the knee. Philadelphia: Lippincott; 1974. p. 145–59.

60. Stark JE, Siegel MJ, Weinberger E, et al. Discoid menisci in children: MR features. J Comput Assist Tomogr 1995;19:608–11.

61. Ryu KN, Kim IS, Kim EJ, et al. MR imaging of tears of discoid lateral menisci. AJR Am J Roentgenol 1998;171:963–7.

62. Wright RW, Boyer DS. Significance of the arthroscopic meniscal flounce sign: a prospective study. Am J Sports Med 2007;35:242–4.

63. Schnarkowski P, Tirman PF, Fuchigami KD, et al. Meniscal ossicle: radiographic and MR imaging findings. Radiology 1995;196:47–50.

64. Kaushik S, Erickson JK, Palmer WE, et al. Effect of chondrocalcinosis on the MR imaging of knee menisci. AJR Am J Roentgenol 2001;177:905–9.

Magnetic Resonance Imaging of the Postoperative Meniscus
Resection, Repair, and Replacement

Robert Downey Boutin, MD[a],*, Russell C. Fritz, MD[b],
Richard A. Marder, MD[c]

KEYWORDS

- Knee MR imaging • Knee arthroscopy • Meniscus tear • Meniscus repair • Postoperative imaging
- Meniscectomy

KEY POINTS

- To correctly interpret magnetic resonance (MR) imaging findings in the postoperative meniscus, physicians must understand the surgical techniques applied to the meniscus: the "3 Rs," namely resection, repair, and replacement, each resulting in a different MR imaging appearance of the postoperative meniscus.
- Resection (most often partial meniscectomy) is by far the most common procedure, but there is an increasing body of literature questioning its clinical efficacy. Consequently, meniscus preservation is increasingly emphasized, and repair techniques may become more common in the coming years.
- Repair techniques generally are subdivided into 3 types: inside-out, outside-in, and all-inside. After surgical repair, the meniscus can be categorized as healed (ie, no fluid signal in the repair), partially healed (ie, fluid signal extending into <50% of the repair site), or not healed (ie, fluid signal extending into >50% of the repair site).
- Meniscus replacement can be performed for postmeniscectomy syndrome in appropriate young to middle-aged patients. In the United States, this usually takes the form of a cadaveric meniscus allograft. In Europe and elsewhere, there is increasing experience with synthetic meniscus implants.

INTRODUCTION

Meniscus surgery is one of the most commonly performed orthopedic procedures, with an estimated 1 million meniscus surgeries[1] and US$4 billion in direct medical expenditures each year.[2]

Magnetic resonance (MR) imaging of the knee commonly is indicated to investigate the cause of unresolved or recurrent pain that can occur in patients after meniscus surgery.

The objectives of this article are to review selected highlights of (1) basic science (normal anatomy and emerging MR imaging techniques), (2) meniscus surgery (indications and techniques), (3) MR imaging protocols (with vs without arthrography), and (4) postoperative MR imaging interpretation (clinical outcomes and diagnostic criteria).

No disclosures.
[a] Department of Radiology, School of Medicine, University of California, Davis, 4860 Y Street, Suite 3100, Sacramento, CA 95817, USA; [b] National Orthopedic Imaging Associates, 1260 South Eliseo Drive, Greenbrae, CA 94904, USA; [c] Sports Medicine, Department of Orthopaedics, University of California, Davis, 2805 J Street, Suite 300, Sacramento, CA 95816, USA
* Corresponding author.
E-mail address: Robert.Boutin@ucdmc.ucdavis.edu

Magn Reson Imaging Clin N Am 22 (2014) 517–555
http://dx.doi.org/10.1016/j.mric.2014.07.007
1064-9689/14/$ – see front matter © 2014 Elsevier Inc. All rights reserved.

BASIC SCIENCE: IMPLICATIONS FOR KNEE MR IMAGING

Like articular (hyaline) cartilage, the fibrocartilaginous meniscus plays several roles, including load bearing, load distribution, joint stability, and joint lubrication. Compared with articular cartilage, the meniscus has a higher collagen content (15%–25% vs 10%–20%), lower proteoglycan content (1%–2% vs 5%–10%), and lower water content (60%–70% vs 68%–85%).[3]

Although the most important principles of meniscus anatomy are covered elsewhere in this issue by Rosas and colleagues, a few basic science concepts regarding the meniscus deserve to be highlighted here to emphasize our evolving understanding of this surprisingly heterogeneous tissue. Indeed, the meniscus structure varies both radially (peripheral to central) and also with depth (superficial to deep). Current research is providing insights into the various constituents within the meniscus, including cells, collagen, vascularity, and innervation.

Meniscus Cells: Do Meniscus Cells Die?

Meniscus cell degeneration and death (apoptosis) is significantly associated with meniscus tears and prognosis for successful meniscus repair.[4]

Meniscus cell (fibrochondrocyte) subpopulations show marked regional variation, with concomitant zonal variation in the surrounding matrix (pericellular and extracellular) that they produce.[5] Indeed, rather than being a homogeneous tissue, recent work indicates that this wedge-shaped tissue varies consistently from the thin, cartilage-like free edge, where compressive forces predominate and proteoglycan content is high, to the thicker, more peripheral region, where circumferential tensile loads predominate and proteoglycan content is low.

In addition to zonal variation in the proteoglycan matrix produced by the cells, there is also a zonal variation in the density of meniscus cells and their phenotypes (chondrocytic inner zone versus fibroblastic outer zone).[6]

MR imaging with T1rho mapping[7,8] and delayed gadolinium enhancement,[9] known to be sensitive to changes in proteoglycan loss in cartilage, recently has been used to show differences between normal and degenerated menisci.

Given that the anatomy and mechanisms that drive meniscus degeneration may be zonally dependent, future treatments such as gene therapy may use a targeted therapeutic approach for inner versus outer zones of the meniscus.

Collagen: Can MR Imaging Evaluate Collagen?

Collagen fibers are primarily responsible for tensile strength. In the classic description, collagen fibers are arranged for transferring vertical (compressive) loads into circumferential hoop stresses. In particular, the hoop stresses are contained via a belt of peripheral circumferential fibers, and these circumferentially oriented fascicles are secured together by radially oriented tie fibers. With aging, there tends to be an increase in connective tissue stiffness related to processes such as elastin degradation and collagen rigidification.[10]

Although the collagen architecture is often presented in a stylized fashion in diagrams, recent work indicates that the highly ordered microstructure is even more complex, and exquisite, than appreciated previously (**Fig. 1**).

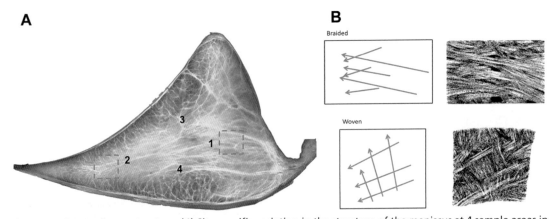

Fig. 1. Meniscus collagen structure. (*A*) Site-specific variation in the structure of the meniscus at 4 sample areas in the body segment: (1) outer third, (2) inner third, (3) femoral surface, and (4) tibial surface. (*B*) Schematic of braided and woven fascicle organizations (*left*) with associated sections from meniscus samples illustrating these arrangements using optical projection tomography (*right*) (scale, 1 mm.). (*From* Andrews SH, Ronsky JL, Rattner JB, et al. An evaluation of meniscal collagenous structure using optical projection tomography. BMC Med Imaging 2013;13(1):21.)

For example, there are 2 major types of collagen fascicle organization: braided and woven.[11]

- The braided fascicle organization is analogous to that seen in rope. With stretching in an axial orientation, the braided fascicles compress against adjacent fascicles, thus increasing stiffness.
- The woven arrangement is analogous to the pattern seen in fabrics or other flat structures that can convert compressive loads into tensile forces in the weave, sharing loads with adjacent supporting structures such as the ligamentous attachments to the tibial plateau. This arrangement may be relevant to normal meniscus movement and abnormal extrusion observed with conventional and dynamic MR imaging techniques.

MR imaging T2 mapping has been used to detect changes in collagen structure and water content, which are associated with degeneration. After meniscus repair, preliminary results suggest that quantitative T2* values correlate with collagen structural integrity, and are sensitive to temporal and zonal differences of meniscus repair.[12–14]

Recent study of the architectural subdivisions within the meniscus conclusively demonstrates the 3-dimensional nature of sheets of collagen tie fibers surrounding blood vessels. These sheets are oriented along the transverse plane of the meniscus, which may explain a propensity for horizontal-cleavage plane tears commonly seen with MR imaging and arthroscopy (**Fig. 2**).[15]

Vascularity: If the Inner Meniscus Is Avascular, How Does It Receive Nourishment?

The geniculate arteries, which are branches of the popliteal artery, supply the meniscus. Although the meniscus is diffusely vascularized during early life, by approximately 10 years of age only the outer 10% to 30% of the meniscus remains vascularized. Indeed, in adults, the inner portion of the meniscus is not only avascular, it is aneural and alymphatic! The inner portion of the meniscus receives nourishment from diffusion or mechanical pumping of synovial fluid, likely via canal-like structures opening deep into the surface of the menisci.[16]

Vascularization of the meniscus is directly related to its healing potential. Well-vascularized, peripheral (red zone) tears have a propensity for healing, whereas tears at the avascular, inner aspect (white zone) of the meniscus are not expected to heal spontaneously. Tears at the transition between the red and white zones are said to be in the red-white zone.

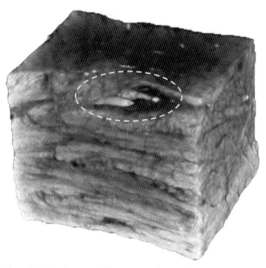

Fig. 2. Meniscus collagen and vessels. Within the meniscus, 2 parallel blood vessels can be seen coursing through an area devoid of collagen fascicles (*ellipse*) using optical projection tomography. (*From* Andrews SH, Ronsky JL, Rattner JB, et al. An evaluation of meniscal collagenous structure using optical projection tomography. BMC Med Imaging 2013;13(1):21.)

In a recent study of 86 peripheral vertical tears,[17] almost all (>94%) tears of the medial meniscus at the posterior meniscocapsular junction healed spontaneously, whereas most (~80%) other peripheral vertical tears did not heal. For the peripheral vertical tears not located at the meniscocapsular junction, however, several MR imaging findings were significantly associated with spontaneous healing: thin tear (width <2 mm), tear visualized on only proton-density (PD)-weighted (but not T2-weighted) imaging, and thin horizontally oriented strands bridging the tear on T2-weighted images. Conversely, a wide gap between torn edges that is filled with fluid signal intensity on T2-weighted images did not heal with nonoperative therapy.

MR imaging performed with intravenous injection of contrast material is not helpful for differentiation of vascularized from nonvascularized zones of the meniscus.[18]

Innervation: If Most of the Meniscus Is Aneural, Do Meniscus Tears Cause Pain?

The primary goals of any meniscus surgery are to help alleviate pain and optimize function. Both pain and function are influenced by meniscus innervation.

The meniscus is well innervated only in vascularized areas.[19,20] Thus, when a tear occurs in the vascularized, innervated area at the meniscus periphery, some pain may result from direct nerve insult and bleeding.

When tears occur at the inner noninnervated meniscus, pain presumably occurs via other mechanisms, such as secondary stimulation of nociceptive fibers in the adjacent subchondral bone, synovium, or joint capsule as sequelae of osteoarticular pathomechanics,[21] in addition to meniscus neovascularity, sensory nerve growth, and perimeniscal synovitis (defined as enhancing synovium >2 mm in thickness on MR imaging),[22] and premature osteoarthritis.

- Symptomatic tears. MR imaging findings significantly associated with knee symptoms include meniscus tears that are vertical or complex, and tears associated with bone marrow edema and joint-capsule thickening.[23] Specific tear types may be associated with particular symptoms at higher frequencies. Examples cited in the literature include: flap tears associated with pain on standing and a catching sensation; posterior root tears associated with popliteal pain; and radial tears in the middle segment associated with nocturnal pain on rolling over in bed.[24]
- Asymptomatic tears. Meniscus tears with a horizontal or oblique configuration on MR imaging are not significantly associated with knee symptoms.

In addition to nociceptors (causing pain), the meniscus also contains several types of mechanoreceptors (converting physical stimuli into electrical nerve impulses) that may be involved in sensorimotor control of the knee.[25]

In the normal medial meniscus, mechanoreceptors may be crucial in a reflex arc that stimulates the semimembranosus to contract, including the segment that pulls the medial meniscus posterior horn posteriorly, thus preventing the meniscus from being trapped and injured with knee flexion.[26] By contrast, derangements and some surgeries involving the meniscus posterior horn may contribute to the inhibition of semimembranosus muscle activation and alter meniscus mobility, thus changing the internal joint forces.[27] In a subset of patients, symptoms of giving way or buckling of the knee may be due to an alteration in stretch-reflex excitability rather than ligamentous laxity.[28]

MENISCUS SURGERY: INDICATIONS AND TECHNIQUES

Nothing has changed so much in knee treatment and surgery as the meniscal treatment algorithms...[29]

Meniscus tears may be managed nonoperatively or operatively, depending on the type of tear and the clinical context (**Box 1**). Besides clinical history, other factors dynamically influence treatment algorithms, including recent sensational advancements in clinical outcomes research, treatment techniques, and musculoskeletal imaging.

Important specific examples of clinical research expected to affect management choices include:

- The recent trials finding lackluster clinical outcomes after meniscectomy for nontraumatic tears, with or without osteoarthritis
- The recent literature on acceptable healing rates for augmented repairs of tears in the red-white zone[30]
- The evolving recommendations that some stable tears be left in situ (sometimes with healing on follow-up MR imaging and second-look arthroscopy)[31–33]

To interpret MR imaging findings in the postoperative meniscus correctly, one must understand the surgical techniques applied to the meniscus. Although treatment algorithms are debated and continue to evolve, there are 3 general surgical strategies (known as the 3 Rs), resection, repair, and replacement (or reconstruction). Each of the 3 techniques results in a different MR imaging appearance for the postoperative meniscus. Repairs and partial replacements are often performed with augmentation techniques to enhance healing, which might promote meniscus regeneration (or rejuvenation), a fourth "R."

Resection

Indications
The general indication for partial meniscectomy is a meniscus tear not amenable to repair. Irreparable tears conventionally include nonperipheral

---

Box 1
Meniscus tears: relevant clinical history

In a patient with a meniscus tear, relevant clinical history includes:

- Age and functional demands
- History of prior meniscus surgery and trauma
- Features of acute injury/trauma
- Significant mechanical symptoms (eg, locking)
- Concomitant injuries (eg, anterior cruciate ligament tear)
- Malalignment
- Articular cartilage status

tears with a horizontal, oblique flap (vertical flap, parrot beak) or a complex configuration, especially nontraumatic tears in middle-aged or older patients (**Fig. 3**).

Technique

The damaged, loose meniscus tissue is removed using arthroscopic instruments until solid tissue is reached; these instruments include manually operated scissors and baskets and mechanical shavers that use suction to draw tissue into a rotating window, which then severs its connection. The remaining meniscus is tapered and contoured, preserving as much meniscus tissue as possible.[34] Debridement of a meniscus tear most often results in partial meniscectomy. Rarely is a complete meniscectomy performed. Unless otherwise specified, the authors use the term "meniscectomy" here to refer to partial resection of the meniscus, because total meniscectomy is so rare in practice.

Repair

Indications

Indications for meniscus repair traditionally have included posttraumatic vertical (longitudinal) peripheral tears located at or near the joint capsule, ideally in younger patients (<40 years).

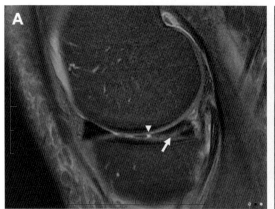
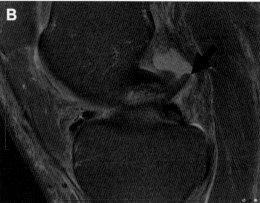
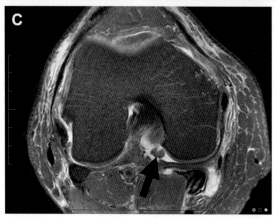

Fig. 3. Missed flap tear in a 61-year-old man. The original scan was read incorrectly as a horizontal tear of the posterior horn of the medial meniscus; a 5 × 16-mm displaced flap was missed by the initial radiologist. Arthroscopic trimming of the free edge was performed 2 weeks later; the displaced flap was not identified or resected. A repeat MR image 3 months later to investigate persistent posterior knee pain revealed a superiorly displaced flap at the posteromedial margin of the medial femoral condyle that was identified by a second radiologist. An additional arthroscopic procedure was then performed to resect this flap. Preoperative fat-suppressed T2-weighted sagittal (*A, B*) and axial (*C*) images reveal a horizontal (*white arrow*) and free-edge radial tear (*arrowhead*) of the posterior horn of the medial meniscus in addition to a 5 × 16-mm superiorly displaced flap (*black arrow*) that was missed by an experienced radiologist. The postoperative fat-suppressed T2-weighted sagittal (*D, E*) and axial (*F*) images reveal evidence of interval free-edge trimming of the posterior horn of the medial meniscus in addition to the superiorly displaced flap (*black arrow*) that was unfortunately missed by the initial radiologist.

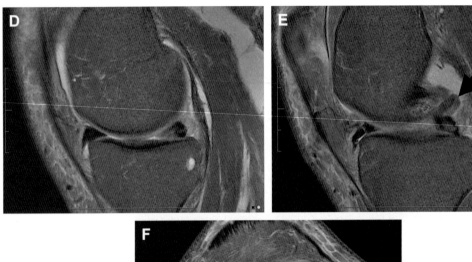

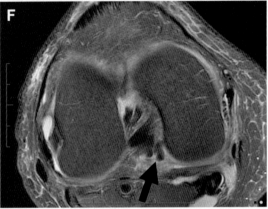

Fig. 3. (*continued*)

Compared with meniscectomy, repair procedures are more technically demanding for the surgeon, cost more (in terms of time and equipment),[35] and traditionally have required longer rehabilitation to allow for successful healing of the repair.[36,37]

Techniques

Repair techniques generally are subdivided into 3 types: inside-out, outside-in, and all-inside. Meniscal repair is analogous to operative repair of a fracture nonunion; the surgeon commonly assesses vascularity of the tear, debrides/rasps the edges, aligns the edges, and applies stable fixation with sutures or bioabsorbable implants at approximately 5-mm intervals, sometimes with biological adjuncts in an attempt to improve healing (**Fig. 4**).

Inside-out The inside-out technique with vertical mattress sutures is the gold standard with which other repair techniques are compared.[38] Although to date it has been the most common technique, comparable results are reported with other techniques that are less technically demanding.[39]

For example, in a review of 767 meniscus repairs involving the red-white zone, clinical healing was reported in 81% (of 470) inside-out repairs and 86% (of 297) all-inside repairs.[30]

The inside-out technique deploys sutures from inside the joint across the meniscus tear and through the capsule to the exterior surface, using a cannulated needle under arthroscopic visualization. To visualize passage of the needles and avoid injury to neurovascular structures adjacent to the knee joint, a 2- to 3-cm length incision with dissection to expose the external joint capsule is necessary.[40]

Outside-in The outside-in technique has evolved since its original description in 1985, with healing rates and functional scores comparable with those of other meniscus repair techniques.[41]

The outside-in technique is most applicable to tears in the anterior and adjacent middle segments of the meniscus. With a recent modification, this technique also can be recommended as an alternative method for repair of the middle segment and the posteromedial or posterolateral corner of the meniscus.[42]

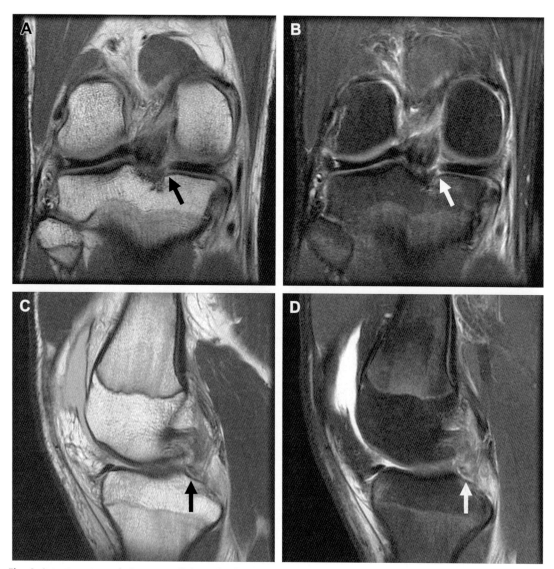

Fig. 4. Intact root repair. Intact medial meniscal posterior root repair in a 14-year-old soccer player with a recurrent injury 12 months after surgery. Preoperative proton-density (PD) (*A*) and fat-suppressed T2-weighted (*B*) coronal images, and PD (*C*) and fat-suppressed T2-weighted (*D*) sagittal images reveal a tear of the posterior root attachment of the medial meniscus (*arrows*). The medial collateral ligament (MCL) and posterior cruciate ligament (PCL) were also torn (not shown). Postoperative PD (*E*) and fat-suppressed T2-weighted (*F*) coronal images, and PD (*G*) and fat-suppressed T2-weighted (*H*) sagittal images reveal an intact repair (*arrowheads*) of the posterior root attachment of the medial meniscus. There was also a recurrent tear of the MCL and the PCL (not shown). Two adjacent drill tracts (*thin arrows*) are seen extending to the intact repair of the posterior root attachment.

All-inside The all-inside technique has progressed dramatically and has become increasingly popular since its first description in 1991.[43]

An all-inside repair technique is suitable for most reparable meniscus tears, especially vertical (longitudinal) posterior horn tears. The all-inside technique also can be combined with other techniques, especially the outside-in method, to repair tears extending the entire axis of the meniscus. In addition, recent innovations may facilitate the repair of radial, horizontal, and root tear patterns that were previously considered difficult or impossible to suture (**Figs. 5** and **6**).[44] Relative contraindications include meniscocapsular separations and anterior horn tears.[45]

Although there are numerous vendors that manufacture different devices, the current fourth generation of all-inside techniques commonly

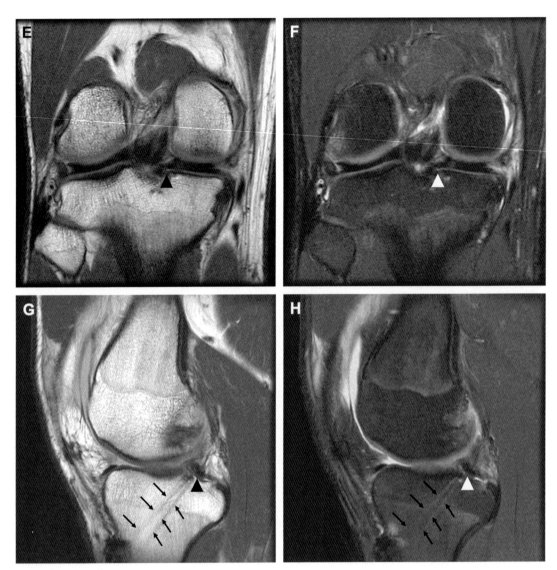

Fig. 4. (continued)

uses an arthroscopic needle to deploy backstop anchors across the meniscus tear to the outer surface of the joint capsule (extra-articularly), followed by a pre-tied sliding-locking knot that compresses the tear margins.[46,47]

Replacement

Indications

Meniscus replacements can be performed via arthroscopic or mini open procedures, particularly when extensive meniscectomy is performed for significant tears that cannot be repaired.

Surgical candidates for synthetic meniscus implants may include skeletally mature, nonobese adults younger than 50 to 55 years with substantial unicompartmental tibiofemoral postmeniscectomy pain, a stable joint, normal alignment (eg, mechanical tibiofemoral angle $\leq 3°$), and the ability to commit to a postoperative physical rehabilitation program. Contraindications generally include advanced chondrosis (eg, International Cartilage Repair Society [ICRS] grade 3 or 4 ipsilateral compartment lesions, <50% joint space narrowing), inflammatory arthritis, and infection.

The algorithm for selecting any particular procedure can vary depending on numerous factors, including the surgeon, geography, and available resources.

- Allograft transplants are most appropriate for extensive meniscus defects.

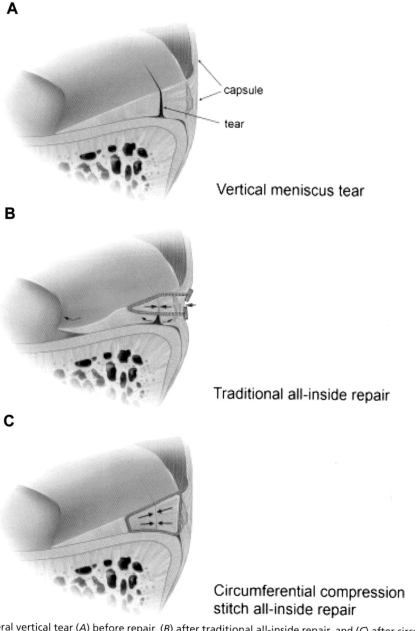

Fig. 5. Peripheral vertical tear (*A*) before repair, (*B*) after traditional all-inside repair, and (*C*) after circumferential compression stitch all-inside repair. Note that with the circumferential compression stitch, the entire tear surface is uniformly compressed from top to bottom and that the capsule remains untethered. (*From* Saliman JD. The circumferential compression stitch for meniscus repair. Arthrosc Tech 2013;2(3):e258; with permission.)

- Partial meniscus implants can be used to fill partial meniscectomy defects, which should be greater than two-thirds of the meniscal width, measuring less than 5 cm, with intact anterior and posterior horn/roots, and a stable rim at the popliteus hiatus. Total meniscus implants are still under clinical investigation; these prostheses are not available outside of clinical trials.

Techniques

Two general techniques are the subjects of intense interest to patients with postmeniscectomy syndrome: (cadaveric) meniscus allograft transplantation and (synthetic) meniscus implantation.

Allograft Meniscal allografts are harvested from human donors and then transplanted, most commonly with attached bone as anchors using

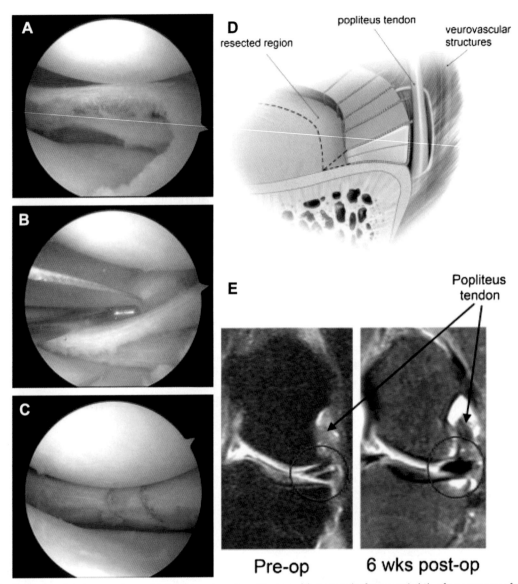

Fig. 6. Horizontal cleavage tear of lateral meniscus in a 28-year-old woman before repair (*A*), after passage of the first stitch around the back of the meniscus at the level of the popliteal hiatus (*B*), and after repair (*C*). (*D*) Drawing showing resected and repaired regions relative to popliteal hiatus. (*E*) Coronal MR images of lateral compartment at level of popliteal hiatus obtained preoperatively (Pre-op) and 6 weeks postoperatively (6 wks post-op), showing excellent early healing of the lateral meniscus horizontal cleavage tear. The postoperative MR image was obtained to guide rehabilitation. The preoperative and postoperative MR scans were obtained from different facilities with slightly different protocols, explaining the difference in contrast within the bone. (*From* Saliman JD. The circumferential compression stitch for meniscus repair. Arthrosc Tech 2013;2(3):e261; with permission.)

double bone plugs or a single bridge of bone placed in a tibial slot technique. In addition, soft-tissue fixation of the allograft to the joint capsule is necessary, but the meniscotibial attachments are not usually reconstructed.

Meniscus allograft transplantation may be performed as an isolated procedure but is more commonly combined with another procedure, such as anterior cruciate ligament (ACL) reconstruction, cartilage repair procedure, or high tibial osteotomy.[48]

Accurate preoperative sizing of the allograft to match the recipient's knee is critical to maximize the likelihood of a successful outcome. For a mismatch of even 10%, significantly increased contact forces occur on the articular cartilage in the setting of an oversized, extruded meniscus allograft or on the transplanted meniscus tissue because of an undersized meniscus allograft.[49] Although sizing is usually performed with radiographs,[50] MR imaging may be more accurate.[51,52]

Implants Unlike cadaveric allografts that require the sacrifice of any normal residual meniscus tissue that a patient might have, the synthetic scaffold implants can be customized to fit the size of a patient's meniscus defect. The surgery for suturing one of these scaffolds into place is similar to repairing a bucket-handle tear (eg, a hybrid of all-inside and outside-in sutures), a less complex process than meniscus allograft transplantation.

The synthetic meniscus scaffolds for partial meniscus replacement are highly porous, acellular, bioresorbable implants manufactured with the aims of supporting ingrowth of meniscus-like tissue, alleviating postmeniscectomy pain, and preventing premature arthrosis.[53–56]

Although the 2 available scaffold products are used in similar ways, they have very different compositions: one is polyurethane-based (Actifit; Orteq Ltd, London, UK)[57] and the other is collagen-based (Menaflex Collagen Meniscus Implant; Ivy Sports Medicine LLC, Gräefelfing, Germany). The collagen-based product is processed type-I collagen from bovine Achilles tendon (97%) that is augmented with glycosaminoglycans to enhance ingrowth of meniscus fibrochondrocytes.

Another implant, currently in clinical trials, is a nonanchored, free-floating, disc-shaped interpositional prosthesis composed of a composite polymer (ie, polycarbonate-urethane reinforced with ultra–high-molecular-weight polyethylene fibers: NUsurface; Active Implants LLC, Driebergen, The Netherlands).[58,59] In contrast to the scaffolds, the target population for this "total meniscus prosthesis" is currently middle-aged adults who have meniscus dysfunction and early osteoarthritis in the medial compartment.[60]

Many other implants have been conceived and patented, such as a partial meniscus patch, coated with a protein cross-linking reagent and biocompatible adhesive to enhance surgical repair,[61] and various complete meniscus implants, typically containing a reinforcing network of fibers embedded in the scaffold.[62]

Augmentation (Regeneration)

With all meniscus repair techniques, there is intense research into augmenting the healing of both peripheral and nonperipheral tears. The fundamental paradigm in regenerative tissue engineering is that 3 factors act in concert to orchestrate a successful outcome: cells (to synthesize new extracellular matrix), scaffolds (for mechanical support of cells), and growth factors (to stimulate cell function).[63,64]

Although specific MR imaging features are not widely reported, some techniques have been used for decades, including fibrin clot augmentation and mechanical stimulation, such as meniscus trephination,[65] meniscus rasping,[66] and synovial rasping.[67] Such techniques may improve the success of meniscus repair substantially.[68] For example, complete radial tears repaired with fibrin clot augmentation reportedly show high rates of healing at follow-up MR imaging and second-look arthroscopy.[69,70] Another study found that intra-articular injection of human stem cells is associated with improved knee pain and meniscus regeneration on MR imaging.[71]

Numerous other substances also may promote healing of fibrocartilage, but specific MR imaging findings are not widely reported. Such agents include platelet-rich plasma, bioadhesives such as those containing chondroitin sulfate,[72] numerous growth factors such as myoblasts expressing recombinant cartilage-derived morphogenetic protein 2,[73] and scaffolds such as gelatin hydrogel scaffold.[74,75] Not all surgical techniques are successful,[76] and MR imaging refinements may allow for objective, noninvasive diagnostic evaluation of surgical techniques at anatomic, cellular, and biochemical levels.

MR IMAGING PROTOCOLS

Regardless of the particular imaging protocol chosen for one's practice, the authors affirm that an optimal MR imaging interpretation has 3 prerequisites:

- A pre–MR imaging "history form" completed by the patient, including the site and duration of symptoms
- An operative note, including the timing and type of surgical procedure
- Preoperative imaging examination(s) for comparison (**Figs. 7** and **8**)

Based on the MR imaging findings, the radiologist can verify independently that prior knee arthroscopy has been performed by looking for validated findings of characteristic fibrosis along portal tracts in and adjacent to the Hoffa fat pad.[77] Less commonly, findings associated with meniscus repair may include susceptibility artifact at the joint line and findings of arthroscopic deep medial collateral ligament pie-crusting release, which is performed for expansion of the medial joint space in the case of a tight medial compartment.[78]

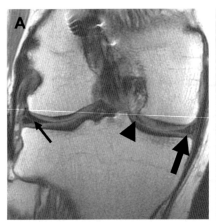
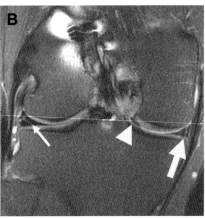

Fig. 7. New meniscus tears. New medial and lateral meniscus tears in a 35-year-old snowboarder with new pain and mechanical symptoms 3 years after an anterior cruciate ligament (ACL) reconstruction. Postoperative PD (*A*) and fat-suppressed T2-weighted (*B*) coronal images reveal an intact ACL graft and a new horizontal tear of the body segment of the lateral meniscus (*small arrows*). There is also a new vertical peripheral tear of the body segment of the medial meniscus (*large arrows*) with a thin 5-mm displaced flap of the posterior horn seen just medial to the medial tibial spine (*arrowheads*). Having access to the baseline scan and the operative history made interpretation of this postoperative scan straightforward. The horizontal tear and the displaced flap were treated with a partial meniscectomies. The vertical peripheral tear was trephined and then repaired.

Choice of Advanced Imaging Technique

The best technique for imaging the postoperative meniscus is a matter of active controversy.

- In some practices,[79] an elaborate algorithm is used before scheduling 1 of 4 types of imaging examination: conventional MR imaging, indirect MR arthrography, direct MR arthrography, or computed tomographic (CT) arthrography. This algorithm includes several variables, including the presence or absence of a joint effusion (ie, minimal vs large), the type of prior meniscus surgery (ie, resection, repair, or replacement), and the extent of any prior partial meniscectomy (ie, more vs less than 25%).
- Other practices focus on the timing of prior meniscus surgery, opting for direct MR arthrography if surgery has been performed within the past 1 to 2 years.
- In the authors' practices, the approach is simpler: we routinely begin with conventional MR imaging.

In particular, preference is to begin with a screening examination of paired fast spin-echo (FSE) PD and fat-suppressed T2 images in all 3 planes. If there is substantial postoperative metallic artifact, the technologist is instructed to perform a metal-artifact reduction protocol that includes optimized FSE PD and FSE inversion recovery pulse sequences (**Fig. 9**). Experience has shown that these conventional MR images do a

good (albeit imperfect) job in evaluating the postoperative knee; arthrographic techniques (also imperfect) are reserved for uncommon cases in which additional problem solving is deemed necessary.

Rationale for Conventional MR Imaging

The accuracy of conventional MR imaging for postoperative menisci is generally less than the accuracy achieved for menisci without previous surgery, and arthrographic techniques can aid in the diagnosis of some meniscus tears.[80–86] However, as discussed by others,[87–90] the authors routinely begin with conventional MR imaging to screen the postoperative knee, for the following reasons:

- Arthrographic techniques are associated with additional time, cost, discomfort, and risk, such as urticaria, vasovagal reaction, anaphylactic reaction, and septic arthritis. Primum non nocere.
- In the United States, the intra-articular administration of gadolinium-based contrast agents is off-label (ie, not specifically approved by the US Food and Drug Administration [FDA]).[91–95]
- With MR arthrography, some tears do not fill with contrast material: the signal contacting the surface of a recurrent meniscus tear may be equal to or less than that of adjacent intra-articular gadolinium contrast material.[96] Of note, when conventional MR imaging

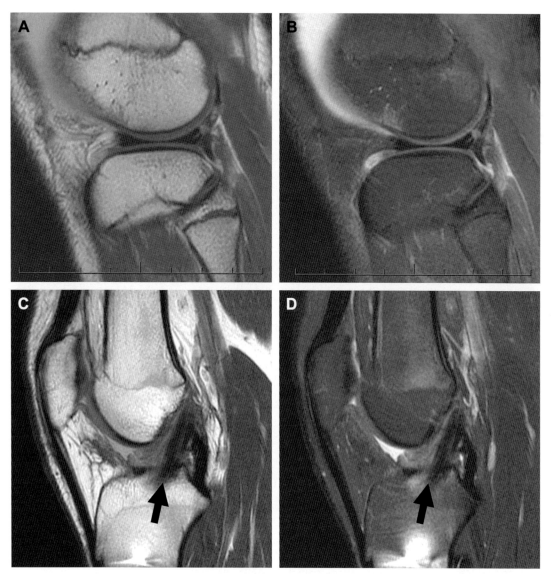

Fig. 8. New tear after surgery. New tear of the posterior horn of the lateral meniscus in a 15-year-old girl with a recurrent injury 1 year after an ACL reconstruction. Preoperative PD (*A*) and fat-suppressed T2-weighted (*B*) sagittal images reveal a normal posterior horn of the lateral meniscus on the initial scan at the time of the acute ACL tear. The lateral meniscus was also normal at the time of ACL reconstruction 4 weeks later. Postoperative PD (*C, E*) and fat-suppressed T2-weighted (*D, F*) sagittal images reveal an intact, but vertically oriented ACL graft (*thick arrow*) and a new tear of the posterior horn of the lateral meniscus (*thin arrows*). Having access to the baseline scan and the operative history made interpretation of this postoperative scan straightforward. This new tear was treated with a partial meniscectomy.

findings are consistent with a meniscus retear, but contrast material does not extend into the meniscus on MR arthrography, a meniscus retear is likely (**Fig. 10**).[97]

- With MR arthrography, it can be difficult to determine whether mild or moderate increased signal intensity in a postoperative meniscus represents contrast material in a tear, unless precontrast MR imaging also is performed, requiring additional time and scheduling challenges.

- With MR arthrography, the imbibition of contrast material into a repaired meniscus tear does not necessarily indicate that the tear is unstable or responsible for symptoms. In fact, some surgeons leave small stable tears alone to maximize meniscus preservation.

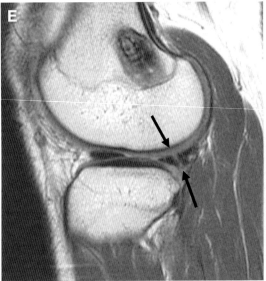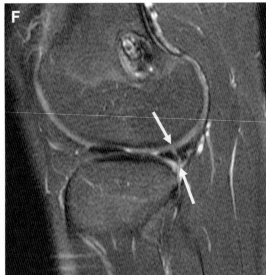

Fig. 8. (*continued*)

- With MR imaging, the development of a parameniscal cyst is a specific, albeit insensitive, finding of a meniscus tear (**Fig. 11**), but these cysts often do not fill with contrast material on arthrographic examinations.
- With a substantial internal derangement, a native joint effusion is often present (defined as anteroposterior distension of the suprapatellar recess by >5 mm or the lateral parapatellar gutter by >10 mm), which tends to mildly increase the accuracy of nonarthrographic MR imaging examinations.
- When less than 25% of the meniscus has been resected, the literature indicates that there is no significant benefit of MR arthrography over MR imaging. Such low-grade partial meniscectomies are much more common than high-grade meniscectomies or meniscus repairs (**Fig. 12**).
- When greater than 25% of the meniscus has been resected or a peripheral tear has been repaired, the literature is not yet definitive as to whether there is a significant difference in accuracy for the diagnosis of a recurrent tear, although there may be an incremental benefit in this population because residual intrasubstance (grade 2) degenerative signal commonly extends to the surface of the meniscus remnant after meniscectomy.
- In contradistinction to small recurrent tears after meniscectomy, a meniscus repair of a large bucket-handle tear or a red-red tear in young active patients may fail dramatically; in such cases, the resulting unstable or

displaced fragment can be readily identified by MR imaging without arthrography (**Fig. 13**).
- Often the source of the patient's pain is not the meniscus itself, but another derangement that is optimally evaluated by conventional MR imaging, rather than with fat-suppressed T1-weighted images with contrast material in the joint; these conditions may include chondrosis, osseous stress reaction, arthrofibrosis, or a ruptured Baker cyst. A combination of internal derangements is well displayed routinely by conventional MR imaging (**Fig. 14**).

POSTOPERATIVE MR IMAGING: OUTCOMES AND INTERPRETATION

Clinical outcomes and common MR imaging findings are summarized here for resection, repair, and replacement using (1) cadaveric meniscus allograft transplantation and (2) synthetic meniscus implantation.

Knowledge of various postoperative outcomes (pre–MR imaging test probability) aids in finding an optimal cut point (decision threshold) on the receiver-operating characteristic (ROC) curve (a plot of test sensitivity plotted on the y-axis versus its false-positive rate plotted on the x-axis).[98,99]

Resection

Outcomes

Maximal preservation of the meniscus is increasingly recognized as an essential goal. It has long been known that high-grade meniscectomy

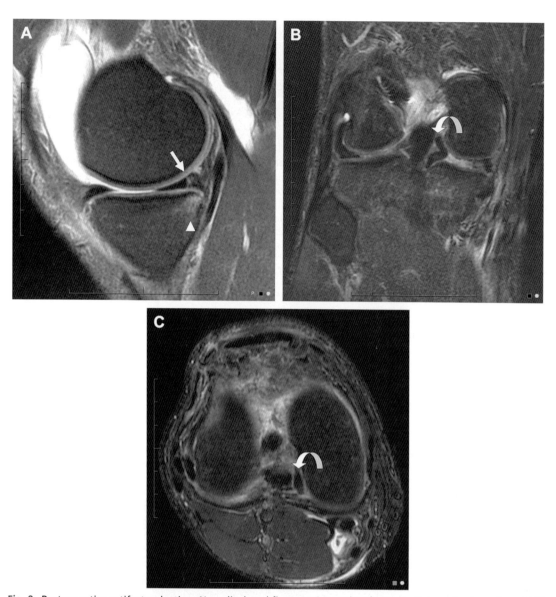

Fig. 9. Postoperative artifact reduction. New displaced flap tear 3 months after a medial meniscal repair and ACL reconstruction in a 28-year-old woman. (*A*) Preoperative fat-suppressed T2-weighted sagittal image of a vertical tear longitudinal ligament (*arrow*) with an adjacent contusion (*arrowhead*). Postoperative short-tau inversion recovery (STIR) coronal (*B*) and axial (*C*) images reveal a superiorly displaced flap (*curved arrow*) seen between the PCL and the medial femoral condyle.

predisposes the knee to osteoarthritis, and there is an increasing body of literature questioning the clinical results of partial meniscectomy.

Level-1 evidence published in high-profile journals indicates that meniscectomy does not significantly benefit most patients with or without radiographic osteoarthritis.[100–104] However, conclusions from these studies are debated fiercely.[105,106] These studies did not focus on whether tears were displaced[107,108] or displaceable,[109,110] as can be assessed by MR imaging

(**Fig. 15**). Displaceable meniscus tears usually have a complex, radial, or longitudinal configuration, and are associated with significantly more symptoms than nondisplaceable meniscus tears.

Research published in the radiology literature indicates that MR imaging can help predict clinical outcome in middle-aged and elderly patients. Worse outcomes after meniscectomy are associated with 5 findings: greater severity of cartilage loss and bone marrow edema in the same

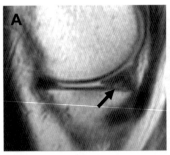
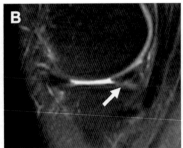
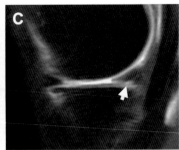

Fig. 10. True positive conventional MR imaging, with false-negative MR arthrography. Recurrent horizontal tear of the posterior horn of the medial meniscus 2 years after a partial meniscectomy in a 42-year-old woman. Postoperative PD (*A*) and fat-suppressed T2-weighted (*B*) sagittal images reveal a new horizontal tear of the posterior horn of the medial meniscus (*arrow*). A fat-suppressed T1-weighted sagittal image (*C*) after an arthrogram 1 week later with dilute gadolinium contrast shows linear increased signal at the site of the tear (*small arrow*), but no definite filling of the tear with high signal intensity that is as bright as the dilute gadolinium contrast within the joint space. The arthrogram was interpreted as negative (although some studies suggest this finding indicates a tear). At arthroscopy 3 weeks later, a new horizontal tear was found and was again treated with a partial meniscectomy.

compartment as the meniscus tear; greater severity of meniscus extrusion; greater overall severity of joint degeneration; a meniscus root tear; and a longer meniscus tear.[111]

MR imaging findings

Diagnosis of recurrent meniscus tears can be challenging, both by clinical evaluation and by MR imaging.

The normal MR imaging appearance after meniscectomy is volume loss and some degree of deformity, commonly free-edge truncation, at the site of resection.

For low-grade partial meniscectomy, defined as less than 25% of the length of the meniscus, the diagnostic criteria and accuracy for conventional MR imaging are similar to those for the unoperated meniscus (**Fig. 16**). Radial tears can be subtle but biomechanically significant (**Fig. 17**). Although radial tears are regarded as more common after meniscus resection than in knees before meniscus surgery (32% vs 14%),[112] superficial contour

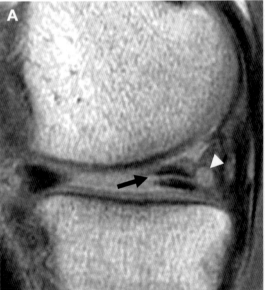
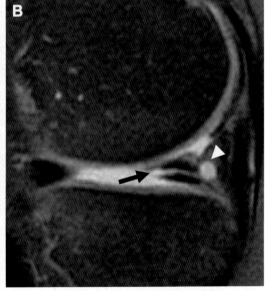

Fig. 11. Recurrent horizontal tear with parameniscal cyst. Recurrent horizontal tear 6 years after a partial meniscectomy with trimming of a free-edge radial tear of the medial meniscus in a 53-year-old golfer. Postoperative PD (*A*) and fat-suppressed T2-weighted (*B*) sagittal images of a horizontal tear of the posterior horn of the medial meniscus (*arrow*) communicating with a tiny parameniscal cyst (*arrowhead*).

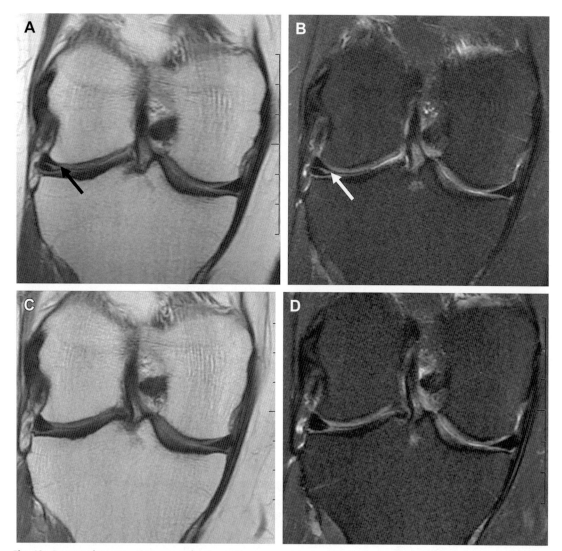

Fig. 12. Expected postmeniscectomy findings. No recurrent tear of the lateral meniscus 5 years after a partial meniscectomy with free-edge trimming of a horizontal tear of the body segment of the lateral meniscus in a 56-year-old physician complaining of vague knee pain. Preoperative PD (*A*) and fat-suppressed T2-weighted (*B*) coronal images reveal a horizontal tear of the body segment of the lateral meniscus (*arrow*). Postoperative PD (*C*) and fat-suppressed T2-weighted (*D*) coronal images reveal an intact meniscal remnant without evidence of a new tear.

irregularities after surgery are sometimes misdiagnosed as a recurrent tear on MR imaging.

For high-grade partial meniscectomy (>25%), the MR imaging diagnostic criteria are modified and the accuracy is significantly lower (**Table 1**). On PD-weighted images, surfacing intermediate signal intensity in the meniscus remnant may be due to a tear containing synovial fluid or fibrovascular tissue but also may be caused by residual grade-2 degenerative signal that abuts the remnant surface after meniscectomy. On T2-weighted images, high signal intensity has high specificity (>90%) for synovial fluid in the cleft of

a tear, but is an insensitive finding (~60%–80%). Given that the essential difference between PD and T2 images is the echo time (TE), the TE can be thought of as regulating the ROC curve: lower TE images are more sensitive in diagnosing meniscus tears, whereas higher TE images are more specific.

Overall accuracy of MR arthrography is generally reportedly in the range of 85% to 92%, which is 10% to 20% higher than conventional MR imaging in some series, but often not statistically significant. CT arthrography after meniscectomy has reported sensitivity and specificity

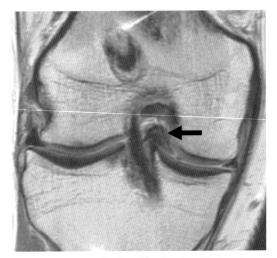

Fig. 13. Recurrent displaced bucket-handle tear. Large recurrent displaced bucket-handle tear in a 29-year-old man who sustained a twisting injury 8 years after an ACL reconstruction and medial meniscal repair. A PD coronal image reveals a large 12-mm wide displaced bucket-handle fragment (*arrow*) seen along the superior aspect of the medial tibial spine adjacent to an intact ACL graft.

of approximately 90%.[113] Unfortunately, the reported accuracies of diagnostic imaging techniques vary widely for retears of the postoperative meniscus.[114,115]

Complications

MR imaging may be helpful in assessing many of the possible complications after meniscus surgery (**Box 2**).[116,117] The self-reported complication rate for meniscectomy (2.8%) is lower than for meniscus repair (7.6%).[118] By comparison, the self-reported complication rates for reconstruction of the ACL (9%) and posterior cruciate ligament (20%) are higher than for meniscus procedures.

Repair

Outcomes

Compared with partial meniscectomy, successful meniscus repair for isolated traumatic tears results in significantly better long-term functional results, such as for osteoarthritis prophylaxis and recovery of sports activity. A meniscus repair may heal completely (50%–60%), heal partially (20%–25%), or fail (15%–25%).

- At long-term follow-up of 81 patients, averaging almost 9 years, no osteoarthritic progress was detectable in 81% after repair, compared with 40% after meniscectomy, and athletes showed a significantly higher level of sports activity after repair in comparison with the athletes after meniscectomy.[119]
- A recent systematic review of meniscus repairs from 13 studies followed for more than 5 years demonstrated clinical failure or

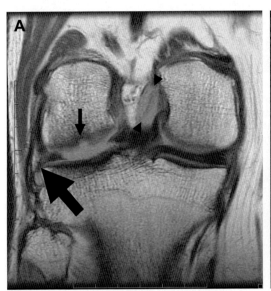
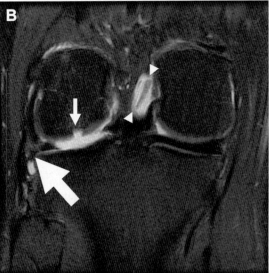

Fig. 14. Recurrent tear with common associated findings. New displaced lateral meniscal flap tear and chondral defect in a 50-year-old man with new pain and mechanical symptoms 5 years after a partial meniscectomy for a lateral meniscal tear. Postoperative PD (*A*) and fat-suppressed T2-weighted (*B*) coronal images reveal a small 4-mm inferolaterally displaced flap of the lateral meniscus (*large arrow*) seen just anterior to the popliteus tendon hiatus, and a chondral defect in the lateral femoral condyle (*small arrow*) with an associated thin chondral loose body in the intercondylar notch (*arrowheads*).

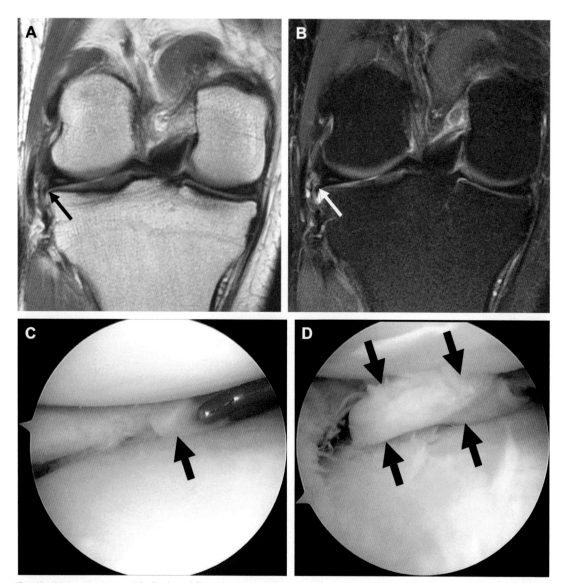

Fig. 15. Recurrent tear with displaced flap. Recurrent tear of the lateral meniscus with a displaced flap 2 years after a partial meniscectomy with trimming of a prior horizontal tear of the posterior horn of the lateral meniscus in a 37-year-old physician complaining of intermittent sharp pain and mechanical symptoms. Postoperative PD (*A*) and fat-suppressed T2-weighted (*B*) coronal images reveal a thin 6-mm inferiorly displaced flap (*arrow*) just anterior to the popliteus tendon. The arthroscopy images from 1 week later show the initial view of the flap (*C, arrow*) and the subsequent view after the flap has been pulled forward into the joint space with a probe (*D, arrows*). This flap was resected, resulting in resolution of the patient's intermittent sharp pain and mechanical symptoms.

reoperation in more than 20% of patients (**Fig. 18**).[120]

Revision meniscus repair can achieve good clinical outcomes. For example, in a recent cohort of 96 patients who underwent a prior meniscus repair, 16 (17%) experienced symptomatic retears (mean, 27 months); subsequently, 5 of these patients had "re-retears" of a resutured meniscus.

From this experience, the investigators ultimately concluded that revision meniscus repair can be performed for a recurrent meniscus tear without degenerative changes.[121]

The healing status of repaired menisci can be assessed with various outcomes measures, including patient pain/function, imaging, and second-look arthroscopy (**Fig. 19**). These end points may be discordant, in part because partially

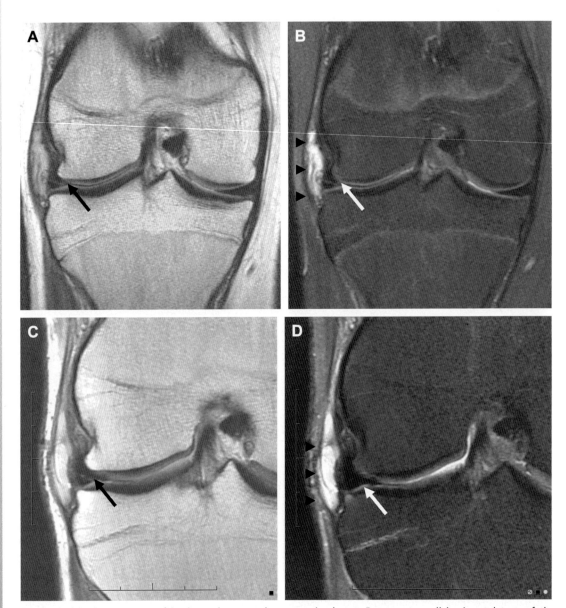

Fig. 16. Delayed recurrence of horizontal tear and parameniscal cyst. Recurrent small horizontal tear of the lateral meniscus with a parameniscal cyst after a partial meniscectomy with trimming of a prior horizontal and free-edge radial tear. This 27-year-old former college baseball player was asymptomatic for 10 years and then presented again complaining of new pain and a tender lateral joint-line soft-tissue mass. Preoperative PD (*A*) and fat-suppressed T2-weighted (*B*) coronal images when the patient was initially seen at age 17 reveal a horizontal tear of the body segment of the lateral meniscus (*arrow*) communicating with a small parameniscal cyst (*arrowheads*). Postoperative PD (*C*) and fat-suppressed T2-weighted (*D*) coronal images reveal a recurrent small horizontal tear (*arrow*) and parameniscal cyst (*arrowheads*) that was again treated with a partial meniscectomy.

healed menisci may or may not be symptomatic.[122]

MR imaging findings

After a repair procedure, the meniscus can be categorized as healed if there is no fluid signal in the repair, partially healed if fluid signal extends into less than 50% of the repair site, or not healed if fluid signal extends into greater than 50% of the repair site (**Figs. 20** and **21**).

Research on MR imaging after meniscus repair is relatively scant, and reported results are disappointing. Perhaps this should not be surprising, given that meniscus repairs represent only about 6% of all patients having knee arthroscopy for meniscus derangements.[123,124]

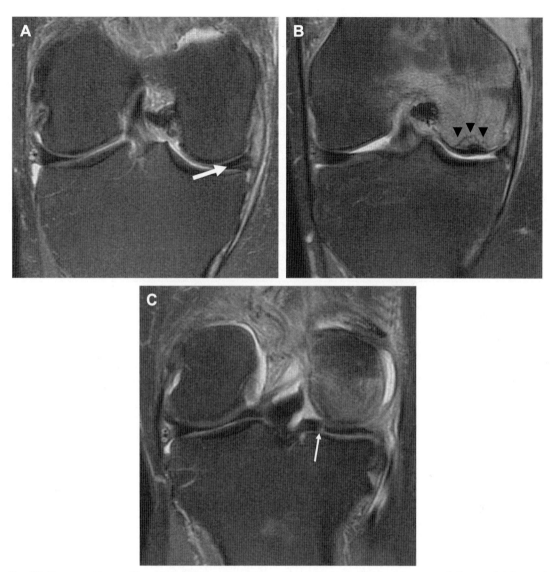

Fig. 17. Recurrent tear with radial configuration. New subchondral insufficiency fracture of the medial femoral condyle and radial tear of the posterior horn of the medial meniscus in a 68-year-old woman 3 months after a partial meniscectomy for a horizontal medial meniscal tear. A preoperative fat-suppressed T2-weighted coronal image (*A*) reveals a horizontal tear of the body segment (*arrow*). Postoperative T2-weighted coronal images (*B, C*) reveal a new subchondral insufficiency fracture of the medial femoral condyle (*arrowheads*) with prominent surrounding bone marrow edema, in addition to a radial tear of the remnant of the posterior horn of the medial meniscus (*arrow*).

With conventional MR imaging, hyperintense signal often persists at the repair site, often for more than 10 years after surgery, and even full-thickness signal abnormalities do not reliably predict recurrent tears.[125–127] This hyperintense signal may be from immature fibrovascular granulation tissue or mature fibrocartilaginous scar tissue. Arthrographic techniques can be useful in these cases,[128,129] but the authors find that conventional MR imaging still is the diagnostic workhorse, commonly showing displaced meniscus fragments, new tears at other locations, and internal derangements not involving the menisci (**Fig. 22**).[88]

Replacement

Allograft

Outcomes Meniscal allograft transplantation has now been performed for 30 years. Studies

Table 1
Diagnostic criteria for meniscus tears on MR imaging or MR arthrography

Diagnosis	MR Imaging Findings
Preoperative meniscus	
Tear	Displaced meniscus fragment, or Not at free edge: definite surfacing signal or distortion on 2 or more images[a], or At free edge: surfacing linear signal may be a vertical cleft (radial tear) or nonvertical (free-edge tear)
Possible tear	Not at free edge: definite surfacing signal or distortion on only one image
Fraying	Superficial, ill-defined, irregular free-edge signal
Postoperative meniscus[b]	
Tear	Displaced meniscus fragment, or Definite surfacing fluid signal[c] on 2 or more images[a], or
Possible tear	Definite surfacing fluid signal on only 1 image, or Linear surfacing fluid signal on only 1 image
Indeterminate[d]	Linear surfacing proton-density signal (but not fluid signal)

[a] In one or more planes, not necessarily contiguous.

[b] At postoperative site/segment. Postoperative meniscus refers to the area operated on, not any other. Criteria for preoperative meniscus can apply to a meniscus segment that has not be operated on and was normal on preoperative MR imaging.

[c] "Fluid signal" refers to high T2 signal on MR imaging or high T1 signal on MR arthrography (isointense with fluid in joint). For the preoperative meniscus, surfacing signal is noted on both proton-density–weighted and T2-weighted images, although variations in meniscus signal and morphology are well described as potential pseudotears (eg, flounce, lateral meniscus posterior horn attachment of the meniscofemoral ligament, lateral meniscus anterior horn root).

[d] May represent postoperative change or recurrent tear. Distortion of meniscus caused by a tear is commonly associated with a displaced fragment.

Data from De Smet AA. MR imaging and MR arthrography for diagnosis of recurrent tears in the postoperative meniscus. Semin Musculoskelet Radiol 2005;9(2):116–24; and De Smet AA, Horak DM, Davis KW, et al. Intensity of signal contacting meniscal surface in recurrent tears on MR arthrography compared with that of contrast material. AJR Am J Roentgenol 2006;187(6):W565–8.

Box 2
Potential complications associated with arthroscopic meniscus surgery

- Synovitis
- Arthrofibrosis
- Chondral damage
- Meniscus damage
- Medial collateral ligament injury
- Nerve injury (saphenous, tibial, peroneal)
- Vascular injury (saphenous vein, lateral geniculate artery, popliteal vessels)
- Deep venous thrombosis
- Infection

Data from Kinsella SD, Carey JL. Complications in brief: arthroscopic partial meniscectomy. Clin Orthop Relat Res 2013;471(5):1427–32. http://dx.doi.org/10.1007/s11999-012-2735-3; and Gwathmey FW Jr, Golish SR, Diduch DR. Complications in brief: meniscus repair. Clin Orthop Relat Res 2012;470(7):2059–66.

generally show significant improvements in pain and functional outcomes in comparison with a preoperative baseline, but a relatively high rate of complications and/or reoperations, as highlighted in the most significant studies to date.

- Clinical results are reported as "fair to excellent" for 75% to 90% based on a review of 39 studies on a total of 1226 allografts and a mean follow-up time of 5.5 years.[130]
- Allograft survival is as high as 95% at 5 years and 70% at 10 years based on one recent report of 172 patients.[131]
- Athletes at the amateur[132] and professional[133] levels may return to their sports in the short term in as many as 75% of cases, based on small short-term studies with at least 36 months of follow-up.
- Reoperations occur in 35% of patients, with 12% requiring conversion to total knee arthroplasty, based on a study of 49 patients with a mean follow-up of almost 13 years.[134] For others

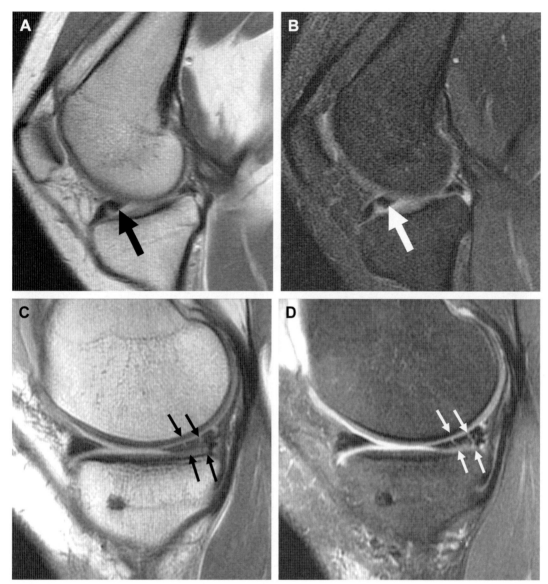

Fig. 18. New vertical tears after successful repair. New complex tear of the posterior horn of the medial meniscus in a 28-year-old tennis player with recurrent pain 1 year after repair of a bucket-handle tear. There was no new acute injury. Preoperative PD (*A*) and STIR (*B*) sagittal images with the knee locked in flexion reveal a displaced bucket-handle fragment (*large arrow*) that was successfully repaired with sutures. Postoperative PD (*C*) and fat-suppressed T2-weighted (*D*) sagittal images reveal 2 adjacent vertical longitudinal tears of the posterior horn of the medial meniscus (*small arrows*).

the outcome is more favorable, with significant improvement in pain and function in addition to generally well preserved joint spaces.

MR imaging findings MR imaging analysis has been performed in more than a dozen studies from 1 to 20 years after allograft surgery. MR imaging correlates well with arthroscopic evaluation of the transplants (**Fig. 23**).

Although MR imaging and second-look arthroscopy provide an objective assessment of gross pathologic findings, the morphologic findings (eg, allograft shrinkage and partial extrusion) do not always correlate with subjective assessments of pain and function by patients. For example, extrusion has been correlated significantly with arthrosis progression, but not clinical outcome metrics, by follow-up at 4 years.[135]

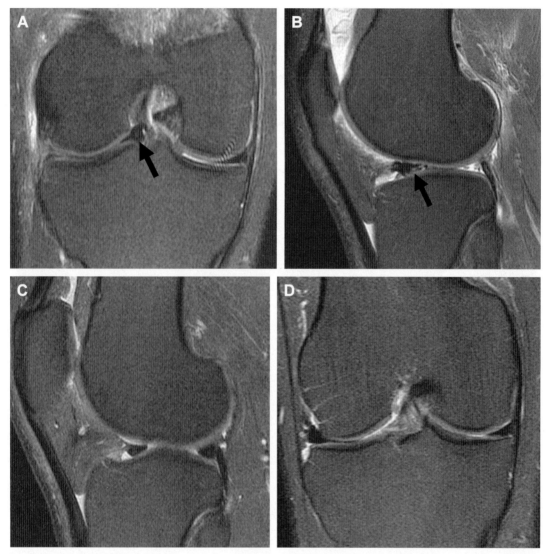

Fig. 19. Successful meniscus repair in a 28-year-old with recurrent pain 2 years after repair of a large displaced bucket-handle tear of the lateral meniscus. Preoperative fat-suppressed T2-weighted coronal (*A*) and sagittal (*B*) images reveal a displaced bucket-handle fragment (*large arrow*) that was successfully reduced and repaired with sutures. Postoperative fat-suppressed T2-weighted sagittal (*C*) and coronal (*D*) images reveal the well-healed repair. Subsequent arthroscopy confirmed that the repair was intact.

Serial MR imaging scans commonly show changes in morphology and signal intensity of the transplanted allograft menisci over the first postoperative year. These changes include progressively increased intrameniscal signal to at least 1 year postoperatively and decreased width and increased thickness of the body segment. However, these findings are not related to clinical outcome.[136,137] Regarding extrusion, a meniscus that extrudes early remains extruded and does not progressively worsen, whereas one that does not extrude early is unlikely to extrude within the first postoperative year.[138]

Complications occur at an average rate of 21% per trial.[48] The most important clinical concern at the time of MR imaging is often progressive high-grade articular cartilage loss; allograft meniscus tears are substantially less common (~10%–15%). Other relatively common postoperative derangements include allograft extrusion, allograft shrinkage, arthrofibrosis, and synovitis, while infection and intra-articular hematoma are less common.[139–142]

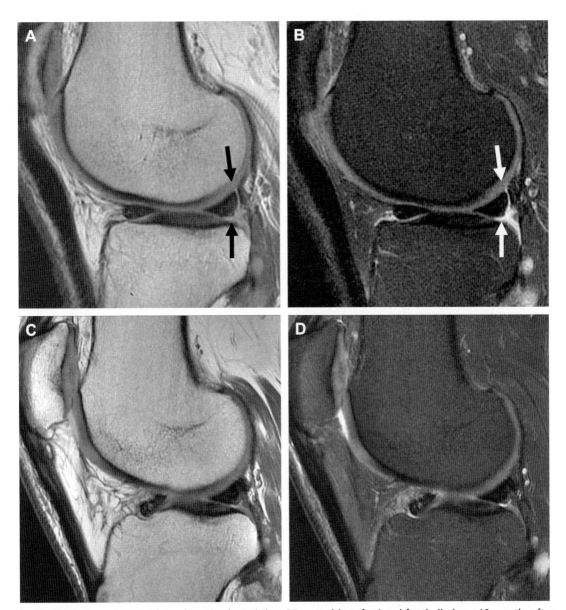

Fig. 20. Healed repair. Intact lateral meniscal repair in a 27-year-old professional football player 10 months after surgery. Preoperative PD (*A*) and fat-suppressed T2-weighted (*B*) sagittal images reveal a vertical peripheral tear of the posterior horn of the lateral meniscus (*arrows*). A postoperative MR scan was performed to document healing before the patient signed a contract with a new team: PD (*C*) and fat-suppressed T2-weighted (*D*) sagittal images reveal an intact repaired meniscus.

Implants

Outcomes and MR imaging findings

The 2 currently available scaffold products (synthetic partial meniscus implants) have shown encouraging early results, without known significant adverse reactions at the time of writing. However, there is a definite need for well-designed randomized trials to confirm the promising preliminary results with a stronger level of evidence.[143]

Polyurethane-based scaffold The polyurethane-based scaffold (Actifit) shows generally good clinical results at early to midterm follow-up, with significant improvements in pain and function scores (**Fig. 24**).[144]

For example, of 52 patients in one study with a 2-year follow-up, there was a 17% incidence of treatment failure, as 9 serious adverse events required reoperation.[145] Of note, on MR imaging

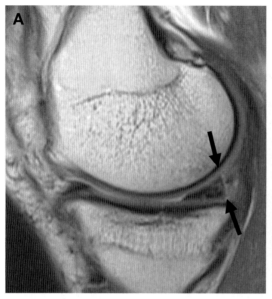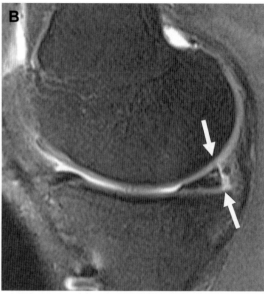

Fig. 21. Failed repair. Failure of healing of a medial meniscal repair in a 24-year-old professional football player 8 months after surgery. Postoperative PD (*A*) and fat-suppressed T2-weighted (*B*) sagittal images reveal a vertical peripheral tear of the posterior horn of the medial meniscus (*arrows*) that has not healed at the site of repair. The extent of the tear was the same as on the preoperative scan (not shown). This scan was performed to determine whether healing had occurred before the signing of a new contract.

this study showed stable or improved ICRS articular cartilage grades in 93% of patients between baseline and 2-year follow-up.

MR imaging shows the scaffold as increased signal intensity on short and long TE pulse sequences, presumably because of the highly porous structure and water content, compared with normal meniscus of low signal intensity (**Fig. 25**).[146] This hyperintensity tends to diminish over the years as the scaffold matures, but never reaches the low signal of normal fibrocartilage.

Serial MR imaging examinations from baseline to 2 years show that limited meniscus extrusion is common preoperatively and increases at an average of 2 mm in the postoperative medial meniscus, but is not correlated with clinical outcomes scores.[147]

Favorable clinical outcomes at minimum 2-year follow-up have been confirmed for patients with MR imaging examinations showing a diffusely hyperintense scaffold and mild to moderate extrusion, in the absence of synovitis (**Fig. 26**).[148]

Collagen-based scaffold The collagen-based scaffold (Menaflex) has a longer performance record, with initial 3-year follow-up data published in the mid-1990s.[149]

- In an analysis of 11 studies with 520 subjects followed postoperatively for 47 ± 40 months,

66% to 70% of patients had satisfactory outcomes, including improved knee function and activity levels, whereas the remainder did not appear to receive any benefit.[150] With implant maturation, the signal intensity tends to decrease over time,[151] although myxoid degeneration is present in most implants.[152]

- In a subsequent study of 25 patients with a minimum 10-year follow-up, results were "good to excellent" in 83%, with a failure rate of 8% and reportedly no complications related to the device.[153] The implant normally decreases in size over time on MR imaging, but joint-space narrowing is minimal or absent.
- In another recent study of 76 patients followed for 12 months postoperatively, significant pain relief and functional improvements also occurred.[154] On MR imaging, the implant usually became partially resorbed (92%), appeared slightly hyperintense (90%), and extruded by more than 3 mm (72%).

Total meniscus implant The total medial meniscus implant (NUsurface) has been reported in 118 patients,[155] with follow-up MR imaging evaluated at 6 weeks and 1 year in 10 patients (**Fig. 27**).[156] At 6 weeks, MR imaging showed

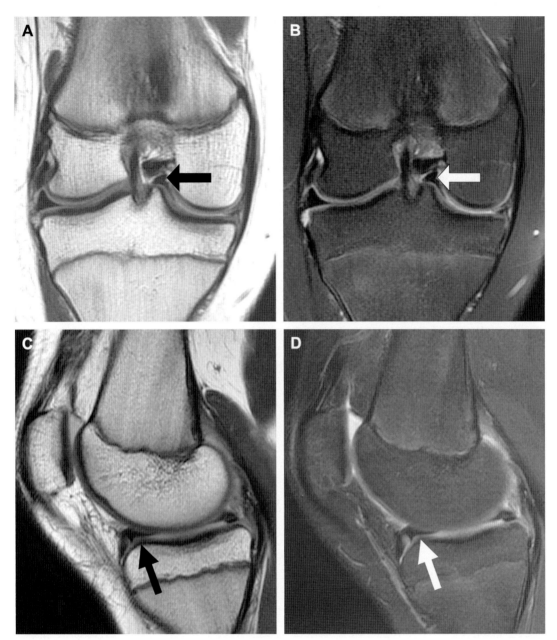

Fig. 22. Successful repair, with new tear at another location. Recurrent tear of the posterior horn of the medial meniscal in a 16-year-old lacrosse player with a recurrent injury 2 years after repair of a bucket-handle tear. Pre-operative PD (*A*) and fat-suppressed T2-weighted (*B*) coronal images, and PD (*C*) and fat-suppressed T2-weighted (*D*) sagittal images reveal a displaced bucket-handle fragment (*large arrows*) that was successfully repaired with sutures. The patient was asymptomatic and returned to sports until a recurrent twisting injury during lacrosse practice. Postoperative PD (*E*) and fat-suppressed T2-weighted (*F*) coronal images, and PD (*G*) and fat-suppressed T2-weighted (*H*) sagittal images reveal an intact repair of the body segment and a recurrent complex tear of the posterior horn of the medial meniscus (*small arrows*).

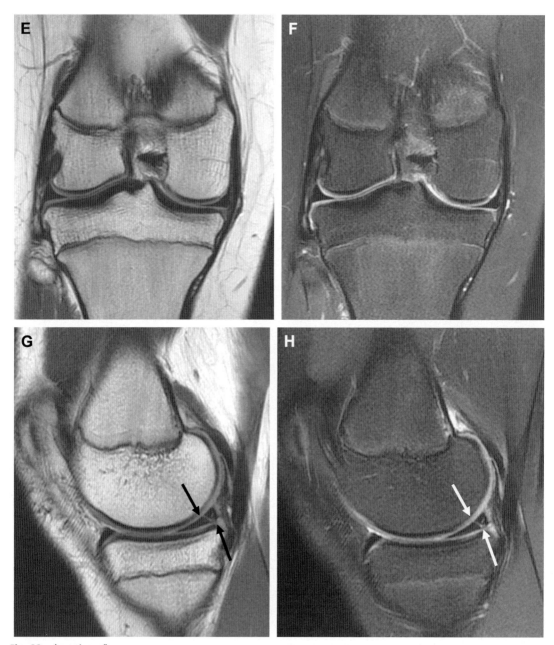

Fig. 22. (continued)

several findings: medial compartment bone marrow edema (9 of 10 patients) and medial pericapsular edema (7 of 10 patients). At 1 year these findings had essentially resolved (except for 1 patient with residual bone marrow edema) and did not correlate with pain scores or altered range of motion.

Where in the world? In the United States the costs of cadaveric meniscus allograft transplantation may be covered by medical insurers, but synthetic meniscus implants are considered investigational.[157]

At present, no partial or total synthetic implants are approved for marketing by the US

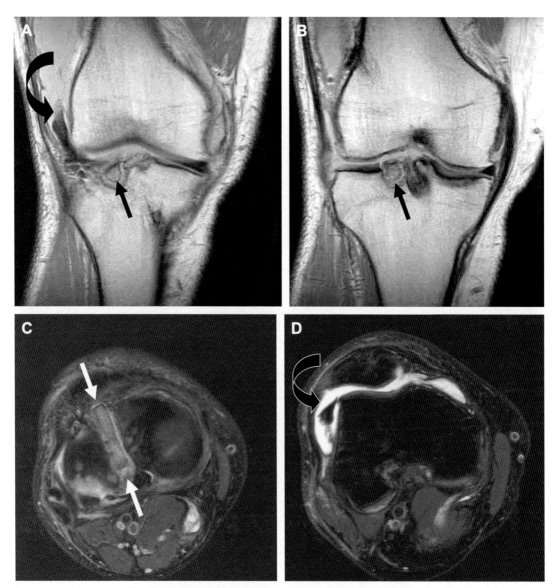

Fig. 23. Meniscal allograft failure. Large displaced meniscal flap tear in a 34-year-old skier 9 months after a lateral meniscal allograft and ACL reconstruction. PD (*A, B*) coronal images and fat-suppressed T2-weighted (*C, D*) axial images reveal a large superiorly displaced flap of the lateral meniscal allograft (*curved arrow*) that occurred after a twisting injury. The allograft bone (*straight arrows*) has not yet incorporated into the lateral tibial plateau.

FDA, although approval was granted to conduct a clinical trial of a total meniscus (NUsurface) in 2014. The FDA did approve the Menaflex collagen meniscus implant in 2008, but rescinded approval in 2010 after more than 120 surgeons had been trained to perform the technique. Medical payers in the United States currently classify meniscus implants as "not reasonable and necessary for the treatment of meniscus injury/tear."[158]

Outside of the United States, both the polyurethane-based (Actifit) and collagen-based (Menaflex) implants are used, most extensively in Europe (eg, Actifit received regulatory clearance for sale in the European Union in 2008).[159]

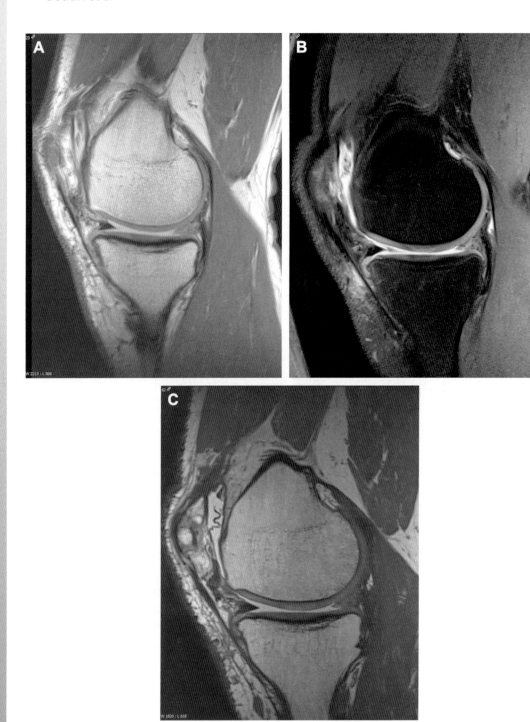

Fig. 24. Meniscus implant in an asymptomatic patient. The patient returned to playing sports and working as a carpenter, and was still asymptomatic at 2 years. Sagittal PD image at 1 month (*A*), and sagittal fat-saturated PD (*B*) and PD SPACE (sampling perfection with application-optimized contrasts using different flip-angle evolution) (*C*) images at 6 months after implantation of a polyurethane meniscus scaffold. Pertinent negatives include the absence of bone marrow edema or an articular cartilage defect. Surfacing hyperintensity should not be misinterpreted as a tear. (*Courtesy of* Wouter C. Huysse, MD. Department of Radiology, Ghent University Hospital, Ghent, Belgium.)

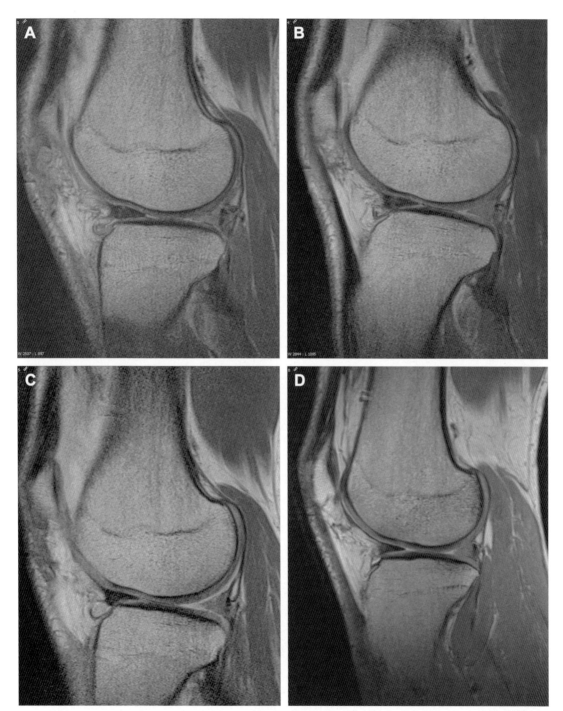

Fig. 25. Meniscus implant from 1 week to 5 years. Sagittal PD image at 1 week (*A*) shows the scaffold is diffusely hyperintense; the native anterior horn and posterior horn peripheral rim remain hypointense. Subsequent serial images show evolution of findings on sagittal PD image at 3 months (*B*), with minimal volume loss and superficial irregular signal at the free edge by 1 year (*C*, sagittal PD). The articular cartilage continues to be preserved on sagittal PD (*D*) and sagittal DESS (double-echo steady-state) with water excitation (*E*) images at 3 years, and on sagittal PD imaging at 5 years (*F*). (*Courtesy of* Wouter C. Huysse, MD. Department of Radiology, Ghent University Hospital, Ghent, Belgium.)

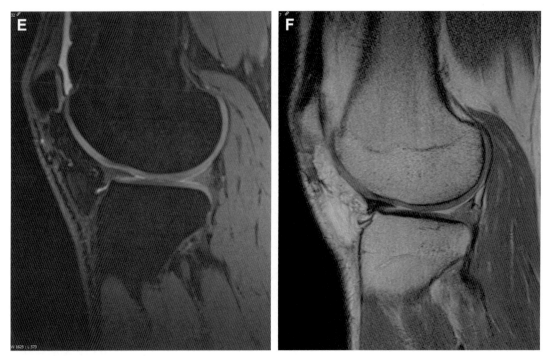

Fig. 25. (*continued*)

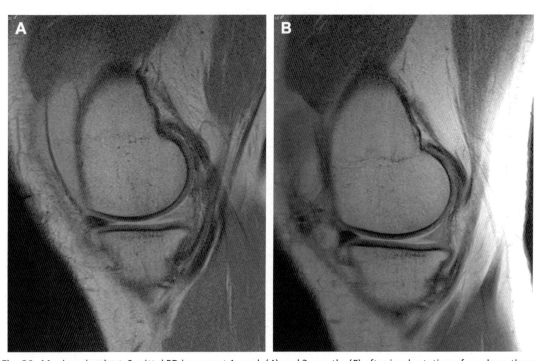

Fig. 26. Meniscus implant. Sagittal PD images at 1 week (*A*) and 3 months (*B*) after implantation of a polyurethane meniscus scaffold showing the expected increased signal intensity of the implant. This patient reported transient pain at 3 months, but improved afterward to become pain-free at 24 months. (*Courtesy of* Wouter C. Huysse, MD. Department of Radiology, Ghent University Hospital, Ghent, Belgium.)

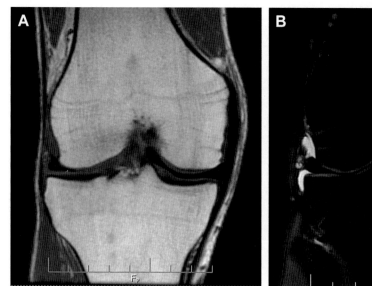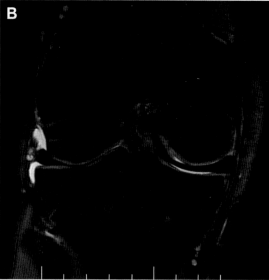

Fig. 27. Total meniscus implant. Coronal T1-weighted (*A*) and fat-suppressed T2-weighted (*B*) MR images of the knee show the normal appearance of a total medial meniscus implant. This nonanchored implant is made of polycarbonate-urethane and polyethylene fibers, and is hypointense on all pulse sequences. (*Courtesy of* Nogah Shabshin, MD. Department of Radiology, Hospital of the University of Pennsylvania, Philadelphia, PA.)

SUMMARY

Meniscus repair is preferable to meniscectomy when practicable. If a partial meniscectomy is performed, maximal meniscus preservation is a high priority. If a high-grade meniscectomy must be performed, meniscus implants may be increasingly used in the future. For all postoperative changes, MR imaging is a powerful tool in identifying appropriate surgical candidates, preoperative planning, and continued follow-up.

REFERENCES

1. Verdonk PCM, Van Laer MEE, Verdonk R. Meniscus replacement: from allograft to tissue engineering. Sports Orthop Traumatol 2008;24(2):78–82. http://dx.doi.org/10.1016/j.orthtr.2008.03.004.
2. Cullen KA, Hall MJ, Golosinskiy A. Ambulatory surgery in the United States, 2006. Natl Health Stat Report 2009;11:1–25.
3. Mow VC, Huiskes R. Basic orthopaedic biomechanics & mechano-biology. 3rd edition. Philadelphia: Lippincott Williams & Wilkins; 2005.
4. Uysal M, Akpinar S, Bolat F, et al. Apoptosis in the traumatic and degenerative tears of human meniscus. Knee Surg Sports Traumatol Arthrosc 2008;16(7):666–9.
5. Sanchez-Adams J, Wilusz RE, Guilak F. Atomic force microscopy reveals regional variations in the Micromechanical properties of the pericellular and extracellular matrices of the meniscus. J Orthop Res 2013;31:1218–25.
6. Fuller ES, Smith MM, Little CB, et al. Zonal differences in meniscus matrix turnover and cytokine response. Osteoarthritis Cartilage 2012;20(1):49–59.
7. Wang L, Chang G, Bencardino J, et al. T1rho MRI at 3T of menisci in patients with acute anterior cruciate ligament (ACL) injury. J Magn Reson Imaging 2014. [Epub ahead of print].
8. Wang L, Chang G, Bencardino J, et al. T1rho MRI of menisci in patients with osteoarthritis at 3 Tesla: a preliminary study. J Magn Reson Imaging 2014;40(3):588–95. http://dx.doi.org/10.1002/jmri.24437.
9. van Tiel J, Kotek G, Reijman M, et al. Delayed gadolinium-enhanced MRI of the meniscus (dGEMRIM) in patients with knee osteoarthritis: relation with meniscal degeneration on conventional MRI, reproducibility, and correlation with dGEMRIC. Eur Radiol 2014;24(9):2261–70.
10. Melnyk M, Luebken FV, Hartmann J, et al. Effects of age on neuromuscular knee joint control. Eur J Appl Physiol 2008;103(5):523–7.
11. Andrews SH, Ronsky JL, Rattner JB, et al. An evaluation of meniscal collagenous structure using optical projection tomography. BMC Med Imaging 2013;13(1):21.
12. Hutchinson ID, Moran CJ, Potter HG, et al. Restoration of the meniscus: form and function. Am J Sports Med 2014;42(4):987–98.

13. Baum T, Joseph GB, Karampinos DC, et al. Cartilage and meniscal T2 relaxation time as noninvasive biomarker for knee osteoarthritis and cartilage repair procedures. Osteoarthritis Cartilage 2013;21(10):1474–84.

14. Koff MF, Shah P, Pownder S, et al. Correlation of meniscal T2* with multiphoton microscopy, and change of articular cartilage T2 in an ovine model of meniscal repair. Osteoarthritis Cartilage 2013;21(8):1083–91.

15. Andrews SH, Rattner JB, Abusara Z, et al. Tie-fibre structure and organization in the knee menisci. J Anat 2014;224(5):531–7.

16. Bird MD, Sweet MB. Canals in the semilunar meniscus: brief report. J Bone Joint Surg Br 1988;70(5):839.

17. Kijowski R, Rosas HG, Lee KS, et al. MRI characteristics of healed and unhealed peripheral vertical meniscal tears. AJR Am J Roentgenol 2014; 202(3):585–92.

18. Hauger O, Frank LR, Boutin RD, et al. Characterization of the "red zone" of knee meniscus: MR imaging and histologic correlation. Radiology 2000; 217(1):193–200.

19. Zimny ML, Albright DJ, Dabezies E. Mechanoreceptors in the human medial meniscus. Acta Anat (Basel) 1988;133(1):35–40.

20. Mine T, Kimura M, Sakka A, et al. Innervation of nociceptors in the menisci of the knee joint: an immunohistochemical study. Arch Orthop Trauma Surg 2000;120(3–4):201–4.

21. Ashraf S, Wibberley H, Mapp PI, et al. Increased vascular penetration and nerve growth in the meniscus: a potential source of pain in osteoarthritis. Ann Rheum Dis 2011;70(3):523–9.

22. Roemer FW, Felson DT, Yang T, et al. The association between meniscal damage of the posterior horns and localized posterior synovitis detected on T1-weighted contrast-enhanced MRI–the MOST study. Semin Arthritis Rheum 2013;42(6):573–81.

23. Zanetti M, Pfirrmann CW, Schmid MR, et al. Patients with suspected meniscal tears: prevalence of abnormalities seen on MRI of 100 symptomatic and 100 contralateral asymptomatic knees. AJR Am J Roentgenol 2003;181:635–41.

24. Kamimura M, Umehara J, Takahashi A, et al. Medial meniscus tear morphology and related clinical symptoms in patients with medial knee osteoarthritis. Knee Surg Sports Traumatol Arthrosc 2014. [Epub ahead of print].

25. Magyar MO, Knoll Z, Kiss RM. Effect of medial meniscus tear and partial meniscectomy on balancing capacity in response to sudden unidirectional perturbation. J Electromyogr Kinesiol 2012;22(3):440–5.

26. Akgun U, Kocaoglu B, Orhan EK, et al. Possible reflex pathway between medial meniscus and semimembranosus muscle: an experimental study in rabbits. Knee Surg Sports Traumatol Arthrosc 2008;16(9):809–14.

27. Saygi B, Yildirim Y, Berker N, et al. Evaluation of the neurosensory function of the medial meniscus in humans. Arthroscopy 2005;21(12):1468–72.

28. Melnyk M, Faist M, Gothner M, et al. Changes in stretch reflex excitability are related to "giving way" symptoms in patients with anterior cruciate ligament rupture. J Neurophysiol 2007;97(1): 474–80.

29. Verdonk R. The meniscus: past, present and future. Knee Surg Sports Traumatol Arthrosc 2011;19: 145–6.

30. Barber-Westin SD, Noyes FR. Clinical healing rates of meniscus repairs of tears in the central-third (red-white) zone. Arthroscopy 2014;30(1):134–46.

31. Lee DW, Jang HW, Lee SR, et al. Clinical, radiological, and morphological evaluations of posterior horn tears of the lateral meniscus left in situ during anterior cruciate ligament reconstruction. Am J Sports Med 2014;42(2):327–35.

32. Shelbourne KD, Gray T. Meniscus tears that can be left in situ, with or without trephination or synovial abrasion to stimulate healing. Sports Med Arthrosc 2012;20(2):62–7.

33. Vermesan D, Prejbeanu R, Laitin S, et al. Meniscal tears left in situ during anatomic single bundle anterior cruciate ligament reconstruction. Eur Rev Med Pharmacol Sci 2014;18(2):252–6.

34. Sihvonen R, Paavola M, Malmivaara A, et al. Finnish Degenerative Meniscal Lesion Study (FIDELITY): a protocol for a randomised, placebo surgery controlled trial on the efficacy of arthroscopic partial meniscectomy for patients with degenerative meniscus injury with a novel 'RCT within-a-cohort' study design. BMJ Open 2013; 3(3). pii:e002510.

35. Musahl V, Jordan SS, Colvin AC, et al. Practice patterns for combined anterior cruciate ligament and meniscal surgery in the United States. Am J Sports Med 2010;38:918–23.

36. Cavanaugh JT, Killian SE. Rehabilitation following meniscal repair. Curr Rev Musculoskelet Med 2012;5:46–58.

37. Lind M, Nielsen T, Faunø P, et al. Free rehabilitation is safe after isolated meniscus repair: a prospective randomized trial comparing free with restricted rehabilitation regimens. Am J Sports Med 2013;41: 2753–8.

38. Ramappa AJ, Chen A, Hertz B, et al. A biomechanical evaluation of all-inside 2-stitch meniscal repair devices with matched inside-out suture repair. Am J Sports Med 2014;42:194–9.

39. Grant JA, Wilde J, Miller BS, et al. Comparison of inside-out and all-inside techniques for the repair of isolated meniscal tears: a systematic review. Am J Sports Med 2012;40:459–68.

40. Nelson CG, Bonner KF. Inside-out meniscus repair. Arthrosc Tech 2013;2:e453–60.

41. Dave LY, Caborn DN. Outside-in meniscus repair: the last 25 years. Sports Med Arthrosc 2012; 20(2):77–85.

42. Cho JH. A modified outside-in suture technique for repair of the middle segment of the meniscus using a spinal needle. Knee Surg Relat Res 2014;26(1): 43–7.

43. Morgan CD. The "all-inside" meniscus repair. Arthroscopy 1991;7(1):120–5.

44. Saliman JD. The circumferential compression stitch for meniscus repair. Arthrosc Tech 2013; 2(3):e257–64.

45. Turman KA, Diduch DR, Miller MD. All-inside meniscal repair. Sports Health 2009;1(5):438–44.

46. Goradia VK. All-inside arthroscopic meniscal repair with meniscal cinch. Arthrosc Tech 2013;2(2): e171–4.

47. Jouve F, Ovadia H, Pujol N, et al. Meniscal repair: technique. In: Beaufils P, Verdonk R, editors. The meniscus. Berlin Heidelberg (Germany): Springer-Verlag; 2010. p. 119–36.

48. Elattar M, Dhollander A, Verdonk R, et al. Twenty-six years of meniscal allograft transplantation: is it still experimental? A meta-analysis of 44 trials. Knee Surg Sports Traumatol Arthrosc 2011;19(2): 147–57.

49. Dienst M, Greis PE, Ellis BJ, et al. Effect of lateral meniscal allograft sizing on contact mechanics of the lateral tibial plateau: an experimental study in human cadaveric knee joints. Am J Sports Med 2007;35(1):34–42.

50. Pollard ME, Kang Q, Berg EE. Radiographic sizing for meniscal transplantation. Arthroscopy 1995;11: 684–7.

51. Prodromos CC, Joyce BT, Keller BL, et al. Magnetic resonance imaging measurement of the contralateral normal meniscus is a more accurate method of determining meniscal allograft size than radiographic measurement of the recipient tibial plateau. Arthroscopy 2007;23(11):1174–9.e1.

52. Shaffer B, Kennedy S, Klimkiewicz J, et al. Preoperative sizing of meniscal allografts in meniscus transplantation. Am J Sports Med 2000;28(4):524–33.

53. Vrancken AC, Buma P, van Tienen TG. Synthetic meniscus replacement: a review. Int Orthop 2013; 37(2):291–9.

54. Spencer SJ, Saithna A, Carmont MR, et al. Meniscal scaffolds: early experience and review of the literature. Knee 2012;19(6):760–5.

55. Rodkey WG. Menaflex (TM) collagen meniscus implant: basic science. In: Beaufils P, Verdonk R, editors. The meniscus. Berlin Heidelberg (Germany): Springer-Verlag; 2010. p. 367–72.

56. Verdonk R, Verdonk P, Heinrichs EL. Polyurethane meniscus implant: technique. In: Beaufils P,

57. Verdonk R, editors. The meniscus. Berlin Heidelberg: Springer-Verlag; 2010. p. 389–94.

57. Heijkants RG, Pennings AJ, de Groot JH, et al. Method for the preparation of new segmented polyurethanes with high tear and tensile strengths and method for making porous scaffolds. United States patent 7,943,678 B2. May 17, 2011. Available at: http://www.google.com/patents/US7943678.

58. Shemesh M, Asher R, Zylberberg E, et al. Viscoelastic properties of a synthetic meniscus implant. J Mech Behav Biomed Mater 2014;29:42–55.

59. Shterling A, Zur G, Linder-Ganz E, et al. Meniscus prosthetic devices with anti-migration features. United States patent 8361147 B2. January 29, 2013. Available at: http://www.google.com/patents/US8361147.

60. ClinicalTrials.gov. Treatment of the medial meniscus with the NUsurface(R) meniscus implant. U.S. National Institutes of Health. Available at: http://clinical-trials.gov/ct2/show/study/NCT01712191. Accessed May 16, 2014.

61. Hedman TP, Slusarewicz P. Crosslinker enhanced repair of knee meniscus. US patent application: 2013/0085569 A1. 2013. Available at: http://www.google.com/patents/US20130085569.

62. Gatt CJ, Merriam AS, Dunn MG. Implantable device and method to replace the meniscus of the knee and other body structures. US patent application: 20140031933 A1. 2014. Available at: http://www.google.com/patents/US20140031933.

63. Taylor SA, Rodeo SA. Augmentation techniques for isolated meniscal tears. Curr Rev Musculoskelet Med 2013;6(2):95–101.

64. Salgado AJ, Oliveira JM, Martins A, et al. Tissue engineering and regenerative medicine: past, present, and future. Tissue engineering of the peripheral nerve: stem cells and regeneration promoting factors. Int Rev Neurobiol 2013;108:1–33.

65. Fox JM, Rintz KG, Ferkel RD. Trephination of incomplete meniscal tears. Arthroscopy 1993;9(4):451–5.

66. Uchio Y, Ochi M, Adachi N, et al. Results of rasping of meniscal tears with and without anterior cruciate ligament injury as evaluated by second-look arthroscopy. Arthroscopy 2003;19(5):463–9.

67. O'Meara PM. Surgical techniques for arthroscopic meniscal repair. Orthop Rev 1993;22(7):781–90.

68. Henning CE, Lynch MA, Yearout KM, et al. Arthroscopic meniscal repair using an exogenous fibrin clot. Clin Orthop Relat Res 1990;(252):64–72.

69. van Trommel MF, Simonian PT, Potter HG, et al. Arthroscopic meniscal repair with fibrin clot of complete radial tears of the lateral meniscus in the avascular zone. Arthroscopy 1998;14(4):360–5.

70. Ra HJ, Ha JK, Jang SH, et al. Arthroscopic inside-out repair of complete radial tears of the meniscus with a fibrin clot. Knee Surg Sports Traumatol Arthrosc 2013;21(9):2126–30.

71. Vangsness CT Jr, Farr J 2nd, Boyd J, et al. Adult human mesenchymal stem cells delivered via intra-articular injection to the knee following partial medial meniscectomy: a randomized, double-blind, controlled study. J Bone Joint Surg Am 2014;96(2):90–8.

72. Simson JA, Strehin IA, Allen BW, et al. Bonding and fusion of meniscus fibrocartilage using a novel chondroitin sulfate bone marrow tissue adhesive. Tissue Eng Part A 2013;19(15–16):1843–51.

73. Zhu WH, Wang YB, Wang L, et al. Effects of canine myoblasts expressing human cartilage-derived morphogenetic protein-2 on the repair of meniscal fibrocartilage injury. Mol Med Rep 2014;9(5): 1767–72.

74. Sarem M, Moztarzadeh F, Mozafari M, et al. Optimization strategies on the structural modeling of gelatin/chitosan scaffolds to mimic human meniscus tissue. Mater Sci Eng C Mater Biol Appl 2013;33(8):4777–85.

75. Narita A, Takahara M, Sato D, et al. Biodegradable gelatin hydrogels incorporating fibroblast growth factor 2 promote healing of horizontal tears in rabbit meniscus. Arthroscopy 2012;28(2):255–63.

76. Kopf S, Birkenfeld F, Becker R, et al. Local treatment of meniscal lesions with vascular endothelial growth factor. J Bone Joint Surg Am 2010;92(16): 2682–91.

77. Discepola F, Park JS, Clopton P, et al. Valid MR imaging predictors of prior knee arthroscopy. Skeletal Radiol 2012;41(1):67–74.

78. Atoun E, Debbi R, Lubovsky O, et al. Arthroscopic trans-portal deep medial collateral ligament pie-crusting release. Arthrosc Tech 2013; 2(1):e41–3.

79. Vance K, Meredick R, Schweitzer ME, et al. Magnetic resonance imaging of the postoperative meniscus. Arthroscopy 2009;25:522–30.

80. Farley TE, Howell SM, Love KF, et al. Meniscal tears: MR and arthrographic findings after arthroscopic repair. Radiology 1991;180:517–22.

81. Applegate GR, Flannigan BD, Tolin BS, et al. MR diagnosis of recurrent tears in the knee: value of intraarticular contrast material. AJR Am J Roentgenol 1993;161:821–5.

82. Van Trommel MF, Potter HG, Ernberg LA, et al. The use of noncontrast magnetic resonance imaging in evaluating meniscal repair: comparison with conventional arthrography. Arthroscopy 1998;14: 2–8.

83. Sciulli RL, Boutin RD, Brown RR, et al. Evaluation of the postoperative meniscus of the knee: a study comparing conventional arthrography, conventional MR imaging, MR arthrography with iodinated contrast material, and MR arthrography with gadolinium-based contrast material. Skeletal Radiol 1999;28:508–14.

84. Ciliz D, Ciliz A, Elverici E, et al. Evaluation of postoperative menisci with MR arthrography and routine conventional MRI. Clin Imaging 2008; 32(3):212–9.

85. Cardello P, Gigli C, Ricci A, et al. Retears of postoperative knee meniscus: findings on magnetic resonance imaging (MRI) and magnetic resonance arthrography (MRA) by using low and high field magnets. Skeletal Radiol 2009;38(2):149–56.

86. Naranje S, Mittal R, Nag H, et al. Arthroscopic and magnetic resonance imaging evaluation of meniscus lesions in the chronic anterior cruciate ligament-deficient knee. Arthroscopy 2008;24(9): 1045–51.

87. De Smet AA. MR imaging and MR arthrography for diagnosis of recurrent tears in the postoperative meniscus. Semin Musculoskelet Radiol 2005;9: 116–24.

88. Toms AP, White LM, Marshall TJ, et al. Imaging the post-operative meniscus. Eur J Radiol 2005;54(2): 189–98.

89. Sanders TG. Imaging of the postoperative knee. Semin Musculoskelet Radiol 2011;15(4):383–407.

90. Gnannt R, Chhabra A, Theodoropoulos JS, et al. MR imaging of the postoperative knee. J Magn Reson Imaging 2011;34(5):1007–21.

91. Saupe N, Zanetti M, Pfirrmann CW, et al. Pain and other side effects after MR arthrography: prospective evaluation in 1085 patients. Radiology 2009; 250(3):830–8.

92. Giaconi JC, Link TM, Vail TP, et al. Morbidity of direct MR arthrography. AJR Am J Roentgenol 2011;196(4):868–74.

93. Hugo PC 3rd, Newberg AH, Newman JS, et al. Complications of arthrography. Semin Musculoskelet Radiol 1998;2:345–8.

94. Craig JG, Vollman A, Zervos MJ, et al. Three cases of joint infection following arthrography including two patients with serious post-operative complications; a warning for us all. Society of Skeletal Radiology Meeting. Miami Beach, FL, March 19, 2012.

95. Haviv B, Thein R, Burg A, et al. Chondrolysis of the hip following septic arthritis: a rare complication of magnetic resonance arthrography. Case Rep Orthop 2013;2013:840681.

96. De Smet AA, Horak DM, Davis KW, et al. Intensity of signal contacting meniscal surface in recurrent tears on MR arthrography compared with that of contrast material. AJR Am J Roentgenol 2006; 187(6):W565–8.

97. Magee T. Accuracy of 3-Tesla MR and MR arthrography in diagnosis of meniscal retear in the postoperative knee. Skeletal Radiol 2014;43(8):1057–64.

98. Obuchowski NA. Receiver operating characteristic curves and their use in radiology. Radiology 2003; 229(1):3–8.

99. Dodd JD. Evidence-based practice in radiology: steps 3 and 4–appraise and apply diagnostic radiology literature. Radiology 2007;242(2):342–54.

100. Vermesan D, Prejbeanu R, Laitin S, et al. Arthroscopic debridement compared to intra-articular steroids in treating degenerative medial meniscal tears. Eur Rev Med Pharmacol Sci 2013;17(23):3192–6.

101. Sihvonen R, Paavola M, Malmivaara A, et al. Arthroscopic partial meniscectomy versus sham surgery for a degenerative meniscal tear. N Engl J Med 2013;369(26):2515–24.

102. Herrlin SV, Wange PO, Lapidus G, et al. Is arthroscopic surgery beneficial in treating non-traumatic, degenerative medial meniscal tears? A five year follow-up. Knee Surg Sports Traumatol Arthrosc 2013;21(2):358–64.

103. Yim JH, Seon JK, Song EK, et al. A comparative study of meniscectomy and nonoperative treatment for degenerative horizontal tears of the medial meniscus. Am J Sports Med 2013;41(7):1565–70.

104. Katz JN, Brophy RH, Chaisson CE, et al. Surgery versus physical therapy for a meniscal tear and osteoarthritis. N Engl J Med 2013;368(18):1675–84.

105. Krych AJ, Carey JL, Marx RG, et al. Does arthroscopic knee surgery work? Arthroscopy 2014;30(5):544–5.

106. Elattrache N, Lattermann C, Hannon M, et al. New England Journal of Medicine article evaluating the usefulness of meniscectomy is flawed. Arthroscopy 2014;30(5):542–3.

107. Dunoski B, Zbojniewicz AM, Laor T. MRI of displaced meniscal fragments. Pediatr Radiol 2012;42(1):104–12.

108. Vande Berg BC, Malghem J, Poilvache P, et al. Meniscal tears with fragments displaced in notch and recesses of knee: MR imaging with arthroscopic comparison. Radiology 2005;234(3):842–50.

109. Boxheimer L, Lutz AM, Zanetti M, et al. Characteristics of displaceable and nondisplaceable meniscal tears at kinematic MR imaging of the knee. Radiology 2006;238:221–31.

110. Amano H, Iwahashi T, Suzuki T, et al. Analysis of displacement and deformation of the medial meniscus with a horizontal tear using a three-dimensional computer model. Knee Surg Sports Traumatol Arthrosc 2014. [Epub ahead of print].

111. Kijowski R, Woods MA, McGuine TA, et al. Arthroscopic partial meniscectomy: MR imaging for prediction of outcome in middle-aged and elderly patients. Radiology 2011;259(1):203–12.

112. Magee T, Shapiro M, Williams D. Prevalence of meniscal radial tears of the knee revealed by MRI after surgery. AJR Am J Roentgenol 2004;182:931–6.

113. Mutschler C, Vande Berg BC, Lecouvet FE, et al. Postoperative meniscus: assessment at dual-detector row spiral CT arthrography of the knee. Radiology 2003;228(3):635–41.

114. Lim PS, Schweitzer ME, Bhatia M, et al. Repeat tear of postoperative meniscus: potential MR imaging signs. Radiology 1999;210(1):183–8.

115. White LM, Schweitzer ME, Weishaupt D, et al. Diagnosis of recurrent meniscal tears: prospective evaluation of conventional MR imaging, indirect MR arthrography, and direct MR arthrography. Radiology 2002;222:421–9.

116. Kinsella SD, Carey JL. Complications in brief: arthroscopic partial meniscectomy. Clin Orthop Relat Res 2013;471(5):1427–32.

117. Gwathmey FW Jr, Golish SR, Diduch DR, et al. Complications in brief: meniscus repair. Clin Orthop Relat Res 2012;470(7):2059–66.

118. Salzler MJ, Lin A, Miller CD, et al. Complications after arthroscopic knee surgery. Am J Sports Med 2014;42(2):292–6.

119. Stein T, Mehling AP, Welsch F, et al. Long-term outcome after arthroscopic meniscal repair versus arthroscopic partial meniscectomy for traumatic meniscal tears. Am J Sports Med 2010;38:1542–8.

120. Nepple JJ, Dunn WR, Wright RW. Meniscal repair outcomes at greater than five years: a systematic literature review and meta-analysis. J Bone Joint Surg Am 2012;94(24):2222–7.

121. Imade S, Kumahashi N, Kuwata S, et al. Clinical outcomes of revision meniscal repair: a case series. Am J Sports Med 2014;42:350–7.

122. Pujol N, Tardy N, Boisrenoult P, et al. Long-term outcomes of all-inside meniscal repair. Knee Surg Sports Traumatol Arthrosc 2013. [Epub ahead of print].

123. Järvinen T, Sihvonen R, Malmivaara A. Arthroscopy for degenerate meniscal tears of the knee. Critical appraisal of evidence on meniscectomy: daunting but necessary. BMJ 2014;348:g2382.

124. Abrams GD, Frank RM, Gupta AK, et al. Trends in meniscus repair and meniscectomy in the United States, 2005-2011. Am J Sports Med 2013;41(10):2333–9.

125. Pujol N, Tardy N, Boisrenoult P, et al. Magnetic resonance imaging is not suitable for interpretation of meniscal status ten years after arthroscopic repair. Int Orthop 2013;37(12):2371–6.

126. Hoffelner T, Resch H, Forstner R, et al. Arthroscopic all-inside meniscal repair–does the meniscus heal? A clinical and radiological follow-up examination to verify meniscal healing using a 3-T MRI. Skeletal Radiol 2011;40(2):181–7.

127. Miao Y, Yu JK, Ao YF, et al. Diagnostic values of 3 methods for evaluating meniscal healing status after meniscal repair: comparison among second-look arthroscopy, clinical assessment, and magnetic resonance imaging. Am J Sports Med 2011;39(4):735–42.

128. Kececi B, Kaya Bicer E, Arkun R, et al. The value of magnetic resonance arthrography in the evaluation of repaired menisci. Eur J Orthop Surg Traumatol 2014. [Epub ahead of print].

129. Popescu D, Sastre S, Garcia AI, et al. MR-arthrography assessment after repair of chronic meniscal tears. Knee Surg Sports Traumatol Arthrosc 2013. [Epub ahead of print].

130. Verdonk P, Van Laer M, EL Attar M, et al. Results and indications. In: Beaufils P, Verdonk R, editors. The meniscus. Berlin Heidelberg: Springer-Verlag; 2010. p. 349–63.

131. McCormick F, Harris JD, Abrams GD, et al. Survival and reoperation rates after meniscal allograft transplantation: analysis of failures for 172 consecutive transplants at a minimum 2-year follow-up. Am J Sports Med 2014;42(4):892–7.

132. Chalmers PN, Karas V, Sherman SL, et al. Return to high-level sport after meniscal allograft transplantation. Arthroscopy 2013;29(3):539–44.

133. Marcacci M, Marcheggiani Muccioli GM, Grassi A, et al. Arthroscopic meniscus allograft transplantation in male professional soccer players: a 36-month follow-up study. Am J Sports Med 2014;42(2):382–8.

134. Vundelinckx B, Vanlauwe J, Bellemans J. Long-term subjective, clinical, and radiographic outcome evaluation of meniscal allograft transplantation in the knee. Am J Sports Med 2014;42(7):1592–9.

135. Kim J, Ha J. Serial assessment of clinical and radiological outcomes after meniscus allograft transplantation with minimum 4-year follow up (abstract). Presented at the 16th ESSKA Congress in Amsterdam, The Netherlands, May 14–17, 2014.

136. Lee DH, Lee BS, Chung JW, et al. Changes in magnetic resonance imaging signal intensity of transplanted meniscus allografts are not associated with clinical outcomes. Arthroscopy 2011;27(9):1211–8.

137. Lee BS, Chung JW, Kim JM, et al. Morphologic changes in fresh-frozen meniscus allografts over 1 year: a prospective magnetic resonance imaging study on the width and thickness of transplants. Am J Sports Med 2012;40(6):1384–91.

138. Lee DH, Kim TH, Lee SH, et al. Evaluation of meniscus allograft transplantation with serial magnetic resonance imaging during the first postoperative year: focus on graft extrusion. Arthroscopy 2008;24(10):1115–21.

139. Monllau JC, Alentorn-Geli E, Pelfort X, et al. Meniscal allograft transplantation: where are we standing? J Transplant Tech Res 2014;4:127.

140. Kim JM, Lee BS, Kim KH, et al. Results of meniscus allograft transplantation using bone fixation: 110 cases with objective evaluation. Am J Sports Med 2012;40(5):1027–34.

141. Yoon KH, Lee SH, Park SY, et al. Meniscus allograft transplantation: a comparison of medial and lateral procedures. Am J Sports Med 2014;42(1):200–7.

142. Verdonk PC, Verstraete KL, Almqvist KF, et al. Meniscal allograft transplantation: long-term clinical results with radiological and magnetic resonance imaging correlations. Knee Surg Sports Traumatol Arthrosc 2006;14:694–706.

143. Papalia R, Franceschi F, Diaz Balzani L, et al. Scaffolds for partial meniscal replacement: an updated systematic review. Br Med Bull 2013;107:19–40.

144. Bouyarmane H, Beaufils P, Pujol N, et al. Polyurethane scaffold in lateral meniscus segmental defects: clinical outcomes at 24 months follow-up. Orthop Traumatol Surg Res 2014;100(1):153–7.

145. Verdonk P, Beaufils P, Bellemans J, et al. Successful treatment of painful irreparable partial meniscal defects with a polyurethane scaffold: two-year safety and clinical outcomes. Am J Sports Med 2012;40(4):844–53.

146. Huysse WC, Verstraete KL, Verdonk PC, et al. Meniscus imaging. Semin Musculoskelet Radiol 2008;12(4):318–33.

147. De Coninck T, Huysse W, Willemot L, et al. Two-year follow-up study on clinical and radiological outcomes of polyurethane meniscal scaffolds. Am J Sports Med 2013;41(1):64–72.

148. Schüttler KF, Pöttgen S, Getgood A, et al. Improvement in outcomes after implantation of a novel polyurethane meniscal scaffold for the treatment of medial meniscus deficiency. Knee Surg Sports Traumatol Arthrosc 2014. [Epub ahead of print].

149. Stone KR, Steadman JR, Rodkey WG, et al. Regeneration of meniscal cartilage with use of a collagen scaffold. Analysis of preliminary data. J Bone Joint Surg Am 1997;79(12):1770–7.

150. Harston A, Nyland J, Brand E, et al. Collagen meniscus implantation: a systematic review including rehabilitation and return to sports activity. Knee Surg Sports Traumatol Arthrosc 2012;20(1):135–46.

151. Genovese E, Angeretti MG, Ronga M, et al. Follow-up of collagen meniscus implants by MRI. Radiol Med 2007;112(7):1036–48.

152. Zaffagnini S, Marcheggiani Muccioli GM, Lopomo N, et al. Prospective long-term outcomes of the medial collagen meniscus implant versus partial medial meniscectomy: a minimum 10-year follow-up study. Am J Sports Med 2011;39(5):977–85.

153. Monllau JC, Gelber PE, Abat F, et al. Outcome after partial medial meniscus substitution with the collagen meniscal implant at a minimum of 10 years' follow-up. Arthroscopy 2011;27(7):933–43.

154. Hirschmann MT, Keller L, Hirschmann A, et al. One-year clinical and MR imaging outcome after partial meniscal replacement in stabilized knees using a collagen meniscus implant. Knee Surg Sports Traumatol Arthrosc 2013;21(3):740–7.

155. Condello V, Arbel R, Agar G, et al. A novel synthetic meniscus implant for the treatment of middle aged patients: results of 118 patients in a prospective, multi-center study. European Federation of National Associations of Orthopaedics and Traumatology Meeting. London, United Kingdom, June 4, 2014.

156. Shabshin N, Elsner J, Asher R, et al. First report on MRI of a novel synthetic meniscus implant: the normal appearance of early remodeling. International Skeletal Society Annual Meeting. Philadelphia, PA. October 1, 2013.

157. BlueCross BlueShield of North Carolina Corporate Medical Policy. Meniscal allografts and other meniscal implants. Available at: www.bcbsnc.com/assets/services/public/pdfs/medicalpolicy/meniscal_allografts_and_other_meniscal_implants.pdf. Accessed May 17, 2014.

158. Centers for Medicare and Medicaid Services. National Coverage Determination (NCD) for Collagen Meniscus Implant (150.12). Available at: http://www.cms.gov/medicare-coverage-database Accessed May 17, 2014.

159. Condello V, Ronga M, Linder-Ganz E, et al. Alternatives to meniscus transplantation outside the United States. In: Farr J, Gomoll AH, editors. Cartilage restoration. New York: Springer; 2014. p. 223–49.

MR Imaging of Cruciate Ligaments

Ali Naraghi, MD[a,b,*], Lawrence M. White, MD[a,c]

KEYWORDS

- Anterior cruciate ligament • Posterior cruciate ligament • Postoperative • MR imaging • Imaging

KEY POINTS

- Magnetic resonance (MR) imaging is highly accurate in assessment of complete tears of cruciate ligaments.
- MR imaging is less accurate in assessment of chronic and partial tears of anterior cruciate ligament and posterior cruciate ligament.
- MR imaging is a useful technique in identifying causes of recurrent symptoms following cruciate ligament reconstruction.

INTRODUCTION

There are more than 200,000 anterior cruciate ligament (ACL) injuries annually in the United States.[1] The incidence of posterior cruciate ligament (PCL) tears is considerably less common, accounting for 3% of all knee injuries in the general population.[2]

A thorough understanding of ACL and PCL anatomy, injury patterns, and reconstructive techniques is a prerequisite to accurate MR interpretation of cruciate ligament injuries and postoperative appearances and these are covered in this article.

NORMAL ANATOMY AND FUNCTION
ACL

The ACL is the major restraint to anterior translation of the tibia relative to the femur. It also provides restraint to rotatory load and contributes to the screw home mechanism of normal knee physiologic motion. The ACL arises from a semilunar region along the medial border of the lateral femoral condyle and inserts onto the proximal tibia, anterior to the tibial spines in close proximity to the anterior root of the lateral meniscus. It consists of 2 anatomically and functionally distinct bundles: the anteromedial (AMB) and posterolateral (PLB) bundles. An intermediate bundle has also been described in the literature.[3]

- The AMB has a more proximal origin and is separated from the more distal origin of the PLB by the bifurcate ridge.[4] The AMB inserts onto the tibia at a point anteromedial to the insertion of the PLB.
- The AMB and PLB parallel each other in the sagittal plane during knee extension but twist around each other during flexion.[5]
- The 2 bundles have reciprocal tensioning characteristics. The AMB is maximally taut during knee flexion, and the PLB is maximally taut in extension and internal rotation.
- The AMB is the predominant restraint to anterior translation of the tibia during knee flexion and the PLB prevents anterior translation during knee extension as well as providing restraint against internal rotation of the tibia.[4]

No Disclosures.

[a] Joint Department of Medical Imaging, University Health Network, Mount Sinai Hospital and Women's College Hospital, University of Toronto, Toronto, Ontario, Canada; [b] Department of Medical Imaging, Toronto Western Hospital, 399 Bathurst Street, Toronto, Ontario M5T 2S8, Canada; [c] Department of Medical Imaging, Toronto General Hospital, 200 Elizabeth Street, Toronto, Ontario M5G 2C4, Canada

* Corresponding author. Department of Medical Imaging, Toronto Western Hospital, 399 Bathurst Street, Toronto, Ontario M5T 2S8, Canada.
E-mail address: ali.naraghi@uhn.ca

Magn Reson Imaging Clin N Am 22 (2014) 557–580
http://dx.doi.org/10.1016/j.mric.2014.07.003

PCL

The PCL is the major restraint to posterior tibial translation, particularly during knee flexion. It consists of the ALB and PMB, functionally aided by the meniscofemoral ligaments.[6]

- The stronger ALB arises anteriorly from the lateral margin of the medial femoral condyle, anterior to the origin of the PMB.
- The 2 bundles insert onto the posterior proximal tibia approximately 1 cm inferior to the articular surface.[7]
- The ALB is maximally taut in flexion and the PMB is maximally taut during knee extension.

IMAGING TECHNIQUES AND PROTOCOL

The exact MR imaging pulse sequences used to image the knee vary among different institutions. The pulse sequences at the authors' institution are illustrated in **Table 1**.

In addition to traditional orthogonal imaging, several oblique acquisitions have also been advocated in the literature for imaging of the ACL.

- Oblique sagittal images may be prescribed along an axis paralleling the lateral border of the lateral femoral condyle.
- Oblique coronal acquisitions, oriented along the longitudinal axis of the ACL or the roof of the intercondylar notch, may assist in depiction of the different components of the ACL and allow for complete visualization of the ACL.[8]
- Oblique axial acquisitions obtained perpendicular to the long axis of the ACL have also been advocated particularly for evaluation of partial tears.[9]

Three-dimensional (3D) isotropic fast spin-echo acquisitions producing high-quality multiplanar reformats in multiple oblique planes (**Fig. 1**) may also be used to evaluate the cruciate ligaments and demonstrate similar diagnostic performance to standard orthogonal 2-dimensional (2D) acquisitions in evaluation of ACL and PCL tears.[10]

IMAGING FINDINGS
Normal Appearances

ACL

- In the sagittal plane, the normal ACL is taut and straight (**Fig. 2A**). It runs parallel, or within 9°, to the roof of the intercondylar notch.[11] On direct sagittal acquisitions, the entirety of the ACL may not be visualized on a single slice.
- On proximal axial images, the proximal ACL has an elongated elliptical appearance (see **Fig. 2B**).[12]
- The normal ACL is of low signal intensity proximally with a more heterogeneous appearance more distally as the ligament fans out toward its tibial attachment.
- The AMB and PLB may be distinguished on the axial and coronal planes (see **Fig. 2C, D**).

PCL

- The PCL has a curved appearance with horizontal (proximal), genu, and vertical (distal) components.
- The PCL is of uniform low signal intensity on all pulse sequences (**Fig. 3**). Slightly increased signal intensity may be visualized at the genu on short TE pulse sequences due to magic angle phenomenon.
- Sagittal images demonstrate the PCL well throughout its entirety. Axial images are particularly well suited for visualization of the vertical component and the coronal images for visualization of the horizontal component.[7]

Table 1
Representative routine pulse sequences used for evaluation of the knee at Joint Department of Medical Imaging, University of Toronto

Pulse Sequence	Plane	TR/TE	ETL	NEX	Matrix	FOV (cm)	Slice Thickness/ Gap (mm)
Proton density	Sagittal oblique	2100/14	6	2	288 × 256	14	4/0
Fat-suppressed T2	Sagittal oblique	3900/75	8	2	256 × 224	14	4/0
Intermediate-weighted	Coronal	4900/34	8	1	512 × 256	14	4/0
Fat-suppressed T2	Axial	3800/70	8	3	256 × 192	14	4/0

Abbreviations: ETL, echo train length; FOV, field of view; NEX, number of excitations; TE, echo time; TR, repetition time.

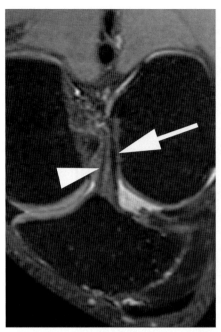

Fig. 1. Coronal oblique reformat from a fat-suppressed isotropic 3D SPACE acquisition demonstrating the entirety of the ACL with distinct visualization of the AMB (*arrowhead*) and PLB (*arrow*).

ACL Tears

Mechanisms of injury

More than 80% of ACL tears occur because of noncontact injuries in sports, where deceleration, cutting, and pivoting are common.[13]

- The most common mechanism of injury is the "pivot shift" injury in which a valgus and axial force is exerted on the flexed knee with concomitant quadriceps loading, anterior tibial translation, and external rotation of the femur.[14]
- A varus force with internal rotation of the tibia can also produce an ACL tear and may be associated with a Segond fracture, an avulsion of the lateral rim of the tibia at the site of the attachment of the lateral capsular ligament (Fig. 4).[15]
- Hyperextension injuries may also result in ACL tears, often with associated PCL or the posterolateral corner injuries.

Depending on the mechanism of injury, associated injuries of the collateral ligaments, menisci, and articular cartilage may be present and impact the stability of the knee joint and the surgical management of patients. The mechanism of ligamentous injury can often be deduced from the bone marrow contusive patterns, aiding in identification of associated injuries.

MR imaging features of ACL injury

MR imaging is highly accurate in evaluation of ACL tears with an overall sensitivity of 83% to 95% and specificity of 95% to 100%. ACL injuries may involve the substance of the ACL, an avulsion of its tibial attachment (Fig. 5), or a peel off lesion of its femoral attachment. Identification of the injury pattern impacts surgical management with intrasubstance ruptures treated by ligament reconstruction and acute osseous avulsions, or peel off lesions, treated by primary fixation.[16]

Primary signs of ACL tear include the following[17,18]:

- Focal discontinuity of the ACL (Fig. 6)
- Diffuse or focal abnormal signal intensity
- A mass-like appearance in the expected location of the ACL
- Abnormal orientation or bowing of the ACL
- Nonvisualization of the ACL (Fig. 7)

Focal discontinuity and diffuse increased signal intensity with enlargement of the ACL are among the most common patterns of ACL injury seen on MR imaging.[17,18] Discontinuity is best appreciated on sagittal and axial images.[18] Thickening and increased signal intensity of the ACL may also be encountered with mucoid degeneration of the ligament, but this often has a striated appearance with intact contiguous ligament fibers visible along its entire length (Fig. 8). A horizontally oriented distal ACL, a vertically oriented proximal ACL, and discontinuity of the ACL have a positive predictive value of 100% for an ACL tear.[17] An angle of greater than 15° between the roof of the intercondylar notch and the ACL or an angle of less than 45° between the distal ACL and the tibia, reflecting horizontal orientation of ACL fibers, are both highly accurate MR imaging findings of complete tears of the ACL.[11] Distal fibers of a torn ACL may flip anteriorly, resulting in mechanical symptoms of a locked knee (Fig. 9).

Secondary signs of ACL injury include (Fig. 10) the following.

Osseous injuries Osseous injury involving the anterior/central aspect of the lateral femoral condyle and the posterior aspect of the lateral tibial plateau is seen with pivot shift injuries. Less commonly, contusive injury of the posterior aspect of the medial tibial plateau and medial femoral condyle may also be visualized. Osseous injury is often associated with meniscal injury in the same compartment and is associated with poorer functional outcome at 1 year.[19]

Anterior translation of the tibia On the midsagittal image through the lateral compartment of the knee, the posterior aspect of the lateral tibial plateau

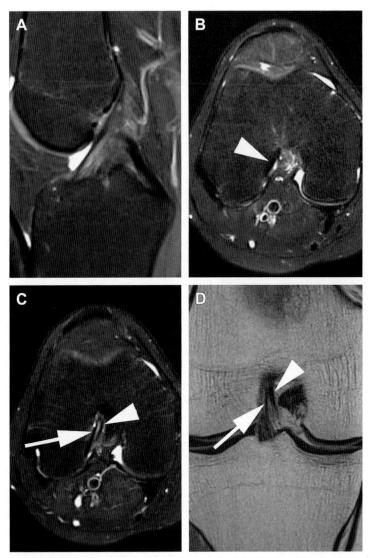

Fig. 2. Sagittal T2 fat-suppressed MR image (*A*) demonstrating a normal taut ACL with normal heterogeneity distally. Axial T2 fat-suppressed MR image (*B, C*) of the proximal and mid point of the normal ACL. Proximally (*B*), the ACL is elliptical and of low signal intensity (*arrowhead* in *B*). More distally (*C*), the 2 separate bundles are visualized with intervening normal increased signal intensity (AMB *arrowhead*, PLB *arrow*). Coronal intermediate weighted MR image (*D*) demonstrating parts of a normal AMB (*arrowhead*) and PLB (*arrow*).

subluxates anteriorly by greater than 5 mm in relation to the posterior aspect of the lateral femoral condyle,[20] with a sensitivity of 86% and specificity of 99% for a complete ACL tear.

Uncovering of the posterior horn of the lateral meniscus Uncovering the posterior horn of the lateral meniscus reflects a posterior displacement of the posterior horn of the lateral meniscus in relation to the posterior aspect of the lateral tibial plateau. Displacement of greater than 3.5 mm has a sensitivity of 44% and a specificity of 94% in the diagnosis of ACL disruption.[11]

Several other signs have also been described in the setting of an ACL tear, including the buckling of the PCL, reduced PCL angle, posterior PCL line, and the posterior femoral line.[11,18] In general, secondary signs are highly specific for the presence of an ACL injury but are of limited sensitivity.[18] Overall, primary signs are the most useful for determining the status of the ACL and the addition of secondary signs are of little added or independent value.[21]

The accuracy of clinical examination and MR imaging evaluation may be diminished in the setting of chronic and partial ACL tears.

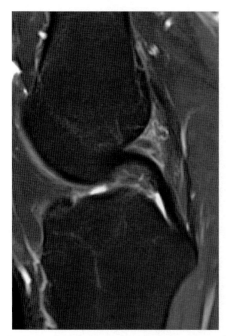

Fig. 3. Sagittal T2 fat-suppressed MR imaging of the knee demonstrating the normal curved appearance of the PCL with the knee imaged in extension. The PCL is of homogeneous low signal intensity.

With chronic complete ACL tears, the ACL remnant may reattach and the true severity of the injury may not be appreciated. Patterns of ACL scarring include the following[22]:

- End-to-end scarring of the torn ACL (**Fig. 11**)
- Scarring of the ACL to the PCL (**Fig. 12**)
- Scarring of the ACL to the roof of the intercondylar notch
- Scarring of the distal remnant onto the anatomic origin of the ACL

Scarring onto the anatomic origin of the ACL, although the least common pattern, has the most significant effect with reduced laxity on clinical examination.[22]

Partial ACL tears

Partial tears comprise up to 30% of all ACL tears.[23] Partial injuries may consist of the following:

- Complete tear of the AMB with either a normal or a partially torn PLB. This pattern is the most common.[9]
- Complete tear of the PLB with either a normal or a partially torn AMB (**Fig. 13**).
- Partial tears of both bundles.

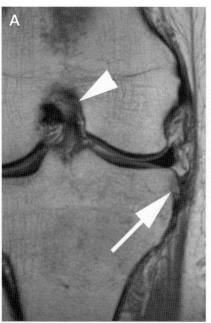
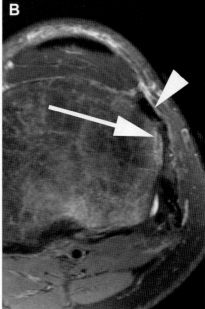

Fig. 4. Coronal intermediate-weighted MR image (*A*) in a 21-year-old woman with an ACL tear (*arrowhead* in *A*) demonstrating a subtle undisplaced Segond fracture (*arrow*). Axial T2 fat-suppressed image (*B*) shows bone marrow edema at the site of the fracture (*arrow*), immediately posterior to the attachment of the iliotibial band (*arrowhead* in *B*).

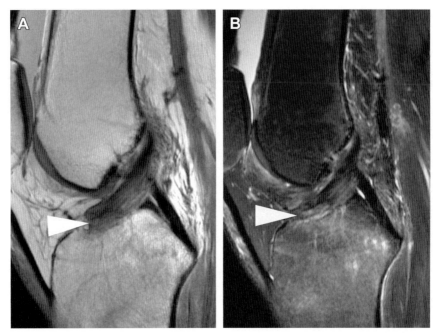

Fig. 5. Sagittal proton density (*A*) and fat-suppressed T2-weighted (*B*) images in an 18-year-old man with an acute knee injury demonstrating a subtle avulsion fracture of the ACL insertion (*arrowheads*).

Although the AMB is commonly injured with higher-energy trauma, the PLB may be injured with lower-energy rotational trauma. Clinically, complete tears of either the AMB or the PLB can be difficult to distinguish from an intact ACL and complete tears of one bundle with a partial tear of the other bundle may be mistaken for a complete tear.[24] Accurate grading and diagnosis of a

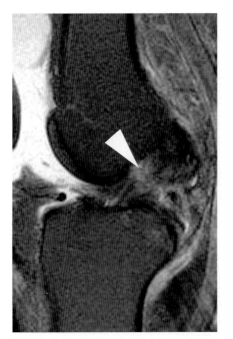

Fig. 6. Fat-suppressed T2-weighted sagittal image in a 46-year-old man a patient with an acute complete ACL tear demonstrating focal discontinuity of the mid ACL (*arrowhead*).

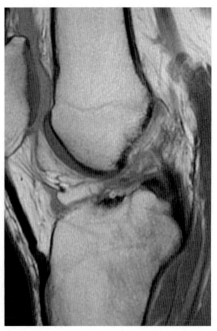

Fig. 7. Sagittal proton density MR image in a 38-year-old woman with a chronic ACL injury with nonvisualization of the ACL.

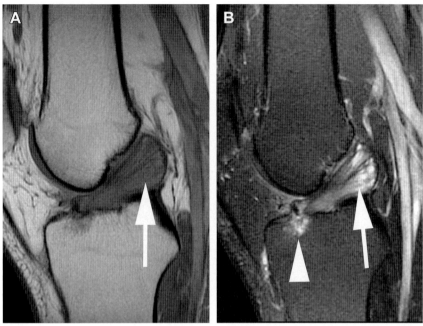

Fig. 8. Sagittal proton density (*A*) and fat-suppressed T2-weighted (*B*) images in a 43-year-old man without history of recent trauma. The ACL is expanded with increased signal intensity (*arrows*) and intact fibers in keeping with mucoid degeneration. Small area of intraosseous increased signal intensity at the ACL insertion (*arrowhead* in *B*) is consistent with reactive edema/intraosseous ganglion cyst formation.

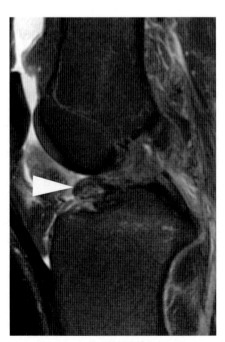

Fig. 9. Sagittal T2 fat-suppressed MR image of a 24-year-old man with an acute rupture of the ACL. The distal ACL fibers have flipped anteriorly (*arrowhead*).

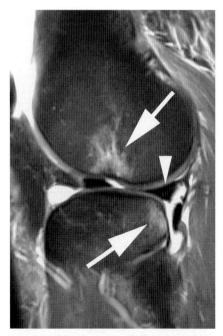

Fig. 10. Sagittal fat-suppressed T2-weighted image in a 23-year-old man with a pivot shift injury and an acute ACL rupture demonstrating multiple secondary signs including anterior translation of the tibia, contusive injury to the lateral femoral condyle, and lateral tibial plateau (*arrows*) and uncovering of the posterior horn of the lateral meniscus (*arrowhead*).

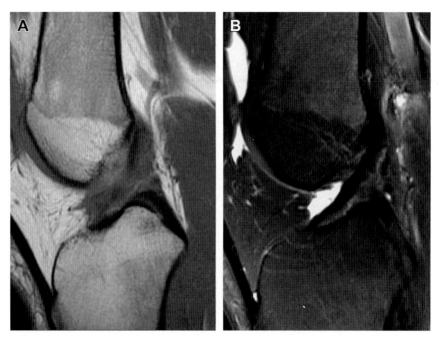

Fig. 11. Sagittal proton density MR image (*A*) in a 32-year-old woman with a high-grade to complete midsubstance tear of the ACL 2 months after injury. There is focal discontinuity of the mid-ACL. Sagittal T2 fat-suppressed MR image (*B*) in the same patient 1 year later shows complete continuity of the ACL with mild deformity and bowing.

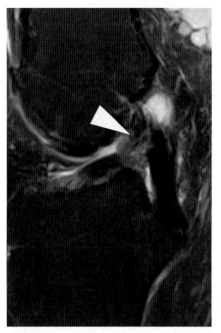

Fig. 12. Sagittal T2 fat-suppressed MR image in a 49-year-old man 4 months after knee injury shows scarring of the ACL to the genu of the PCL (*arrowhead*). The distal ACL fibers are horizontally oriented in keeping with a complete tear.

partial tear is of clinical significance because selective bundle reconstructions may be undertaken and risk of progression to ACL insufficiency is related to the grade of initial ligament injury sustained. With less than 25% of the ligament disrupted, there is a 12% risk of insufficiency as opposed to an 86% risk when greater than 75% of the ligament is injured.[25]

Accuracy of MR imaging for identification of partial ACL tears is significantly diminished in comparison with complete tears, with sensitivities and specificities of 62% to 81% and 19% to 97%, respectively,[26,27] and accuracy rates as low as 25% to 53%.[28] 3T MR imaging has a sensitivity, specificity, and accuracy of 77%, 97%, and 95%, respectively.[29] Diagnostic performance of axial oblique images, with a sensitivity and specificity of 87%,[9] is better than orthogonal acquisitions, but this difference is not significant. Similarly, 3D isotropic acquisitions show no significant difference from standard 2D pulse sequences in the diagnosis of partial ACL injuries.[10]

Signs that indicate partial tears include the following[27–30]:

- Attenuation of the ACL
- Hyperintense intrasubstance signal with identification of intact fibers

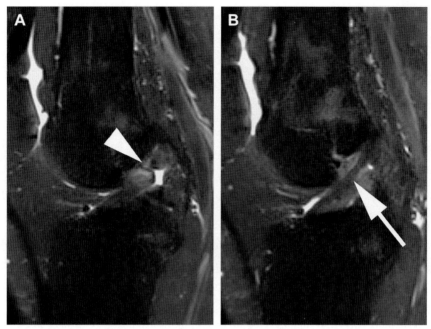

Fig. 13. Sagittal isotropic fat-suppressed 3D SPACE acquisition (*A, B*) in a 33-old woman with a complete tear of the PLB of the ACL. There is focal discontinuity of the PLB (*arrowhead* in *A*). The AMB remains intact with mild signal changes and mild focal thickening consistent with a partial tear (*arrow* in *B*).

- Posterior/inferior bowing of the ACL
- Distortion of the ACL without obvious discontinuity

Given that surgical treatment depends on the grade of injury, it is worthwhile to stratify ACL injuries as stable (normal ligament or stable partial tears) or unstable (unstable partial or complete tears) based on MR imaging (**Fig. 14**). In one study using axial images, the visualization of a single bundle, an ill-defined mass-like appearance, and nonvisualization of the ACL had 100% sensitivity and 96% specificity for unstable tears. An elliptical ACL, attenuation of the ligament, and presence of isolated intrasubstance signal correlated with stable ACLs.[12] Secondary signs of ACL insufficiency are more commonly seen with unstable tears, but these signs have a low sensitivity (specificity 100%, sensitivity 23%).[30]

PCL Tears

Mechanism of PCL injury
Overall, 45% of PCL injuries are related to road traffic accidents, with athletic injuries accounting for approximately 40% of injuries.[31]

- Dashboard injury with an anterior blow to the proximal tibia, forcing the tibia posteriorly relative to the femur, is a common mechanism

of injury in motor vehicle accidents. Because of the high-energy nature of this mechanism, there is a higher incidence of associated concomitant ligamentous and posterior capsular injuries.
- In the athletic population, a fall on a flexed knee and hyperflexion injuries are common mechanisms. A hyperflexion injury may cause isolated injury to the anterolateral bundle with the posteromedial bundle remaining intact.[32] The posterior capsule may be spared from injury with this mechanism.[7]
- Hyperextension injuries tend to be a less common cause of PCL rupture.[31] Severe hyperextension injury may be associated with ACL tears and posterolateral corner or posteromedial corner injuries.

Clinically, integrity of the PCL is assessed by the posterior drawer test. Because the tibia may be posteriorly subluxated at rest, in the setting of PCL disruption, an ACL pseudolaxity may be detected clinically and at arthroscopy.[32]

MR imaging features of PCL injury
Multiligamentous injuries involving the PCL are more common than isolated PCL tears.[7] The PCL may be injured through its substance or at its tibial (**Fig. 15**) and femoral attachments (**Fig. 16**). Midsubstance tears are most common.

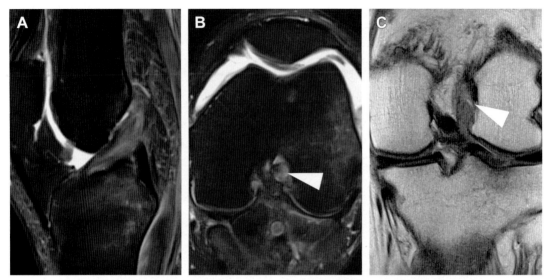

Fig. 14. T2 fat-suppressed sagittal (*A*), axial (*B*), and coronal intermediate-weighted (*C*) MR image of a 36-year-old woman with a high-grade partial tear of the ACL and grade III laxity on clinical examination. The ACL is expanded with increased signal intensity on T2-weighted images with an amorphous appearance on the axial image (*arrowhead* in *B*). Focal discontinuity is identified on the coronal image (*arrowhead* in *C*).

MR imaging signs of PCL tear include the following[7,33]:

- Focal disruption of the PCL (**Fig. 17**).
- Amorphous increased signal intensity with disruption of one or both margins of the

ligament (**Fig. 18**). Increased signal intensity on proton density images is more common than on T2-weighted images.
- Nonvisualization of the PCL.
- Abnormal thickening of the PCL distal to the genu with an anteroposterior diameter of

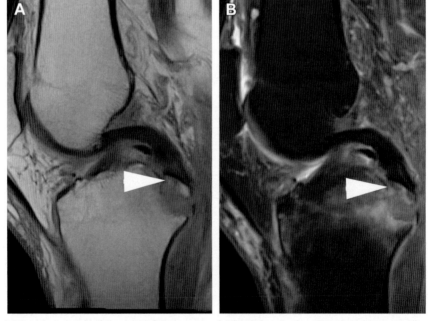

Fig. 15. Sagittal proton density (*A*) and T2 fat-suppressed (*B*) MR images in a 22-year-old man with a knee injury demonstrating an avulsion fracture of the tibial insertion of the PCL with a small bony fragment (*arrowheads*) best visualized on the proton density image, with adjacent bone marrow edema on T2-weighted images.

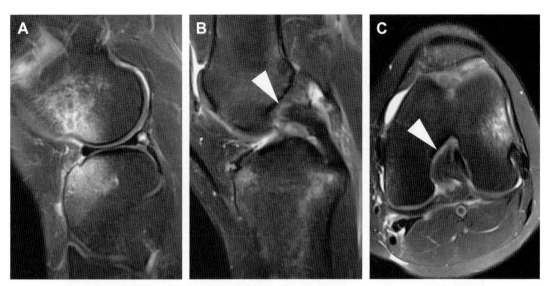

Fig. 16. Sagittal (*A, B*) and axial (*C*) T2 fat-suppressed MR images of the PCL in a 21-year-old man with hyperextension injury demonstrating a tear of the femoral attachment of the PCL (*arrowheads*). Anterior femoral condyle and tibial impaction fractures/contusive injuries (*A*) are noted in keeping with a hyperextension injury and anterior joint compressive loading.

greater than 7 mm has a sensitivity of 94% and a specificity of 92% for PCL tears[34] and is seen irrespective of the location of the tear.

In approximately 47% to 62% of cases, the PCL may be partially torn.[34,35]

- Intrasubstance fluid signal intensity on T2-weighted images is only seen in 19% of partial tears.[34]
- A striated appearance in the setting of a partial tear is more common with up to 71% of cases demonstrating this appearance.[34]

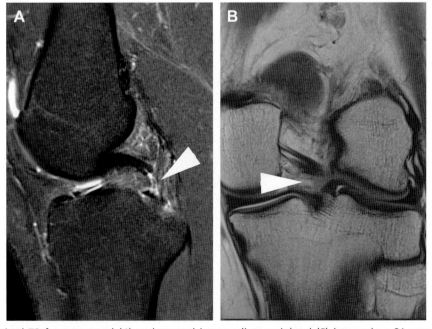

Fig. 17. Sagittal T2 fat-suppressed (*A*) and coronal intermediate-weighted (*B*) images in a 21-year-old athlete 2 years after injury showing nonvisualization and complete discontinuity of the PCL distal to the genu (*arrowheads*).

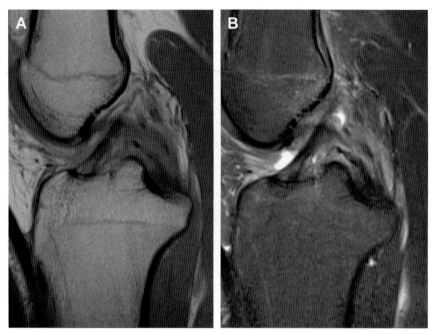

Fig. 18. Sagittal proton density (*A*) and T2 fat-suppressed (*B*) MR images of a 39-year-old man with a complete PCL tear demonstrating intrasubstance intermediate signal intensity and discontinuity of the PCL on both pulse sequences.

Intrasubstance mucoid degeneration of the PCL also can demonstrate a striated "tram-track" appearance with thickening mimicking a tear.[36] A distinguishing feature is the presence of intact low signal intensity margins to the PCL in the setting of mucoid degeneration.

The PCL has a propensity for healing and a previously injured PCL may be mistaken for a normal ligament, particularly when imaged more than 6 months following injury.[33,37] In one study, 28% of chronic PCL injuries demonstrated a near normal MR imaging appearance, with 44% showing continuity but residual morphologic deformity of the ligament (**Fig. 19**).[37] Patients with posterolateral corner injuries and those with greater than 12 mm of posterior displacement of the tibia on stress radiography are less likely to demonstrate continuity of PCL fibers on follow-up imaging.[33]

ACL RECONSTRUCTION

Single bundle ACL reconstruction, reconstructing the anatomy of the AMB, is the most common type of ACL reconstruction. However, 15% to 25% of patients with single bundle procedures have continued pain and instability after reconstruction[38] and therefore double bundle reconstructions, individually reconstituting the anatomic courses of the AMB and PLB, have been advocated.[4]

Graft material may include autograft or allograft. The commonest choices for autograft are bone-patellar tendon-bone (BPTB) and hamstring tendons. With BPTB grafts, the central third of the patellar tendon as well as bone plugs from the inferior patella and tibial tuberosity are harvested. BPTB graft reconstructions have the advantage of firm fixation and increased strength but may be associated with postoperative anterior knee pain and an increased incidence of arthrofibrosis.[39] With hamstring grafts, the distal semitendinosus and gracilis tendons are classically harvested, sutured together side-by-side and then folded on themselves to yield a 4-strand graft construct. Graft fixation may be achieved by interference screws, surgical staples, cross-pins, or endobuttons. These fixation devices may be metallic or bioabsorbable. Allograft material is more varied in source and can include BPTB, hamstrings, tibialis posterior, and Achilles tendons. Synthetic graft material has fallen out of favor because of increased incidence of synthetic graft complications and foreign body reactions (**Fig. 20**).

Normal MR Imaging: ACL Reconstruction

The normal ACL graft demonstrates uniform low signal intensity in the immediate postoperative period and is of uniform caliber.[40] With a hamstring graft, the individual graft construct strands may be visualized with a small amount of intervening fluid.

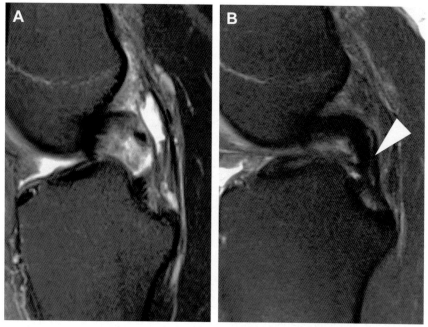

Fig. 19. Sagittal T2 fat-suppressed MR image (*A*) in a 26-year-old man 6 weeks following a knee injury demonstrating a complete tear of the PCL. Follow-up T2 fat-suppressed MR image (*B*) 8 months later demonstrates continuity of the PCL with mild residual deformity and signal change consistent with some interval healing (*arrowhead*).

Between 3 and 12 months postoperatively, the graft undergoes a process of remodeling and revascularization known as "ligamentization."[41] During this period, the graft may demonstrate increased MR signal intensity on T1-weighted and T2-weighted images.[42] The graft typically demonstrates low signal intensity by 18 months postoperatively, although small foci of intermediate

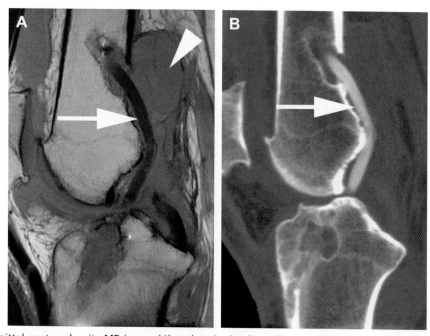

Fig. 20. Sagittal proton density MR image (*A*) and sagittal reformatted CT (*B*) in a 46-year-old man with prior synthetic ACL reconstruction demonstrating uniform low signal intensity and high attenuation of the synthetic graft (*arrows*). There is abnormal soft tissue posteriorly (*arrowhead*), consistent with synovitis and foreign body reaction. Erosive change and slight widening of the tunnels also noted.

to high signal intensity may be visualized in normal grafts beyond this time point in the absence of impingement or graft laxity.[43,44]

Patellar tendon graft harvest sites typically demonstrate a central longitudinal defect within the patellar tendon (**Fig. 21**), which fills in with scar tissue by 2 years postoperatively. Persistent thickening of the patellar tendon with uniform low signal intensity is seen as a normal postoperative finding.[45] Similarly, scar tissue may be seen at the site of the hamstring graft harvest site, illustrating features of normal tendon reconstitution postoperatively.

ACL reconstruction tunnel positioning is critical in providing stability and avoiding graft impingement. Isometric graft positioning depends on the position of the femoral tunnel.

- The optimal opening of the femoral tunnel corresponds to the junction of the roof of the intercondylar notch and the posterior femoral cortex on sagittal MR images.
- On coronal images, the femoral tunnel opening should be located at the 10 to 11 o'clock position (right knee) or 1 to 2 o'clock position (left knee).
- With double bundle ACL grafts, the femoral tunnel for the AMB is ideally located at the 10 to 11 o'clock (right knee) or 1 to 2 o'clock (left knee). The PLB should be at 9 to 10 o'clock (right knee) or 2 to 3 o'clock (left knee) of the intercondylar notch.[46]
- In the sagittal plane, with the knee in extension, the tibial tunnel should be located such that the anterior margin of the ACL graft should run parallel and posterior to a line drawn along the roof of the intercondylar notch (Blumensaat's line) (**Fig. 22**).[47]
- In the coronal plane, the lateral edge of the tibial tunnel should be in line with the lateral tibial spine and the graft should be ideally oriented with an angle of 60 to 65° to the joint line (**Fig. 23**).[47] Increased vertical orientation of the graft may predispose to PCL impingement (**Fig. 24**) and possible rotational instability of the joint.[48]
- In double bundle reconstruction, the center of the AMB tibial tunnel should be at the junction of the anterior and middle thirds of the tibia with the center of the PLB just posterior to the midpoint of the tibia (**Fig. 25**).[46]

MR imaging of Postoperative Complications: ACL Reconstructions

Clinically, patients with postoperative complications following ACL reconstruction may present with pain, symptoms of recurrent instability as a result of poor femoral tunnel positioning (**Fig. 26**), improper graft tensioning, failure of graft fixation,

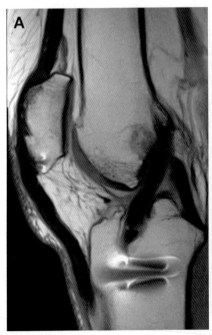
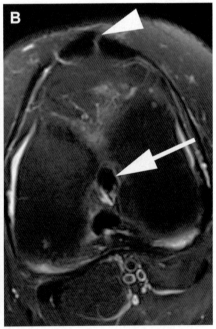

Fig. 21. Sagittal proton density (*A*) and axial T2 fat-suppressed MR image after BPTB reconstruction in a 33-year-old man. The graft demonstrates uniform low signal intensity on both sequences (*arrow in B*). There is normal postoperative thickening of the patellar tendon with a central defect (*arrowhead in B*).

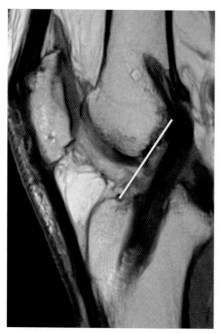

Fig. 22. Sagittal proton density MR image of a 40-year-old woman with BPTB ACL reconstruction. Optimal femoral tunnel positioning is noted with the opening of the femoral tunnel at the junction of the roof of the intercondylar notch and the posterior femoral cortex. The tibial tunnel and anterior margin of the graft are located posterior to Blumensaat line (*white line*).

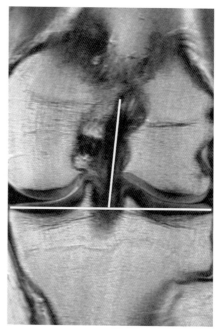

Fig. 24. Coronal intermediate-weighted MR image in a 29-year-old woman demonstrating a vertically oriented graft with an abnormal angle of 83° relative to the joint line.

graft stretching, or graft tearing, or with loss of terminal extension as a result of graft impingement or scarring.

Graft tear

MR imaging has shown a sensitivity of 36% and a specificity of 80% for detection of an ACL graft tear (complete and partial tears vs intact graft),[49] although one study using conventional MR imaging showed 100% accuracy.[50] The sensitivity and specificity for detection of full-thickness graft disruption are 50% and 100%, respectively.[49] MR arthrography has shown a sensitivity of 100% and specificity of 89% to 100% for graft tears.[51] Primary signs of graft injury include graft discontinuity, focal change in the caliber of the graft, increased signal intensity within the graft, and posterior-inferior bowing of the graft (**Fig. 27**). Graft discontinuity on coronal and sagittal images has the highest specificity for full-thickness tears and graft continuity has 100% negative predictive value for a tear.[49] A graft with no evidence of thinning or caliber change has 100% specificity and positive predictive value in excluding a full-thickness tear. Focal or diffuse signal change within the graft has limited reliability in identifying graft tears and may be seen in intact and biomechanically stable grafts.[44] Posterior and inferior bowing of a graft construct may be seen in the setting of graft tearing as well as

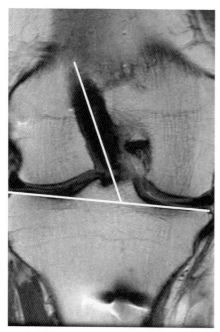

Fig. 23. Coronal intermediate-weighted MR image demonstrating a coronal angle of 67° between the graft and the joint line.

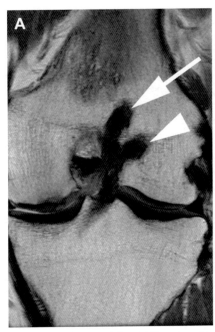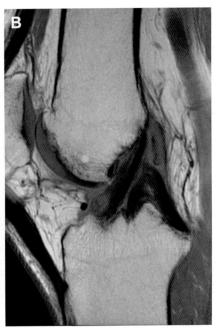

Fig. 25. Coronal intermediate-weighted (*A*) and sagittal proton density (*B*) MR image of a 39-year-old woman with double bundle ACL reconstruction of the left knee. The AMB tunnel is seen at the 1 to 2 o'clock position (*arrow*) and the PLB tunnel is seen at 2 to 3 o'clock position (*arrowhead*). On sagittal images, the AMB is seen anteriorly with tibial attachment at the junction of anterior to middle third of the tibia and the PLB is seen more posteriorly with tibial attachment just posterior to the midpoint of the tibia. Small area of focal scar and granulation tissue is seen anterior to the AMB.

with graft stretching and laxity. The diagnostic accuracy of MR imaging for detection of partial graft tears is poor with a focal change in caliber of the graft as the most useful sign observed (**Fig. 28**).[49]

Similar to the native ACL, secondary signs of ACL graft tearing may be seen at imaging. However, such secondary signs are of limited sensitivity for detection of graft tears, although specificity remains high.[49] Secondary signs of ACL graft insufficiency and joint instability may also be seen in the presence of morphologically intact grafts. Such findings may be reflective of instability because of graft stretching, although similar findings can also be seen in the absence of clinical knee laxity.[52]

Graft impingement

ACL graft impingement may cause loss of knee joint extension and predispose to graft tearing over time. Development of graft impingement is predominantly related to positioning of the tibial tunnel. If the anterior wall of the tibial tunnel is located anterior to the Blumensaat line, the graft is at risk of roof impingement.[53] This roof impingement is manifested at MR imaging as mechanical abutment and focal deviation in the course of the ACL graft by the anterior margin of the intercondylar shelf. With mechanical impingement, areas of

increased signal intensity may be seen within the distal two-thirds of the graft.[53] However, isolated increased signal intensity within the graft may also be seen in normal asymptomatic individuals as well as during "ligamentization." In the setting of focal increased intrasubstance graft signal, images should be carefully scrutinized for other supportive evidence of graft impingement, such as tibial tunnel malpositioning, notch osteophytes, and contact between the graft and the roof of the intercondylar notch (**Fig. 29**).

Arthrofibrosis

Arthrofibrosis following ACL reconstruction may be diffuse, surround the graft, or manifest with a focal nodular fibrotic mass anterior to the graft (Cyclops lesion). Arthrofibrosis is present in 1% to 10% of ACL reconstructions, may be of variable size, and may lead to loss of terminal extension similar to that seen with graft impingement.[54] Arthrofibrosis is characterized by intermediate-low T1-signal and T2-signal intensity owing to the combination of fibrotic, osseous, and synovial tissue (**Fig. 30**).[55] MR imaging has a sensitivity and specificity of 85% for detection of these complications following ACL surgery.[54] Surgeons sometimes contend that "arthrofibrosis" is a clinical diagnosis implying global stiffness of the

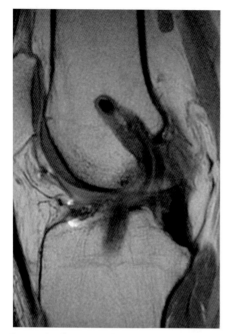

Fig. 26. Sagittal proton density MR image in a 46-year-old man with anterior positioning of the femoral tunnel and presenting with instability 1 year after ACL reconstruction with a hamstring graft. The femoral tunnel is located almost at the midway point of the roof of the intercondylar notch. Two separate strands of the hamstring graft are visualized. The graft demonstrates posterior bowing.

joint; as such, one may be well advised to describe focal forms of this complication as "focal scarring." "Cyclops lesion" is an appropriate name for the focal nodular form extending from the anterior margin of the graft.

Ganglion cyst formation and tunnel widening
A small amount of longitudinal fluid signal intensity within a hamstring ACL graft can be a normal postoperative finding at MR imaging. However, more significant focal cystic accumulations of fluid may be encountered within a graft and within the tibial tunnel (**Fig. 31**). Such graft cysts are more common with hamstring grafts and may be seen in the absence of a graft tear. Small cysts tend to be asymptomatic but larger cysts may protrude into the subcutaneous tissue adjacent to the tibia. Tunnel widening may also be seen in the absence of ganglion cyst formation with proposed causes, including mechanical attrition and tunnel widening due to repetitive graft cycling and motion within osseous tunnels during physiologic knee joint function, or less commonly due to inflammatory granulomatous reactions.

Hardware failure
Hardware complications consist of malpositioning, fracture, and dislodgement. Hardware failure in the early postoperative period may lead to loss of graft fixation and instability. Once an ACL graft

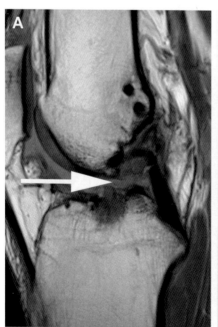
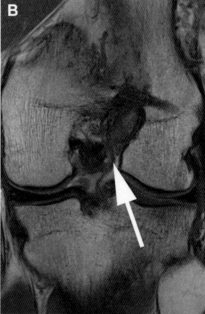

Fig. 27. Sagittal proton density (*A*) and coronal intermediate-weighted (*B*) MR image in a 40-year-old man with recurrent trauma after ACL reconstruction. The sagittal image demonstrates complete discontinuity of the graft (*arrow* in *A*) with a tiny redundant strand visualized on the coronal image (*arrow* in *B*).

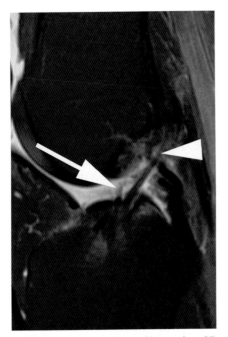

Fig. 28. Sagittal T2 fat-suppressed image in a 27-year-old woman 5 years after ACL reconstruction with a high-grade partial tear of the ACL graft. The graft is attenuated (*arrowhead*) and demonstrates discontinuity distally (*arrow*).

construct has been firmly embedded, stability may not be compromised, but dislodged or fractured fixation hardware components can lead to intra-articular bodies and mechanical joint symptoms (**Fig. 32**).

PCL Reconstruction

PCL reconstruction is far less commonly undertaken than ACL reconstruction, especially in cases of isolated PCL injury. PCL reconstruction is typically performed following multiligamentous injuries, or isolated complete PCL injuries with continued symptomatic instability despite conservative treatment.[56] Identification of other associated ligamentous injuries of the joint is critical to clinical management decisions in the setting of a PCL tear. PCL reconstruction may be performed with a single bundle technique, anatomically reconstructing the ALB of the native PCL, or less commonly, as a double bundle procedure. The choice of graft material is similar to that used for the ACL.

Normal MR imaging: PCL reconstruction

A PCL reconstruction femoral tunnel is typically situated along the anterior aspect of the PCL footprint along the anterior quarter of the intercondylar

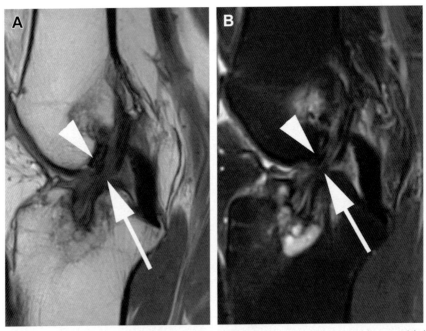

Fig. 29. Sagittal proton density (*A*) and T2 fat-suppressed (*B*) MR image in a 50-year-old man with limited knee extension 4 years after revision ACL reconstruction demonstrating multifactorial graft impingement. There is increased intrasubstance signal change within the graft secondary to impingement. Focal caliber change of the graft is seen consistent with a partial tear (*arrow*). The anterior wall of the tibial tunnel is located slightly anterior to Blumensaat line and there is a roof osteophyte abutting the graft at the site of the graft caliber change (*arrowhead*). The old femoral tunnel is seen midway along the roof of the intercondylar notch.

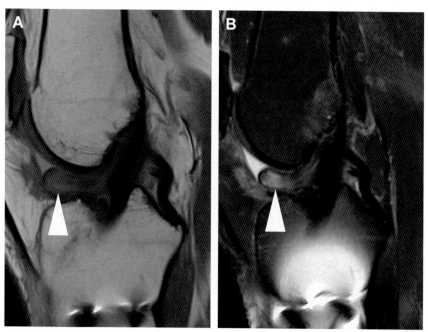

Fig. 30. Sagittal proton density (*A*) and T2 fat-suppressed (*B*) MR image in a 25-year-old woman 2 years after ACL reconstruction presenting with limited extension. There is abnormal intermediate-low signal intensity tissue along the anterior surface of the graft extending anteriorly toward Hoffa fat (*arrowheads*) consistent with a Cyclops lesion.

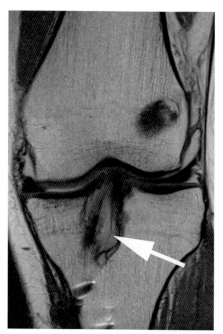

Fig. 31. Coronal intermediate-weighted MR image in a 42-year-old woman with hamstring ACL reconstruction showing a tibial tunnel ganglion cyst (*arrow*) with slight widening of the tibial tunnel.

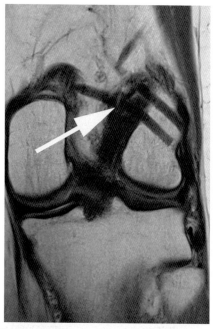

Fig. 32. Coronal intermediate-weighted image in a 32-year-old woman, 5 years following ACL reconstruction demonstrating fixation with 2 bioabsorbable cross-pins. Both pins protrude into the soft tissues medially and the more inferior pin is angulated (*arrow*), consistent with a pin fracture. The patient was asymptomatic with no evidence of instability.

notch on sagittal images and at 1 o'clock (right knee) or 11 o'clock (left knee) on coronal images.[57,58] Tibial graft fixation may be achieved by using either a tibial tunnel or a tibial inlay procedure with a BPTB graft. Tibial tunnel fixation is achieved arthroscopically, but the angulation of the graft at the opening of the tunnel results in a "killer turn," which may predispose to focal graft stress and attrition over time, with potential ultimate graft failure (**Fig. 33**). Tibial inlay fixation, avoiding the killer turn, is carried out by a combined arthroscopic and open technique and consists of graft bone plug fixation to the posterior cortex of the proximal tibia through a unicortical window. The normal PCL graft undergoes a similar "ligamentization" process as the ACL, but at 12 to 24 months postoperatively, it demonstrates uniform low signal intensity (**Fig. 34**).[59] It may have a curved or straight morphologic contour.

MR imaging of postoperative complications: PCL reconstructions

Postoperative complications of PCL most commonly relate to recurrent instability. Recurrent instability may be seen in the presence of a torn graft or a graft that appears intact on MR imaging.[60] Excessive posterior positioning of the

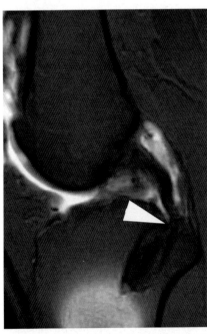

Fig. 33. Sagittal T1-weighted fat-suppressed MR arthrogram in a 43-year-old man with PCL reconstruction using a tibial tunnel fixation technique demonstrating an intact graft with the typical angulation of the graft at entry point into the tibial tunnel (*arrowhead*), which may predispose to graft attrition and tear.

femoral tunnel or anterior positioning of the tibial tunnel may contribute to instability. MR imaging signs of a disrupted PCL graft are similar to that of the ACL with increased signal intensity and discontinuity of graft construct fibers (**Figs. 35** and **36**).

PEARLS, PITFALLS, AND VARIANTS

- Primary MR imaging signs are most useful for evaluation of ACL tears.
- Chronic and partial ACL tears, and PCL tears, may heal with relatively normal appearances on MR imaging.
- Accuracy results for MR imaging detection of partial tears of the native ACL and PCL, and partial tears following cruciate ligament reconstruction, are limited.
- Mucoid degeneration of the cruciates, particularly the PCL, may mimic the imaging appearance of a partial ligament tear.
- Identification of associated ligamentous injuries is critical in assessment of patients with cruciate ligament injury.

WHAT THE REFERRING CLINICIAN NEEDS TO KNOW

- Grade of cruciate injuries: complete versus partial (high grade vs low grade).
- Presence of possible associated cruciate avulsion fractures.
- Status of menisci and hyaline articular cartilage: the status of the ACL and PCL may be accurately assessed clinically in the setting of complete tears. Identification of concomitant meniscal and particularly chondral injuries, which are more problematic to diagnose clinically, impacts on treatment decision-making and is a critical role for MR imaging following cruciate ligament injury.
- The status of other ligamentous structures: integrity of other ligamentous structures in the knee may contribute to overall stability of the articulation and determination of whether a patient with cruciate ligament injury is treated conservatively or surgically.
- Cause of a symptomatically "locked knee": patients with cruciate ligament injuries may present with a locked knee. Identification of the cause (meniscal vs flipped ACL fibers vs pseudolocking) is important in emergent treatment of such patients.
- Cause of postreconstruction loss of terminal knee extension: identification of the cause of loss of terminal extension (graft impingement vs focal fibrosis) following ACL reconstruction

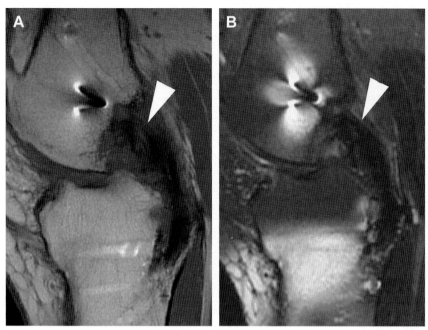

Fig. 34. Sagittal proton density (*A*) and fat-suppressed T2-weighted MR images (*B*) in a 41-year-old man following PCL reconstruction demonstrating thickening of the graft on both pulse sequences (*arrowheads*) with increased signal intensity on the proton density images. The knee was clinically stable.

is important information in planning possible patient management or revision surgical intervention.

- Measurement of tunnel width before revision surgery: assessment of tunnel width and identification of possible tunnel widening before revision graft reconstruction is important in determination of bone stock loss and the possible need for prerevision bone grafting.

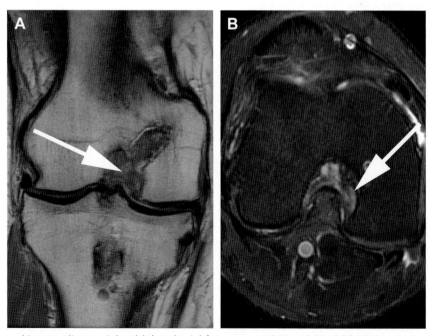

Fig. 35. Coronal intermediate-weighted (*A*) and axial fat-suppressed T2-weighted (*B*) MR images in a 39-year-old man with a prior multiligamentous knee injury. The PCL graft is not visualized in the intercondylar notch (*arrows*), consistent with a complete rupture. The patient also has a ruptured ACL graft.

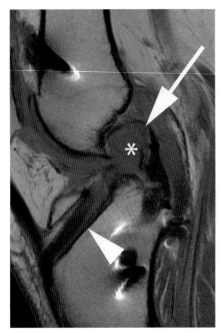

Fig. 36. Sagittal proton density MR image in a 29-year-old man with prior multiligamentous knee reconstruction demonstrating a very high grade and functionally complete tear of the proximal PCL graft (*arrow*). Part of the ACL tibial tunnel is demonstrated (*arrowhead*). Intermediate signal intensity within the intercondylar notch (*asterisk*) represented extensive focal fibrosis.

SUMMARY

MR imaging is the imaging modality of choice for the detection of cruciate ligament injuries with a high sensitivity and specificity for detection of complete tears. However, accuracy of MR imaging in the presence of chronic tears and partial tears is more limited.

REFERENCES

1. Paterno MV, Rauh MJ, Schmitt LC, et al. Incidence of contralateral and ipsilateral anterior cruciate ligament (ACL) injury after primary ACL reconstruction and return to sport. Clin J Sport Med 2012;22(2):116–21.

2. Miyasaka KC, Daniel DM, Stone ML, et al. The incidence of knee ligament injuries in the general population. Am J Knee Surg 1991;4:43–8.

3. Amis AA, Dawkins GP. Functional anatomy of the anterior cruciate ligament. Fibre bundle actions related to ligament replacements and injuries. J Bone Joint Surg Br 1991;73(2):260–7.

4. Muller B, Hofbauer M, Wongcharoenwatana J, et al. Indications and contraindications for double-bundle ACL reconstruction. Int Orthop 2013;37(2):239–46.

5. Steckel H, Starman JS, Baums MH, et al. Anatomy of the anterior cruciate ligament double bundle structure: a macroscopic evaluation. Scand J Med Sci Sports 2007;17(4):387–92.

6. Kusayama T, Harner CD, Carlin GJ, et al. Anatomical and biomechanical characteristics of human meniscofemoral ligaments. Knee Surg Sports Traumatol Arthrosc 1994;2(4):234–7.

7. Sonin AH, Fitzgerald SW, Hoff FL, et al. MR imaging of the posterior cruciate ligament: normal, abnormal, and associated injury patterns. Radiographics 1995;15(3):551–61.

8. Hong SH, Choi JY, Lee GK, et al. Grading of anterior cruciate ligament injury. Diagnostic efficacy of oblique coronal magnetic resonance imaging of the knee. J Comput Assist Tomogr 2003;27(5):814–9.

9. Ng AW, Griffith JF, Hung EH, et al. MRI diagnosis of ACL bundle tears: value of oblique axial imaging. Skeletal Radiol 2013;42(2):209–17.

10. Kijowski R, Davis KW, Woods MA, et al. Knee joint: comprehensive assessment with 3D isotropic resolution fast spin-echo MR imaging–diagnostic performance compared with that of conventional MR imaging at 3.0 T. Radiology 2009;252(2):486–95.

11. Gentili A, Seeger LL, Yao L, et al. Anterior cruciate ligament tear: indirect signs at MR imaging. Radiology 1994;193(3):835–40.

12. Roychowdhury S, Fitzgerald SW, Sonin AH, et al. Using MR imaging to diagnose partial tears of the anterior cruciate ligament: value of axial images. AJR Am J Roentgenol 1997;168(6):1487–91.

13. Viskontas DG, Giuffre BM, Duggal N, et al. Bone bruises associated with ACL rupture: correlation with injury mechanism. Am J Sports Med 2008;36(5):927–33.

14. Quatman CE, Quatman-Yates CC, Hewett TE. A 'plane' explanation of anterior cruciate ligament injury mechanisms: a systematic review. Sports Med 2010;40(9):729–46.

15. Gottsegen CJ, Eyer BA, White EA, et al. Avulsion fractures of the knee: imaging findings and clinical significance. Radiographics 2008;28(6):1755–70.

16. Ahn JH, Han KY, Yu IS, et al. Arthroscopic treatment for tibial "Peel off" tears in anterior cruciate ligament-case report. Eur J Orthop Surg Traumatol 2013;23(Suppl 2):S251–5.

17. Barry KP, Mesgarzadeh M, Triolo J, et al. Accuracy of MRI patterns in evaluating anterior cruciate ligament tears. Skeletal Radiol 1996;25(4):365–70.

18. Robertson PL, Schweitzer ME, Bartolozzi AR, et al. Anterior cruciate ligament tears: evaluation of multiple signs with MR imaging. Radiology 1994;193(3):829–34.

19. Kijowski R, Sanogo ML, Lee KS, et al. Short-term clinical importance of osseous injuries diagnosed at MR imaging in patients with anterior cruciate ligament tear. Radiology 2012;264(2):531–41.

20. Vahey TN, Hunt JE, Shelbourne KD. Anterior translocation of the tibia at MR imaging: a secondary sign of anterior cruciate ligament tear. Radiology 1993;187(3):817–9.

21. Brandser EA, Riley MA, Berbaum KS, et al. MR imaging of anterior cruciate ligament injury: independent value of primary and secondary signs. AJR Am J Roentgenol 1996;167(1):121–6.

22. Nakase J, Toratani T, Kosaka M, et al. Roles of ACL remnants in knee stability. Knee Surg Sports Traumatol Arthrosc 2013;21(9):2101–6.

23. Tjoumakaris FP, Donegan DJ, Sekiya JK. Partial tears of the anterior cruciate ligament: diagnosis and treatment. Am J Orthop (Belle Mead NJ) 2011;40(2):92–7.

24. Lintner DM, Kamaric E, Moseley JB, et al. Partial tears of the anterior cruciate ligament. Are they clinically detectable? Am J Sports Med 1995; 23(1):111–8.

25. Noyes FR, Mooar LA, Moorman CT 3rd, et al. Partial tears of the anterior cruciate ligament. Progression to complete ligament deficiency. J Bone Joint Surg Br 1989;71(5):825–33.

26. Yao L, Gentili A, Petrus L, et al. Partial ACL rupture: an MR diagnosis? Skeletal Radiol 1995; 24(4):247–51.

27. Umans H, Wimpfheimer O, Haramati N, et al. Diagnosis of partial tears of the anterior cruciate ligament of the knee: value of MR imaging. AJR Am J Roentgenol 1995;165(4):893–7.

28. Van Dyck P, De Smet E, Veryser J, et al. Partial tear of the anterior cruciate ligament of the knee: injury patterns on MR imaging. Knee Surg Sports Traumatol Arthrosc 2012;20(2):256–61.

29. Van Dyck P, Vanhoenacker FM, Gielen JL, et al. Three tesla magnetic resonance imaging of the anterior cruciate ligament of the knee: can we differentiate complete from partial tears? Skeletal Radiol 2011;40(6):701–7.

30. Van Dyck P, Gielen JL, Vanhoenacker FM, et al. Stable or unstable tear of the anterior cruciate ligament of the knee: an MR diagnosis? Skeletal Radiol 2012;41(3):273–80.

31. Schulz MS, Russe K, Weiler A, et al. Epidemiology of posterior cruciate ligament injuries. Arch Orthop Trauma Surg 2003;123(4):186–91.

32. Lee BK, Nam SW. Rupture of posterior cruciate ligament: diagnosis and treatment principles. Knee Surg Relat Res 2011;23(3):135–41.

33. Mariani PP, Margheritini F, Christel P, et al. Evaluation of posterior cruciate ligament healing: a study using magnetic resonance imaging and stress radiography. Arthroscopy 2005;21(11): 1354–61.

34. Rodriguez W Jr, Vinson EN, Helms CA, et al. MRI appearance of posterior cruciate ligament tears. AJR Am J Roentgenol 2008;191(4):1031.

35. Sonin AH, Fitzgerald SW, Friedman H, et al. Posterior cruciate ligament injury: MR imaging diagnosis and patterns of injury. Radiology 1994;190(2):455–8.

36. McMonagle JS, Helms CA, Garrett WE Jr, et al. Tram-track appearance of the posterior cruciate ligament (PCL): correlations with mucoid degeneration, ligamentous stability, and differentiation from PCL tears. AJR Am J Roentgenol 2013;201(2):394–9.

37. Jung YB, Jung HJ, Yang JJ, et al. Characterization of spontaneous healing of chronic posterior cruciate ligament injury: analysis of instability and magnetic resonance imaging. J Magn Reson Imaging 2008;27(6):1336–40.

38. Bach BR Jr, Tradonsky S, Bojchuk J, et al. Arthroscopically assisted anterior cruciate ligament reconstruction using patellar tendon autograft. Five- to nine-year follow-up evaluation. Am J Sports Med 1998;26(1):20–9.

39. Marrale J, Morrissey MC, Haddad FS. A literature review of autograft and allograft anterior cruciate ligament reconstruction. Knee Surg Sports Traumatol Arthrosc 2007;15(6):690–704.

40. Howell SM, Clark JA, Blasier RD. Serial magnetic resonance imaging of hamstring anterior cruciate ligament autografts during the first year of implantation. A preliminary study. Am J Sports Med 1991;19(1):42–7.

41. Boynton MD, Fadale PD. The basic science of anterior cruciate ligament surgery. Orthop Rev 1993;22(6):673–9.

42. Vogl TJ, Schmitt J, Lubrich J, et al. Reconstructed anterior cruciate ligaments using patellar tendon ligament grafts: diagnostic value of contrast-enhanced MRI in a 2-year follow-up regimen. Eur Radiol 2001;11(8):1450–6.

43. Trattnig S, Rand T, Czerny C, et al. Magnetic resonance imaging of the postoperative knee. Top Magn Reson Imaging 1999;10(4):221–36.

44. Saupe N, White LM, Chiavaras MM, et al. Anterior cruciate ligament reconstruction grafts: MR imaging features at long-term follow-up–correlation with functional and clinical evaluation. Radiology 2008;249(2):581–90.

45. Svensson M, Kartus J, Ejerhed L, et al. Does the patellar tendon normalize after harvesting its central third?: a prospective long-term MRI study. Am J Sports Med 2004;32(1):34–8.

46. Casagranda BU, Maxwell NJ, Kavanagh EC, et al. Normal appearance and complications of double-bundle and selective-bundle anterior cruciate ligament reconstructions using optimal MRI techniques. AJR Am J Roentgenol 2009;192(5):1407–15.

47. Howell SM, Hull ML. Checkpoints for judging tunnel and anterior cruciate ligament graft placement. J Knee Surg 2009;22(2):161–70.

48. Simmons R, Howell SM, Hull ML. Effect of the angle of the femoral and tibial tunnels in the coronal plane

and incremental excision of the posterior cruciate ligament on tension of an anterior cruciate ligament graft: an in vitro study. J Bone Joint Surg Am 2003; 85-A(6):1018–29.

49. Horton LK, Jacobson JA, Lin J, et al. MR imaging of anterior cruciate ligament reconstruction graft. AJR Am J Roentgenol 2000;175(4):1091–7.

50. Rak KM, Gillogly SD, Schaefer RA, et al. Anterior cruciate ligament reconstruction: evaluation with MR imaging. Radiology 1991;178(2):553–6.

51. McCauley TR, Elfar A, Moore A, et al. MR arthrography of anterior cruciate ligament reconstruction grafts. AJR Am J Roentgenol 2003;181(5):1217–23.

52. Naraghi AM, Gupta S, Jacks LM, et al. Anterior cruciate ligament reconstruction: MR imaging signs of anterior knee laxity in the presence of an intact graft. Radiology 2012;263(3):802–10.

53. Howell SM, Berns GS, Farley TE. Unimpinged and impinged anterior cruciate ligament grafts: MR signal intensity measurements. Radiology 1991; 179(3):639–43.

54. Recht MP, Piraino DW, Cohen MA, et al. Localized anterior arthrofibrosis (cyclops lesion) after reconstruction of the anterior cruciate ligament: MR imaging findings. AJR Am J Roentgenol 1995; 165(2):383–5.

55. Bradley DM, Bergman AG, Dillingham MF. MR imaging of cyclops lesions. AJR Am J Roentgenol 2000;174(3):719–26.

56. Levy BA, Dajani KA, Whelan DB, et al. Decision making in the multiligament-injured knee: an evidence-based systematic review. Arthroscopy 2009;25(4):430–8.

57. Harner CD, Hoher J. Evaluation and treatment of posterior cruciate ligament injuries. Am J Sports Med 1998;26(3):471–82.

58. Christel P. Basic principles for surgical reconstruction of the PCL in chronic posterior knee instability. Knee Surg Sports Traumatol Arthrosc 2003;11(5): 289–96.

59. Mariani PP, Adriani E, Bellelli A, et al. Magnetic resonance imaging of tunnel placement in posterior cruciate ligament reconstruction. Arthroscopy 1999;15(7):733–40.

60. Sherman PM, Sanders TG, Morrison WB, et al. MR imaging of the posterior cruciate ligament graft: initial experience in 15 patients with clinical correlation. Radiology 2001;221(1):191–8.

Posterolateral and Posteromedial Corner Injuries of the Knee

Daniel Geiger, MD[a], Eric Y. Chang, MD[b,c],
Mini N. Pathria, MD[c], Christine B. Chung, MD[b,c],*

KEYWORDS

• Knee • Posterolateral • Posteromedial • Corner • Injuries

KEY POINTS

- Posterolateral and posteromedial corners of the knee are complex anatomic regions; detailed knowledge of anatomic structures and relationships is necessary for appropriate assessment at imaging.
- Association between untreated posterolateral and posteromedial corner injuries of the knee and failure of central support structure reconstruction has been established. Accurate diagnosis and characterization of these injuries will improve clinical and surgical outcome.
- Posterolateral and posteromedial corner injuries of the knee may be difficult to diagnose clinically. Classic magnetic resonance imaging patterns allow noninvasive diagnosis that can guide management.

INTRODUCTION

The posterolateral (PLC) and posteromedial (PMC) corners of the knee are anatomic units composed of a complex arrangement of structures. As referenced in their names, they extend both posteriorly[1] and along the lateral and medial aspects of the knee, respectively (**Fig. 1**). As the posterior extension of the lateral and medial supporting structures, they act in conjunction with the central supporting ligaments (anterior and posterior cruciate ligaments) to provide static (capsular and noncapsular ligaments) and dynamic (musculotendinous units and their aponeuroses) articular stability.[2,3] The delineation of fine anatomic detail in these regions and identification of delicate structures are particularly challenging at imaging because of composite anatomy, orientation, and small size of their components. Pathology might be overlooked or misdiagnosed without clear knowledge of the regional morphology, biomechanics, and specific patterns of injury. Moreover, PLC and PMC injuries uncommonly occur in an isolated fashion, more often associated with concomitant injuries that may dominate the clinical picture. Untreated PLC injuries can lead to chronic posterolateral instability[4,5] and PMC deficiencies may cause persistent valgus instability[6]; both conditions lead to poor outcome of anterior cruciate ligament (ACL) and posterior cruciate ligament (PCL) reconstruction. It is therefore imperative, in

Disclosure: The authors declare that they have no conflict of interest.

This manuscript was previously published in: Chung CB, Geiger D, Pathria M, et al. Posterolateral and Posteromedial Corner Injuries of the Knee. Radiol Clin N Am 2013;51(3):413-32.

[a] Department of Radiological, Oncological and Pathological Sciences, Sapienza University of Rome, Viale Regina Elena 324, Rome 00161, Italy; [b] VA Healthcare San Diego, 3350 La Jolla Village Drive, La Jolla, CA 92161, USA; [c] Department of Radiology, University of California-San Diego, 408 Dickinson Street, San Diego, CA 92103–8226, USA
* Corresponding author.
E-mail address: cbchung@ucsd.edu

Magn Reson Imaging Clin N Am 22 (2014) 581–599
http://dx.doi.org/10.1016/j.mric.2014.08.001

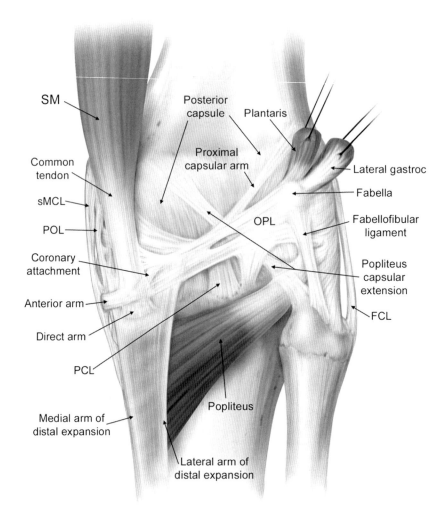

Fig. 1. Posterior aspect of the knee after removal of medial and lateral gastrocnemius muscles and neurovascular structures. SM, semimembranosus muscle; sMCL, superficial medial collateral ligament; FCL, fibular (lateral) collateral ligament; lateral gastroc, lateral gastrocnemius; OPL, oblique popliteal ligament; PCL, posterior cruciate ligament; POL, posterior oblique ligament. (*From* LaPrade RF, Morgan PM, Wentorf FA, et al. The anatomy of the posterior aspect of the knee. An anatomic study. J Bone Joint Surg Am 2007;89(4):758–64; with permission.)

a postinjury or preoperative setting, to provide the referring physician with an accurate description (when possible) of the PLC and PMC structures. The characterization of structural alteration at imaging will allow a reference for clinical evaluation that can guide surgical approach and interrogation, facilitating optimal treatment, and thereby improving patient outcome. Magnetic resonance imaging (MRI) currently is the gold standard imaging strategy in the evaluation of the soft tissues; therefore, the authors focus mainly on this technique. Ultrasound scan has been established as a complementary technique.[7] Plain films and computed tomography play a role in the evaluation of osseous lesions (bony avulsions, cortical stress changes related to chronic injury). This article discusses the anatomy, basic biomechanics, and

common injuries of the PLC and PMC complexes, presenting the reader with a systematic approach for their evaluation.

POSTEROLATERAL CORNER OF THE KNEE
Anatomy, Biomechanics, and Mechanism of Injuries to the Posterolateral

Seebacher and colleagues[8] in 1982 introduced a three-layered approach in the anatomic description of the lateral supporting structures of the knee, using a similar three-layer concept previously assumed in their description of the medial side supporting structures (**Fig. 2**).[9] In Seebacher's original description of the lateral supporting structures, the *superficial layer (I)* consists of the iliotibial tract and its expansion anteriorly and the biceps

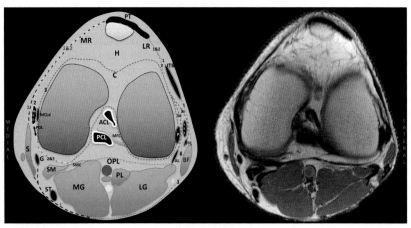

Fig. 2. Axial diagram (*left*) shows layers and anatomic components at the level of the joint line with a corresponding axial T2-weighted MRI (*right*). 1 = first layer, 2 = second layer, 3 = third layer, 3s = third layer (superficial lamina), 3d = third layer (deep lamina), AL, arcuate ligament; BF, biceps femoris and its tendon; C, capsule and H, Hoffa's fat pad; FFL, fabellofibular ligament; G, gracilis muscle tendon; g, lateral inferior genicular artery; ITB, iliotibial band; LCL, lateral collateral ligament; LG, lateral gastrocnemius muscle; LR, lateral retinaculum; MCL, medial collateral ligament; MCLd, deep medial collateral ligament; MFL, meniscofemoral ligament (Humphrey's); MG, medial gastrocnemius muscle; MR, medial retinaculum; OPL, oblique popliteal ligament; P, popliteus muscle tendon; PL, plantaris muscle; POL, posterior oblique ligament; PT, patellar tendon; S, sartorius muscle and its tendon; SM, semimembranosus muscle tendon; SMC, semimembranosus tendon (capsular arm); ST, semitendinosus muscle tendon.

femoris tendon (BFT) and its expansion posteriorly. The peroneal nerve lies deep to it, posterior to the BFT. The *middle layer (II)* is incomplete and consists of the lateral patellar retinaculum anteriorly and the 2 patellofemoral ligaments posteriorly. The proximal patellofemoral ligament joins the lateral intermuscular septum, the distal patellofemoral ligament attaches to the fabella (when present) or at the femoral insertion of the posterolateral joint capsule or lateral head of the gastrocnemius. Included in the middle layer is the patellomeniscal ligament, which travels from the patella to the lateral meniscus, reaching inferiorly the lateral tibial tubercle of Gerdy, running deep to the iliotibial tract. The *deepest layer (III)* is composed of the lateral extent of the joint capsule and is attached to the edges of the tibia and femur. Posterior to the overlying iliotibial tract, the capsule divides into 2 laminae (superficial and deep). The superficial lamina travels superficial to the lateral collateral ligament and ends posteriorly at the fabellofibular ligament. The deeper lamina travels deep to the lateral collateral ligament, passes along and attaches to the edge of the lateral meniscus, giving rise to the coronary ligament and ultimately reaching the arcuate ligament. The deep and superficial laminae of the posterolateral capsule are always separated from each other with the lateral inferior genicular artery, considered an anatomic landmark, between them (see **Fig. 2**). Further cadaveric,[10] MRI[11–18] and ultrasound

scan[7,19] evaluations of specific PLC anatomy followed Seebacher's original work to delineate the imaging counterpart of his anatomic description. Because of the increasing interest in the anatomy and biomechanics of the PLC corner of the knee in the orthopedic literature, the need for standardization and a systematic approach to the nomenclature of the lateral complex structures and PLC has been addressed.[20,21] For a systematic approach to these structures we consider the superficial layer (first layer) comprising the lateral fascia, iliotibial band and biceps femoris tendon. The middle layer (second layer) comprises the patellar retinaculum, and patellofemoral and patellomeniscal ligaments. The deep layer (third layer) consists of the *lateral collateral ligament* (fibular collateral ligament), the *lateral coronary ligament* (lateral meniscotibial ligament), the *arcuate ligament*, the *popliteus tendon-muscle unit*, the *popliteofibular ligament*, the *fabellofibular ligament*, and the lateral joint capsule with its attachment to the lateral meniscus edge. The deep layer is the most anatomically variable of the 3 layers and the one constituting the posterolateral corner of the knee complex.[20] We briefly describe the components of the third inner layer and their anatomic relations.

The lateral collateral ligament (fibular collateral ligament), is an extracapsular structure, has a tubular shape, and measures approximately 3–4 mm in diameter and 7 cm in length. It originates from the lateral femoral condyle, arising from a small depression posterior to the lateral femoral epicondyle and 2 cm proximal to the joint line. It courses distally and posteriorly to attach to the posterior portion of the lateral aspect of the fibular head (see **Fig. 1**).

The lateral coronary ligament (or meniscotibial portion of the midthird lateral capsular ligament or lateral meniscotibial ligament) attaches the lateral meniscus to the lateral tibial plateau and functions as a meniscal stabilizer. The lateral coronary ligament is composed of short confluent ligamentous bands attached to the peripheral portion of the meniscal body and to the lateral tibia several millimeters inferior to the articular surface, occasionally resulting in a small synovial recess.[22,23]

The arcuate ligament has an inverted Y shape. The 2 superior arms consist of a lateral limb (upright), coursing upward along the joint capsule and extending to the lateral femoral condyle, and a medial limb (arcuate), crossing over the popliteal tendon, attaching to the posterior capsule, and merging with the oblique popliteal ligament. The lower limb attaches to the fibular head.[24] The arcuate ligament lies deep to the lateral inferior genicular artery, and its presence is variable, ranging from 24% to 80% in previous studies.[8,25,26]

The popliteus muscle originates from the lateral aspect of the lateral femoral condyle, attaches to the posterior horn of the lateral meniscus via the popliteomeniscal fascicles (anteroinferior, posterosuperior, posteroinferior) and to the apex of the fibula via the popliteofibular fascicles, extending distally to the posteromedial aspect of the tibial shaft (see **Fig. 1**). The popliteus muscle is always present, whereas the posteroinferior popliteomeniscal fascicle may be absent.[26,27]

The popliteofibular ligament originates at the level of the musculotendinous junction of the popliteus muscle and courses distally and laterally to insert on the fibular styloid. The popliteofibular ligament is a wide tendinous band, approximately the same width or wider than the popliteus tendon,[28–31] and is reportedly present in between 94% and 98% of the population.[25,26] The proximal myotendinous portion of the popliteus muscle and the popliteofibular ligament originating from it form an inverted Y-shaped structure. Therefore, the 3 arms of the inverted Y are the superior portion of the popliteus myotendinous unit, the popliteofibular ligament, and the inferior portion of the popliteus myotendinous unit distal to the origin of the popliteofibular ligament.

The fabellofibular ligament is the distal edge of the capsular arm of the short head of the biceps femoris muscle, and, as such, is present in all knees. Usually, it is a delicate structure but is more robust in appearance when the bony fabella is present but less consistent and more subtle in nature when a cartilaginous fabellar analog is present. We would like to reinforce the concept addressed from LaPrade[21] regarding the presence of at least a fabellar cartilaginous analog in every knee. When the fabella is present, the fabellofibular ligament arises from the lateral margin of the fabella, and, when absent, it originates from the posterior aspect of the supracondylar process of the femur.[32] Extending from the fabella or the fabellar analog, the fabellofibular ligament extends toward the fibula, parallel to the lateral collateral ligament, and inserts distally on the lateral aspect of the tip of the fibular head styloid process, posterior to the fibular insertion of the biceps femoris tendon (see **Fig. 1**). Previous studies addressed the variable presence of the fabellofibular ligament, ranging from 51%–87%.[8,26]

Biomechanically the PLC structures resist varus and external rotation forces. With regard to varus forces the lateral collateral ligament is considered the major stabilizer, with a minor contribution from the posterior cruciate ligament and the posterolateral capsule; a minor secondary contribution is made from the anterior cruciate ligament. In relation to external rotation forces, the lateral collateral ligament, popliteofibular ligament, fabellofibular ligament, capsular attachment of the short head of the biceps femoris muscle, and the popliteus tendon play a fundamental role in resisting stress. A role of the PLC in resisting posterior translation of the tibia has been addressed, establishing the popliteomeniscal fascicles as stabilizers of the posterior horn of the lateral meniscus. Isolated injuries of the PLC tend to be rare and commonly occur in conjunction with cruciate ligament lesions. The association of lateral collateral ligament and deep PLC structure injuries increases varus angulation and tibial external rotation, also causing anteroposterior instability of the knee. Deep PLC lesions (preserved lateral collateral ligament), in conjunction with anterior cruciate ligament deficiency, increase anterior translation of the tibia without causing external rotation of the tibia or varus angulation of the joint. When deep PLC structures fail and lateral collateral ligament and anterior cruciate ligament injuries are present, anterior and varus instability with external rotation of the tibia occur. Deep PLC structure deficiency, with lateral collateral ligament and posterior cruciate ligament injury, cause posterior translation, varus angulation, and external rotation of the tibia.[33–42] Posterolateral corner injuries are frequently associated with acute posterior cruciate ligament tears and have been reported in 62% of patients.[43] Therefore, when a posterior cruciate ligament injury is observed, particular attention should be paid to the PLC area. Injuries of the PLC are less common than injuries of the PMC, but because this anatomic area is subject to a greater stress during motion than the medial side, they tend to be more disabling.[13] PLC injuries most commonly occur via a direct blow to the anteromedial aspect of the proximal tibia in the fully extended knee, with the force directed in a posterolateral direction, but can also occur from a hyperextension injury with external rotation.[41,44] Anterior rotatory dislocations (varus stress and hyperextension) and posterior rotatory dislocations (varus stress, posteriorly directed blow to proximal tibia and flexion), are also common mechanisms of injury,[20,45] the latter known as a "dashboard injury." An undetected PLC injury can lead to chronic instability and failure of efforts to reconstruct the central supporting structures because of deficiency of PLC in resisting biomechanical stress.[34,46–49] Testing of the PLC resistance to stress involves varus and external rotation stress tests at different degrees of flexion.[35] The posterolateral rotation test (dial test) is one commonly used for posterolateral instability, assessing increasing external rotation of the tibia in relation to the femur at 30° of knee flexion.

INJURIES TO THE POSTEROLATERAL COMPLEX
Soft-tissues Injuries of the Posterolateral

Lateral collateral ligament (fibular collateral ligament)
Alterations to the lateral collateral ligament are a common feature of PLC injuries. In vitro studies addressed the role of the lateral collateral ligament (LCL) as a restraint to PLC instability and varus angulation in static testing. Nielsen and colleagues[50] noted an increase in varus joint opening with marked posterolateral rotatory instability when an LCL lesion is associated with a posterolateral capsule transection rather than an LCL injury alone. Grood and coworkers[51] addressed the increase of varus angulation at partial knee flexion when a PCL injury is combined with an LCL injury. Gollehon and colleagues[52] showed the principal role of the LCL and PLC deep ligament complex in preventing varus and external rotation of the tibia and the increase of varus rotation and posterior translation in combined injuries of the LCL, PCL, and deep lateral complex. However, LaPrade and Terry[33] evaluated 71 patients presenting with a PLC knee injury and signs of instability but at surgery found an injured LCL in only 23% of the knees. Based on this finding,

they suggest that an LCL injury should not be the sole determining factor when diagnosing PLC injuries. Lateral collateral ligament injuries consist of structural alterations that include thickening, tears, soft-tissue avulsions from the femoral attachment, and soft-tissue avulsions (with or without a bony component) from the fibular head. LCL injuries are best visualized in the axial and coronal plane at MRI examination (**Fig. 3**).[5,13,53]

Popliteus muscle and its tendon
Injuries to the popliteus muscle can be intra-articular (at the femoral insertion or at the level of the popliteal hiatus) or extra-articular (muscular or myotendinous portion) in nature, the latter being more frequent. An avulsion at the femoral attachment may appear as an irregular contour of its tendon at the level of the popliteal hiatus with surrounding edema. Partial tears of the myotendinous junction present with increased T2 signal at the level of the muscle-tendon junction on fat suppressed, fluid-sensitive sequences at MRI examination. Complete tendon tears may present as an interruption of the muscle belly appearing as a masslike lesion with surrounding edema.[13] Enlargement of the muscle belly or disruption of muscle fibers may be apparent. Only 8% of all popliteus injuries occur in an isolated fashion,[54]

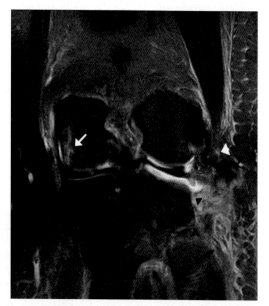

Fig. 3. Coronal proton density (PD) image with fat saturation (FS) of the knee in a patient after reduction of a knee dislocation shows a displaced arcuate fracture fragment (*black arrow*). Additionally, there is disruption of the midportion of the LCL (*white arrowhead*), avulsion of the lateral meniscotibial ligament (soft tissue Segond injury, *black arrowhead*), and a bone contusion at the peripheral aspect of the medial femoral condyle (*white arrow*).

with isolated cases of muscle or tendon lesions reported in skiers,[55] football,[55–57] soccer,[58,59] rugby,[60] and polo players.[61] Lesions of the popliteus muscle are usually combined with injuries to other knee structures.[13] Brown and colleagues,[54] in their MRI analysis of popliteus injuries (n = 24), reported combined injuries in 92% of cases, with involvement of its muscular portion in 96% of patients. Associated injuries included ACL (17%) or PCL (29%) tears, combined medial (46%) or lateral (25%) meniscal injuries, and medial (8%) or lateral (4%) collateral ligament lesions. Bone bruises or fractures were reported in 33% of patients. Popliteus muscle injuries are best evaluated on the axial and coronal planes (**Fig. 4**), and diagnosis of abnormalities on MR imaging plays a fundamental role in the diagnosis of an injury to the popliteus muscle because of the difficulty in assessing this structure at arthroscopy.[53,62]

Popliteofibular ligament

Visualization and assessment of the popliteofibular ligament can be challenging on MRI. Standard imaging planes (coronal, sagittal, and axial) may depict the structure, but visualization is not always optimal because of its oblique orientation and the delicate nature of the structure; coronal and sagittal planes are in our practice the most useful planes for assessment (**Fig. 5**). Some advocate the use of a coronal oblique plane, oriented parallel to the direction of the popliteus tendon, with one study showing visualization of the popliteofibular tendon improving from 8% to 53% of the knees.[63] Another study compared coronal oblique fat-saturated T2 with isotropic three-dimensional water excitation double-echo steady state (WE-DESS) sequences. The latter sequence improved the identification of the popliteofibular ligament from 71% to 91% of cases.[64]

Injuries to the popliteofibular ligament consist of ligamentous disruption, avulsion from the fibular insertion, partial tearing, and intrasubstance degeneration in the form of signal alteration within the tendon.[53] Surgical reconstruction of a disrupted popliteofibular ligament has been found to be beneficial in patients with posterolateral external rotatory instability of the knee.[65]

Arcuate ligament

The variable presence and subtlety of the arcuate ligament makes assessment difficult[24,66] and makes recognizing injuries of the arcuate ligament complex a challenging proposition. The anatomy of the arcuate ligament is debated[39] and can be considered a thickening of the posterolateral capsule. On sagittal images, the arcuate ligament is best identified on images on which the popliteus tendon and fibular tip are both visualized. The straight limb of the arcuate can be found superficial to the popliteus tendon as a delicate linear low-signal structure attaching to the fibular tip (**Fig. 6**). Dedicated imaging of the PLC in the coronal oblique plane may significantly improve visualization of the arcuate ligament, with an increase from 10% to 46% reported by Yu and colleagues[63] compared with standard coronal imaging.

Increased signal at the level of the posterolateral capsule on fat-saturated fluid-sensitive images should raise concern for capsular disruption and the possibility of associated injury or tear of the arcuate ligament (**Fig. 7**).[53] Injury to the posterolateral capsule has been suggested as one reason why PLC injuries can occasionally present without a significant knee joint effusion.[67] Baker and coworkers[68] operated on 13 patients with acute PCL injuries and posterolateral instability of the knee, identifying tears of the arcuate ligament complex in all 13. Their results suggest that surgical repair of the arcuate ligament complex improves patient outcome in PCL injuries with posterolateral instability,[68] emphasizing the importance of evaluating this structure on preoperative imaging.

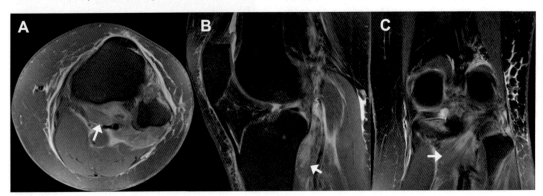

Fig. 4. Axial (*A*), sagittal (*B*), and coronal (*C*) PD FS images show a strain (grade II lesion) at the level of the myotendinous junction of popliteus (*white arrows*) and extensive circumferential soft tissue edema.

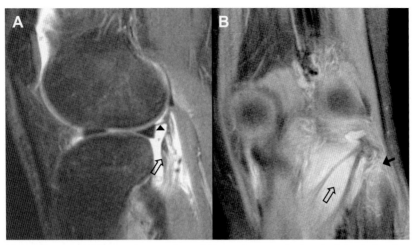

Fig. 5. Sagittal (A) and coronal (B) T2 FS images show diffuse edema at the level of the PLC and surrounding the myotendinous junction of popliteus compatible with a high-grade strain (*open arrows*). A partial tear of the popliteofibular ligament is present (*black arrow*). The posterosuperior popliteomeniscal fascicle is intact (*black arrowhead*).

Fabellofibular ligament

The fabellofibular ligament is best visualized on MRI in the coronal plane and is located posteriorly to the lateral collateral ligament and at the far posterior tip of the fibular styloid.[12] Yu and colleagues[63] compared visualization of the fabellofibular ligament in the coronal oblique plane with the standard coronal plane imaging and reported an increase in visualization from 34% to 48% on coronal oblique images. The fabellofibular ligament was seen in only 4% in the sagittal plane. Injuries of the fabellofibular ligament include degeneration, tearing and avulsion from the fibular tip (see **Fig. 7**). Avulsion of the fabellofibular ligament can be associated with an avulsive injury of the direct arm of the short head of the biceps femoris tendon.[5,14,53] The inferior lateral genicular artery is a branch of the popliteal artery, which can be used as an anatomic landmark in evaluating the fabellofibular ligament, as it passes around the posterior joint capsule laterally, running anterior to the fabellofibular ligament and posterior to the popliteofibular ligament.[39]

Soft tissue Segond injury (lateral meniscotibial capsular injury)

The soft tissue Segond injury is a soft-tissue avulsion injury described by LaPrade and colleagues,[12] consisting of disruption of the conjoined tibial attachment of the anterior arm of

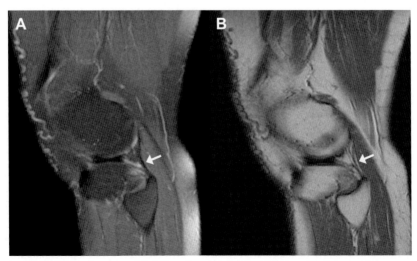

Fig. 6. Sagittal proton density images with (A) and without fat saturation (B) show an intact arcuate ligament (lateral limb) (*arrows*).

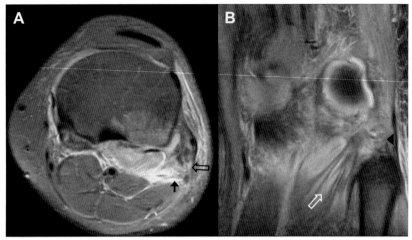

Fig. 7. Axial (*A*) and coronal (*B*) PD FS images show edema in the expected location of the arcuate (*black arrow*) and fabellofibular (*open black arrow* and *black arrowhead*) ligaments, without clearly identified ligaments suggesting injury of these structures. There is also high T2 signal within the muscle belly and around the myotendinous junction of the popliteus compatible with a grade II strain (*open white arrow*).

the short head of the biceps femoris muscle and the meniscotibial portion of the midthird lateral capsular ligament, with associated proximal retraction or thickening (see **Fig. 3**; **Fig. 8**).

Myotendinous injuries of the lateral head of gastrocnemius

The proximal myotendinous portion of the lateral gastrocnemius muscle is commonly not included in the classic list of the specific anatomic structures composing the PLC.[8] However, different factors determine its participation in knee stability provided by the posterolateral corner structures. Based on several anatomic relationships, it is clear that this structure serves as an important secondary dynamic stabilizer of the PLC. This is supported by its involvement in accommodating the fabella

(or its cartilaginous equivalent) with its attachment to the fabellofibular ligament. Furthermore, the lateral gastrocnemius reinforces the meniscofemoral capsule and is firmly attached to the lateral femoral condyle at the level of the supracondylar process. Clinically, the stabilizing role of the lateral gastrocnemius is recognized in PLC reconstruction, including advancement procedures.[4,69]

Injuries to the gastrocnemius muscle usually involve the distal myotendinous junction of the medial gastrocnemius (tennis leg).[70] Although primary injuries of the lateral gastrocnemius are rare, the lateral gastrocnemius should be evaluated carefully in cases of posterolateral corner injury because of the secondary stabilizing role of this structure. The lateral gastrocnemius is usually best seen on sagittal images.[12,15,53]

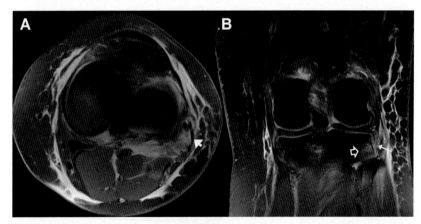

Fig. 8. Axial (*A*) and coronal (*B*) PD FS images show a distal biceps femoris tendon injury (*short white arrow*) and an avulsion of the lateral meniscotibial ligament (*white arrow*) with subjacent bone marrow edema (*open white arrow*), falling in the spectrum of a soft tissue Segond injury.

Osseous Alterations Associated with Posterolateral Injuries

Arcuate fracture

This injury is an avulsion fracture at the level of the fibular head (**Fig. 9**). If a pattern of diffuse fibular head edema is present at MRI examination, the injury usually involves the distal lateral collateral ligament insertion and the distal insertion of the biceps femoris tendon to the fibula (LCL and BFT distally form the conjoint tendon). When edema is localized at the medial aspect of the fibular head, the arcuate ligament or popliteofibular insertions are usually involved. Plain films (arcuate sign) and computed tomography (CT) show the bony avulsion at the fibular tip; MRI has a role in depicting ligamentous injuries.[15,71,72] The authors advocate the presence of fibular edema at the level of the fibular head on MRI as a diagnostic clue. In their MRI evaluation of 19 knees presenting with an arcuate sign at conventional radiographic examination, Juhng and colleagues,[71] reported a tear of the posterolateral capsule in 67% of the cases and an injury to the cruciate ligaments in 89% (16 knees) of the cases: 9 knees with a combined ACL and PCL injury, 4 knees with isolated ACL, and 3 knees with isolated PCL injuries. A bone bruise or fracture was present in all cases, with 50% showing an anteromedial femoral condyle bone bruise and 28% showing the same feature at the anteromedial tibia. A meniscal tear was present on the medial or lateral side in 28% and 22% of the cases, respectively. An injury of the popliteus muscle was evident in 33% of the cases, and all patients had a joint effusion. Huang and coworkers,[72] in their MRI evaluation of 13 knees presenting with an arcuate sign on plain film, found that in 85% of the patients the avulsed bony fragment from the fibula originated either

from the attachment of the popliteofibular ligament or the attachment of the popliteofibular, arcuate, and fabellofibular ligaments at the posterosuperior aspect of the fibular styloid process. All patients presented with both PCL and medial collateral ligament (MCL) injury, but no ACL injuries were reported. A popliteus tendon tear was present only in one case, and 77% of the cases had an injury to the arcuate ligament complex, although integrity of the arcuate, popliteofibular, and fabellofibular ligaments could not be fully assessed. The medial meniscus was injured in 38% of the knees and the lateral meniscus in 46%, with arthroscopic confirmation. Bone marrow edema was present in 38% of the patients (anterior lateral tibial plateau, medial tibial plateau, lateral femoral condyle, medial femoral condyle, patella, posterior tibial plateau and fibular head).[72]

Segond fracture

First described in 1879 by Dr Segond,[73] this injury is classically described as a bony avulsion at the tibial attachment of the midthird lateral capsular ligament (**Fig. 10**).[10,12,14,74,75] The midthird lateral capsular ligament is a thickening of the lateral joint capsule that attaches to the lateral femoral condyle and lateral tibia with capsular attachments to the lateral meniscus. It is the lateral equivalent of the deep medial collateral ligament.[21] Its tibial attachment is just posterior to Gerdy's tubercle.[14] The avulsion may also involve the anterior arm of the short head of the biceps femoris that joins the midthird lateral capsular ligament at the tibial insertion. Different studies found its association with ACL injuries, meniscal tears, and damage to the PLC structures. Dietz and colleagues,[76] in a study on 20 knees, reported a concomitant ACL injury (confirmed at arthroscopy

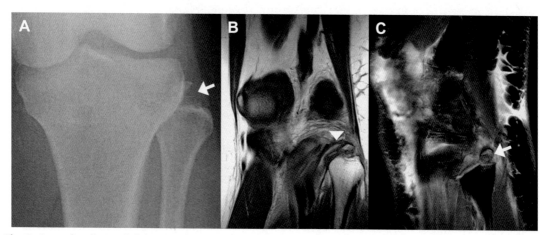

Fig. 9. Frontal radiograph (*A*) coronal PD weighted (*B*) and sagittal T2-weighted FS images (*C*) show an arcuate avulsion fracture (*white arrows*) displaced toward the popliteofibular ligament (*white arrowhead*).

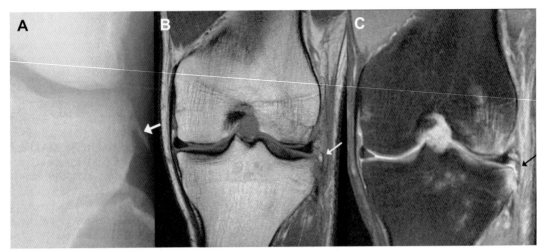

Fig. 10. Frontal radiograph (*A*) coronal T1 (*B*) and coronal T2-weighted FS (*C*) images show a displaced Segond fracture (*white and black arrows*) with surrounding soft tissue and marrow edema.

or physical examination) in 75% of the cases, whereas Goldman and colleagues,[77] in their study on 9 knees, reported an associated ACL injury in 100% of their patients with arthrographic and surgical confirmation. Campos and colleagues[78] suggested the involvement of the iliotibial band and the anterior oblique band of the lateral collateral ligament as important factors in the pathogenesis of the Segond fracture. In their patient population (n = 17) they reported an association with ACL injuries (94%), bone contusions (82%), meniscal tears (53%), PLC injuries (35%), MCL tears (35%), and popliteus tendon injuries (23%).

Anteromedial femoral bone bruise

The presence of a bone bruise in the anterior aspect of the medial femoral condyle on MRI has been associated with PLC knee injuries in the literature (**Fig. 11**). Ross and colleagues[67] reported a bone contusion in the anterior aspect of the medial femoral condyle in 100% of the knees presenting with a complete lateral complex injury (grade III), although their study was small, only containing 6 patients. Varus force and knee hyperextension are commonly involved, both considered common mechanisms of PLC injuries. Therefore, if an anteromedial femoral condylar bone bruise is present on MRI, it is a diagnostic clue that requires a careful evaluation of the PLC complex.

Avulsion of Gerdy's tubercle

The iliotibial band inserts into Gerdy's tubercle on the lateral tibia, and its avulsion can be seen in conjunction with PLC injuries. Isolated injuries

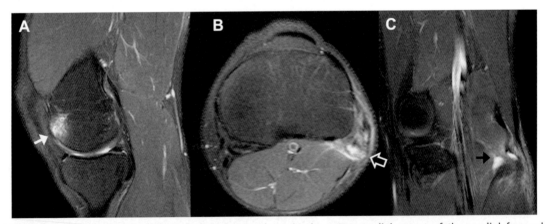

Fig. 11. Sagittal T2-weighted FS image (*A*) shows edema in the anteromedial aspect of the medial femoral condyle (*white arrow*). Axial (*B*) and coronal (*C*) PD FS images from the same patient show edema in the posterolateral corner with high-grade tear of the LCL at the fibular attachment (*open white arrow*), and a high-grade injury of the plantaris muscle (*black arrow*).

of the iliotibial band are infrequent. Ross and colleagues,[67] reported an avulsed iliotibial band in 50% of the knees (6 knees) presenting with a PLC complex injury. Hayes and colleagues[79] developed a mechanism-based classification of complex knee injuries (100 cases) based on patterns of bone marrow edema and ligament injuries seen on MRI and recognized 10 patterns, with injuries based on pure varus force accounting for just 1% (medial tibia and femoral condyle "coup-contrecoup" impactions with ITB and LCL injuries).

This mechanism is rarely seen because varus positioning is normally associated with an internally rotated flexed knee,[79] and additional structures beyond the iliotibial band are usually involved, with concomitant ACL lesions commonly present.[13,80] In their evaluation of avulsion fractures of the lateral femoral condyle in children, Sferopoulos and colleagues[81] reported 2 cases of avulsive fracture of the Gerdy's tubercle. Both of these were sport-related injuries from a direct blow to the medial aspect of the knee while playing football. MRI (**Fig. 12**), CT, and plain radiographs are all able to demonstrate this injury.[81]

Fracture of tibial plateau rim (anterior aspect of the medial plateau)

Fractures of the peripheral anterior margin of the medial tibial plateau have been associated with PLC injuries, and their presence is a useful indicator to raise awareness of a potential PLC injury. Bennett and colleagues[82] evaluated 16 patients with clinically suspected posterolateral corner injuries using MRI and found a tibial plateau fracture in 35%; of these, 83% were at the level of the anterior rim of the medial tibial plateau.

Components of the *Posterolateral Corner Complex*	Suggested Imaging Planes for MR Visualization
Lateral collateral ligament	Axial and coronal
Lateral coronary ligament	Coronal
Arcuate ligament	Sagittal
Popliteus myotendinous unit	Axial
Popliteofibular ligament	Coronal, *coronal oblique*[a] and sagittal
Fabellofibular ligament	Coronal and *coronal oblique*[a]
Lateral joint capsule	Axial and coronal

[a] Dedicated imaging plane usually not included in routine MRI protocols.

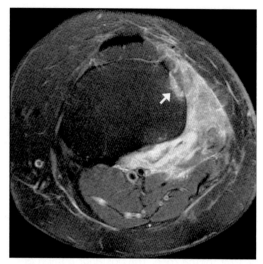

Fig. 12. Axial T2 FS image shows bone marrow edema localized at the level of Gerdy's tubercle (*white arrow*) consistent with an avulsive injury, with extensive edema around the PLC and lateral aspect of the knee.

POSTEROMEDIAL CORNER OF THE KNEE
Anatomy, Biomechanics, and Mechanism of Injuries to the Posteromedial

In 1979, Warren and Marshall[9] introduced the concept of a three-layer approach in the evaluation of the medial supporting structures of the knee, dividing those structures in a *superficial layer (I)*, *intermediate layer (II)*, and *capsule proper (III)* (see **Fig. 2**). In their original description, the superficial layer consists of fascial extensions, made by the deep (crural) fascia that invests the sartorius muscle. Posteriorly, it consists of a thin fascial sheet overlying the 2 heads of the gastrocnemius and the popliteal fossa structures. Serving as a support structure to muscle bellies and neurovascular structures in the popliteal region, it may be reinforced by fascial fibers originating from the sartorius, vastus medialis, and fascia at the level of the popliteal fossa. Anteriorly, layer I connects to layer II to form the medial patellar retinaculum. A fatty tissue layer lies between the superficial layer and the structures deep to it. Anteriorly and distally, the superficial layer joins the tibial periosteum at the level of the sartorius muscle insertion. The gracilis and semitendinosus muscles can be identified more distally as distinct structures with layer I lying superficial and layer II deep to them. The intermediate layer consists of the fibers of the MCL, also called the superficial medial collateral ligament or tibial collateral ligament. At the level of the posteromedial aspect of the knee, the intermediate layer (II) joins the capsule proper (III) and the tendon sheath of the semimembranosus muscle, forming the posteromedial corner pouch surrounding the medial femoral condyle (see **Fig. 2**).[9,83–85] The capsule proper, the deepest of the 3 layers, attaches to the medial meniscus and to the articular margins. Anatomic descriptions of the medial side of the knee describe the MCL as having an anterior vertical component and a posterior oblique component (see **Fig. 1**).[86] The vertical anterior portion measures 1.5 cm in width and 10–11 cm in length, attaching proximally to the medial femoral epicondyle about 5 cm above the joint line, and attaching distally to the medial aspect of the tibial metadiaphysis around 6–7 cm below the joint line. Its distal attachment lies deep to the semitendinosus and gracilis tendons.[83,85,87,88] The intermediate layer (II) and the deeper capsule proper (III) unite posteriorly with the anterior margin of the superficial MCL and the PMC of the knee. The posterior portion of the MCL originates at the proximal attachment of the medial collateral ligament and extends distally in a posterior oblique fashion (at 25° with respect to the anterior vertical portion) to reach the posteromedial aspect of the knee, forming an envelope about the semimembranosus tendon.[88] The posterior oblique portion of the MCL gained its own discrete anatomic consideration in an article from Hughston and Eilers[89] describing the posterior oblique ligament (POL), introducing the concept of the posteromedial corner. To be more specific, the POL has its proximal origin at the adductor tubercle of the medial femoral condyle while the MCL proper (anterior portion) originates around 1 cm anterior and distal to it. The POL also attaches to the medial meniscus at the posteromedial corner of the knee while the superficial MCL does not. The POL comprises 3 arms: the central or tibial arm, attaching to the medial meniscus; the superior or capsular arm, attaching to the posterior joint capsule and proximal portion of the oblique popliteal ligament; and a distal arm, attaching both to the sheath of the semimembranosus tendon and distally to the tibial insertion of the semimembranosus.[89] The MCL includes a deep thickened component called the deep medial collateral ligament (or deep medial capsular ligament), divided into a meniscofemoral component proximally and a meniscotibial component distally. A bursa separates the deep and superficial fibers of the MCL.

The anatomic structures that comprise the PMC of the knee and participate in its function as a restraint to anteromedial rotary instability (AMRI) are the *distal semimembranosus myotendinous complex*, the *POL*, the *medial portion of the oblique popliteal ligament* (OPL), the *meniscotibial ligament* (distal portion of the deep MCL), and the *posterior horn of the medial meniscus*.[90,91]

The distal semimembranosus myotendinous complex consists of 5 distal insertional arms dividing at the level of the joint line: the direct (principal), capsular, anterior (tibial or reflected), inferior (popliteal) arms, and the OPL expansion.[92] The direct arm travels anteriorly and inserts just below the joint line at the tibial tubercle on the posterior aspect of the medial tibial condyle passing beneath the anterior arm. The anterior arm extends anteriorly, under the posterior oblique ligament to attach to the medial aspect of the proximal tibia just beneath the medial collateral ligament. The inferior arm travels more distally than the direct and anterior arms, passing beneath the POL and the MCL to attach just above the tibial attachment of the MCL. The capsular arm has a deep location and coalesces with the capsular portion of the oblique popliteal ligament. A sixth arm, inserting at the posterior third of the lateral meniscus, has been described in 43% of cases by Kim and colleagues.[93]

The OPL is a lateral extension of the semimembranosus tendon that surrounds the posteromedial joint capsule, extending in a superolateral oblique direction as the largest structure in the posterior knee. The OPL is therefore a component of both the PMC and PLC of the knee and contributes to the posterior joint stabilizers, forming part of the popliteal fossa (see **Fig. 1**; **Fig. 13**). LaPrade and colleagues[1] elegantly showed its anatomic relationships, describing it as a broad fascial band crossing the posterior aspect of the knee in an oblique direction. Medially, the OPL arises from the confluence of the lateral expansion of semimembranosus distally and the capsular arm of the POL proximally. Laterally, the OPL attaches to an osseous or cartilaginous fabella, to the meniscofemoral portion of the posterolateral joint capsule and the plantaris muscle. There is also a fibrous attachment to the lateral aspect of the PCL facet.

Flandry and Perry[94] have described the biomechanics of the medial supporting structures of the knee with emphasis to the posteromedial corner. With its 5 arms attaching to bone, capsule, medial meniscus, ligaments, and tendon sheaths, the semimembranosus muscle acts as the main dynamic stabilizer of the PMC. If a structure of the PMC fails, the semimembranosus muscle activates itself, eventually developing intrinsic muscle spasm and articular instability. When the semimembranosus muscle contracts, flexion and internal rotation occur, increasing tension in the adjacent ligaments and contributing to joint stability. The semimembranosus also produces traction on the posterior horn of the medial meniscus, reducing the incidence of meniscal injuries caused by compression of the medial femoral condyle. The semimembranosus muscle causes tension on the oblique popliteal

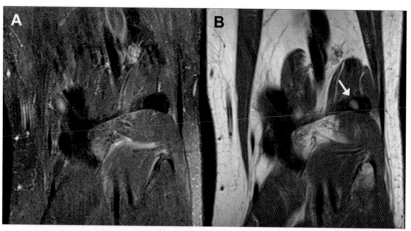

Fig. 13. Coronal FS PD (*A*) and non FS PD (*B*) images show the normal anatomy of the oblique popliteal ligament. Note its attachment to the fabella at the posterolateral aspect of the knee (*arrow*).

ligament and therefore participates in lateral capsular stability. The natural tendency of the POL is to be lax when the knee is flexed and tight when the knee extends. The above mechanism is therefore extremely important, because most knee injuries occur during knee flexion.[40,41] With respect to patterns of injury, patients with symptomatic AMRI almost always have involvement of the POL (99%), with the injury to the semimembranosus (70%) and peripheral meniscal detachment (30%) occurring less frequently.[90] When a grade III MCL injury is present, in conjunction with an anterior cruciate ligament (ACL) injury and medial meniscal tear, a specific pattern of injury has been described, the so-called *O'Donoghue's unhappy triad*.[95] The latter pattern of injury may be associated with PMC injuries. There is a strong association between PMC and ACL injuries,[90] and if those lesions do not occur together, usually an intact PMC compensates for the ACL deficiency to maintain stability. Combined PCL and MCL injuries are uncommon, and likewise a combination of PCL and lateral support structure injury is rare. Combined ACL-PCL injuries with medial supporting structure involvement occur with equal or greater frequency than on the contralateral side.[6,96–99] Usually an isolated MCL injury is treated conservatively, but the presence of a simultaneous posteromedial corner injury may require surgical intervention because of the potential for AMRI. An accurate evaluation of the PMC at imaging is imperative to guide the clinical and surgical management.

INJURIES TO THE POSTEROMEDIAL
Soft-tissue Injuries of the Posteromedial

Semimembranosus insertion injuries
Injuries to the distal semimembranosus insertion occur in up to 70% of posteromedial corner

injuries[90] and include avulsion fracture at its tibial attachment, partial or complete tendon tears, and tendinosis (**Figs. 14** and **15**). Chan and colleagues[100] reviewed the radiographs and MRI studies of 10 patients with posteromedial tibial plateau injuries, including 5 fractures of the posteromedial tibial plateau and 5 distal semimembranosus insertional injuries, and found an ACL tear in 100% of patients.

Avulsion fractures usually occur at the insertion of the direct arm and may appear as a bone bruise with a fracture line on MRI examination. Partial tears and strains are common and usually involve the capsular arm. At MRI, partial tears and strains manifest as altered signal within an otherwise intact tendon. Complete tears of the semimembranosus, although uncommon, present as a discontinuity of the tendon itself, and are best seen on axial and sagittal images. Tendinosis caused by chronic stress is seen as thickening of the tendon insertion. If the capsular arm of the semimembranosus tendon is involved, signal alteration with eventual thickening may be seen at the level of the posterior medial capsular region, contiguous with the POL, and better seen on axial images.[91] The presence of fluid distending the joint capsule may facilitate evaluation of these deep structures. If fluid is absent, the capsular arm appears as a flat structure on the posterior aspect of the medial tibial plateau, indistinguishable from the nearby direct arm, in continuity anteriorly with the anterior arm and posteriorly with the OPL. The anterior arm is better seen on peripheral medial sagittal images, curving anteriorly with an almost horizontal course, and on coronal images as a round hypointense structure adjacent to the medial tibia, passing under the MCL. The direct arm is usually not visible on MRI. The inferior arm may be seen anteriorly as a low signal intensity structure that extends below the joint line.[92]

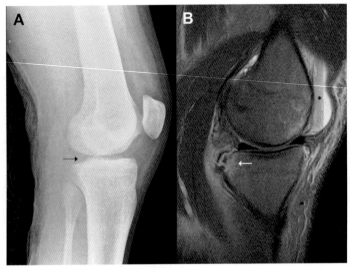

Fig. 14. Lateral radiograph (*A*) and sagittal T2-weighted MR with fat saturation (*B*) show an insertional avulsion injury of the distal semimembranosus tendon, involving both the capsular and direct arms. Note the small bony avulsed fragment (*black arrow*) and resulting bone marrow edema (*white arrow*). A lipohemarthrosis is also evident as a sequela of knee trauma (*asterisk*).

Posterior oblique ligament (POL) injuries

As previously mentioned, POL injuries have been found in 99% of surgically treated patients presenting with medial-sided knee injuries and AMRI.[90] Wijdicks and colleagues[101] in their biomechanic cadaveric study on 24 knees, directly evaluated the changes in tensile forces of the POL in an injury state and its relation to the MCL. They applied a valgus and external rotation moment to the knee after sectioning the MCL (superficial and deep) and found a significant load increase to the POL compared with a knee with an intact MCL condition. This finding reinforces the concept that in cases of reconstruction or surgical repair, all injured medial knee structures should be restored to reproduce the force relationships between them. Petersen and colleagues,[102] in another kinematic cadaveric study on 10 knees, addressed the importance of the POL as a restraint to posterior tibial translation in PCL-deficient knees, therefore emphasizing the need to specifically evaluate it in cases of combined injuries to PMC structures and the PCL. House and colleagues,[91] recommended applying the same grading system used for medial collateral ligament injuries to POL injuries (grade I, microscopic tear; grade II, partial tear; grade III, complete tear). POL injuries comprise sprains, partial tears, and complete tears, and are best visualized on axial and coronal planes (**Fig. 16**).

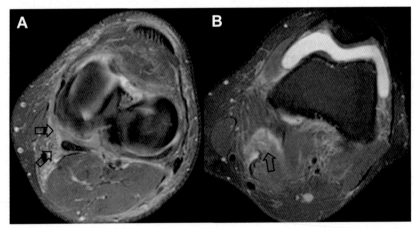

Fig. 15. Axial T2 FS images (*A, B*) show prominent edema within the myotendinous junction of the distal semimembranosus (*black open arrows*) consistent with a strain.

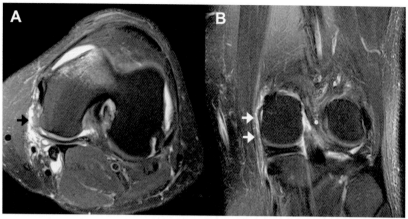

Fig. 16. Axial PD FS image (*A*) shows an irregular POL with surrounding edema consistent with disruption (*black arrow*). Coronal PD FS image (*B*) from a different patient shows an acute on chronic POL injury characterized by thickening of the ligament proximally and partial thickness tearing at femoral attachment with surrounding edema (*white arrows*).

Medial meniscocapsular lesions

The posterior third of the medial meniscus contributes to the dynamic stabilizing function of the PMC because of its intimate anatomic relations with the deep structures, which act as a restraint to posterior translation of the medial femoral condyle on the tibia. Its firm attachment to the tibia is important and guaranteed in part by the meniscotibial portion of the deep MCL. Meniscal instability may put the PMC under stress, therefore making it more prone to injury.[91] MRI can detect injuries to both the meniscotibial and meniscofemoral portions of the deep MCL, which can be seen as disruption, thickening, or bony avulsion. When a bony avulsion is appreciated at the level of the meniscotibial ligament insertion, the specific lesion is called a reverse *Segond fracture* (**Fig. 17**), which is associated with posterior cruciate ligament rupture.[66,103]

Injuries to the oblique popliteal ligament (OPL)

The OPL is the largest structure along the posterior aspect of the knee[1] (see **Figs. 1** and **13**), and its anatomic contribution to the PMC complex has been established. Morgan and colleagues[104] did an in vitro cadaveric study on 20 knees and defined the role of the OPL as the primary ligamentous restraint to knee hyperextension, describing its participation in genu recurvatum (knee hyperextension) development. The OPL should therefore be carefully assessed on MRI when evaluating the posteromedial corner of the knee.[1,104] On axial and sagittal planes, the OPL appears as a thin

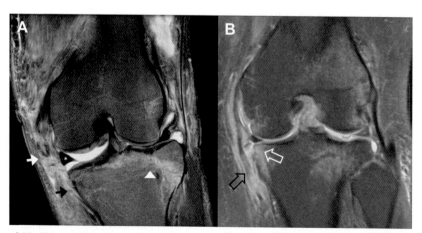

Fig. 17. Coronal PD FS image (*A*) shows disruption of the MCL at the distal midportion (*white arrow*) with associated injury of the meniscotibial fibers of the deep MCL (*black arrow*) and a floating medial meniscus (*asterisk*). An osteochondral impaction fracture of the lateral tibial plateau is also present (*white arrowhead*). Coronal PD FS image (*B*) from a different patient shows a meniscotibial avulsion fracture (Reverse Segond fracture) (*open white arrow*) and a disrupted MCL distally (*open black arrow*).

deep structure of low signal intensity, indistinguishable in most cases from the posterior capsule, but continuous with the semimembranosus tendon.[92] Injuries to the OPL may manifest as irregularity of this fascialike structure, with encircling edema in the deep posteromedial aspect of the knee. On axial imaging, this finding is appreciable on fluid-sensitive sequences at the level of the joint line.

Components of the Posteromedial Corner Complex	Suggested Imaging Planes for MRI Visualization
Distal semimembranosus myotendinous complex	Sagittal and axial
POL	Axial
OPL	Axial and sagittal
Meniscotibial ligament	Coronal
Posterior horn of medial meniscus	Sagittal

SUMMARY

The posterolateral and posteromedial corners of the knee represent challenging anatomic regions in musculoskeletal imaging. Plain films and CT are helpful in the assessment of osseous involvement. However, MRI is the imaging modality of choice because of its intrinsic ability to evaluate soft tissue structures, although ultrasound scan can be used as a complementary technique. High field strength MRI is becoming the standard in high-end musculoskeletal imaging services and will lead to future technologic advances that will enhance the visualization of even the most delicate anatomic components. The ability of the musculoskeletal radiologist to see more, demands a deeper understanding of complex anatomy and specific injury patterns, particularly in those anatomic areas in which anatomy does not follow classical imaging planes and is confined in a narrow space. The posterolateral and posteromedial corner of the knee fall into this category. The underestimation and misinterpretation of reporting injuries in these specific areas can result in a poor patient outcome. For example, chronic posterolateral instability for untreated PLC injuries[4,5] and valgus instability for PMC deficiencies[6] can cause reconstruction of the central supporting structures to fail long term. Therefore, a full appreciation of PMC and PLC structures is of primary importance in the MRI evaluation of the knee to generate a relevant, pertinent, and exhaustive report that will guide the clinical or surgical management of these patients and improve patient outcome.

REFERENCES

1. LaPrade RF, Morgan PM, Wentorf FA, et al. The anatomy of the posterior aspect of the knee. An anatomic study. J Bone Joint Surg Am 2007; 89(4):758–64.
2. Hughston JC, Andrews JR, Cross MJ, et al. Classification of knee ligament instabilities. Part I. The medial compartment and cruciate ligaments. J Bone Joint Surg Am 1976;58(2):159–72.
3. Hughston JC, Andrews JR, Cross MJ, et al. Classification of knee ligament instabilities. Part II. The lateral compartment. J Bone Joint Surg Am 1976; 58(2):173–9.
4. Hughston JC, Jacobson KE. Chronic posterolateral rotatory instability of the knee. J Bone Joint Surg Am 1985;67(3):351–9.
5. Pacholke DA, Helms CA. MRI of the posterolateral corner injury: a concise review. J Magn Reson Imaging 2007;26(2):250–5.
6. Tibor LM, Marchant MH Jr, Taylor DC, et al. Management of medial-sided knee injuries, part 2: posteromedial corner. Am J Sports Med 2011; 39(6):1332–40.
7. Barker RP, Lee JC, Healy JC. Normal sonographic anatomy of the posterolateral corner of the knee. AJR Am J Roentgenol 2009;192(1):73–9.
8. Seebacher JR, Inglis AE, Marshall JL, et al. The structure of the posterolateral aspect of the knee. J Bone Joint Surg Am 1982;64(4):536–41.
9. Warren LF, Marshall JL. The supporting structures and layers on the medial side of the knee: an anatomical analysis. J Bone Joint Surg Am 1979; 61(1):56–62.
10. Terry GC, LaPrade RF. The posterolateral aspect of the knee. Anatomy and surgical approach. Am J Sports Med 1996;24(6):732–9.
11. Veltri DM, Warren RF. Anatomy, biomechanics, and physical findings in posterolateral knee instability. Clin Sports Med 1994;13(3):599–614.
12. LaPrade RF, Gilbert TJ, Bollom TS, et al. The magnetic resonance imaging appearance of individual structures of the posterolateral knee. A prospective study of normal knees and knees with surgically verified grade III injuries. Am J Sports Med 2000; 28(2):191–9.
13. Recondo JA, Salvador E, Villanua JA, et al. Lateral stabilizing structures of the knee: functional anatomy and injuries assessed with MR imaging. Radiographics 2000;20(Spec No):S91–102.
14. Haims AH, Medvecky MJ, Pavlovich R Jr, et al. MR imaging of the anatomy of and injuries to the lateral and posterolateral aspects of the knee. AJR Am J Roentgenol 2003;180(3):647–53.
15. Harish S, O'Donnell P, Connell D, et al. Imaging of the posterolateral corner of the knee. Clin Radiol 2006;61(6):457–66.

16. Malone WJ, Koulouris G. MRI of the posterolateral corner of the knee: normal appearance and patterns of injury. Semin Musculoskelet Radiol 2006; 10(3):220–8.

17. Bolog N, Hodler J. MR imaging of the posterolateral corner of the knee. Skeletal Radiol 2007; 36(8):715–28.

18. De Maeseneer M, Shahabpour M, Vanderdood K, et al. Posterolateral supporting structures of the knee: findings on anatomic dissection, anatomic slices and MR images. Eur Radiol 2001;11(11): 2170–7.

19. Sekiya JK, Swaringen JC, Wojtys EM, et al. Diagnostic ultrasound evaluation of posterolateral corner knee injuries. Arthroscopy 2010;26(4): 494–9.

20. Davies H, Unwin A, Aichroth P. The posterolateral corner of the knee. Anatomy, biomechanics and management of injuries. Injury 2004;35(1):68–75.

21. LaPrade RF. Posterolateral knee injuries: anatomy, evaluation and treatment. New York: Thieme; 2006.

22. El-Khoury GY, Usta HY, Berger RA. Meniscotibial (coronary) ligament tears. Skeletal Radiol 1984; 11(3):191–6.

23. Bikkina RS, Tujo CA, Schraner AB, et al. The "floating" meniscus: MRI in knee trauma and implications for surgery. AJR Am J Roentgenol 2005; 184(1):200–4.

24. Munshi M, Pretterklieber ML, Kwak S, et al. MR imaging, MR arthrography, and specimen correlation of the posterolateral corner of the knee: an anatomic study. AJR Am J Roentgenol 2003; 180(4):1095–101.

25. Sudasna S, Harnsiriwattanagit K. The ligamentous structures of the posterolateral aspect of the knee. Bull Hosp Jt Dis Orthop Inst 1990;50(1): 35–40.

26. Watanabe Y, Moriya H, Takahashi K, et al. Functional anatomy of the posterolateral structures of the knee. Arthroscopy 1993;9(1):57–62.

27. Peduto AJ, Nguyen A, Trudell DJ, et al. Popliteomeniscal fascicles: anatomic considerations using MR arthrography in cadavers. AJR Am J Roentgenol 2008;190(2):442–8.

28. Maynard MJ, Deng X, Wickiewicz TL, et al. The popliteofibular ligament. Rediscovery of a key element in posterolateral stability. Am J Sports Med 1996;24(3):311–6.

29. Shahane SA, Ibbotson C, Strachan R, et al. The popliteofibular ligament. An anatomical study of the posterolateral corner of the knee. J Bone Joint Surg Br 1999;81(4):636–42.

30. Wadia FD, Pimple M, Gajjar SM, et al. An anatomic study of the popliteofibular ligament. Int Orthop 2003;27(3):172–4.

31. McCarthy M, Camarda L, Wijdicks CA, et al. Anatomic posterolateral knee reconstructions require a popliteofibular ligament reconstruction through a tibial tunnel. Am J Sports Med 2010; 38(8):1674–81.

32. Diamantopoulos A, Tokis A, Tzurbakis M, et al. The posterolateral corner of the knee: evaluation under microsurgical dissection. Arthroscopy 2005;21(7): 826–33.

33. LaPrade RF, Terry GC. Injuries to the posterolateral aspect of the knee. Association of anatomic injury patterns with clinical instability. Am J Sports Med 1997;25(4):433–8.

34. LaPrade RF, Resig S, Wentorf F, et al. The effects of grade III posterolateral knee complex injuries on anterior cruciate ligament graft force. A biomechanical analysis. Am J Sports Med 1999;27(4): 469–75.

35. Covey DC. Injuries of the posterolateral corner of the knee. J Bone Joint Surg Am 2001;83-A(1): 106–18.

36. Fanelli GC, Larson RV. Practical management of posterolateral instability of the knee. Arthroscopy 2002;18(2 Suppl 1):1–8.

37. LaPrade RF, Bollom TS, Wentorf FA, et al. Mechanical properties of the posterolateral structures of the knee. Am J Sports Med 2005;33(9):1386–91.

38. Stannard JP, Brown SL, Farris RC, et al. The posterolateral corner of the knee: repair versus reconstruction. Am J Sports Med 2005;33(6): 881–8.

39. Moorman CT 3rd, LaPrade RF. Anatomy and biomechanics of the posterolateral corner of the knee. J Knee Surg 2005;18(2):137–45.

40. Resnick D, Kang HS, Petterklieber ML. Internal derangements of joints. 2nd edition. Philadelphia: Saunders Elsevier; 2007.

41. DeLee JC, Drez JD, Miller MD. Orthopaedic sports medicine: principles and practice. 3rd edition. Philadelphia: Saunders Elsevier; 2009.

42. Malone WJ, Verde F, Weiss D, et al. MR imaging of knee instability. Magn Reson Imaging Clin N Am 2009;17(4):697–724, vi–vii.

43. Fanelli GC, Edson CJ. Posterior cruciate ligament injuries in trauma patients: part II. Arthroscopy 1995;11(5):526–9.

44. Baker CL Jr, Norwood LA, Hughston JC. Acute posterolateral rotatory instability of the knee. J Bone Joint Surg Am 1983;65(5):614–8.

45. Fanelli GC, Orcutt DR, Edson CJ. The multiple-ligament injured knee: evaluation, treatment, and results. Arthroscopy 2005;21(4):471–86.

46. O'Brien SJ, Warren RF, Pavlov H, et al. Reconstruction of the chronically insufficient anterior cruciate ligament with the central third of the patellar ligament. J Bone Joint Surg Am 1991;73(2):278–86.

47. Chen FS, Rokito AS, Pitman MI. Acute and chronic posterolateral rotatory instability of the knee. J Am Acad Orthop Surg 2000;8(2):97–110.

48. Harner CD, Vogrin TM, Hoher J, et al. Biomechanical analysis of a posterior cruciate ligament reconstruction. Deficiency of the posterolateral structures as a cause of graft failure. Am J Sports Med 2000;28(1):32–9.

49. Freeman RT, Duri ZA, Dowd GS. Combined chronic posterior cruciate and posterolateral corner ligamentous injuries: a comparison of posterior cruciate ligament reconstruction with and without reconstruction of the posterolateral corner. Knee 2002;9(4):309–12.

50. Nielsen S, Rasmussen O, Ovesen J, et al. Rotatory instability of cadaver knees after transection of collateral ligaments and capsule. Arch Orthop Trauma Surg 1984;103(3):165–9.

51. Grood ES, Stowers SF, Noyes FR. Limits of movement in the human knee. Effect of sectioning the posterior cruciate ligament and posterolateral structures. J Bone Joint Surg Am 1988;70(1):88–97.

52. Gollehon DL, Torzilli PA, Warren RF. The role of the posterolateral and cruciate ligaments in the stability of the human knee. A biomechanical study. J Bone Joint Surg Am 1987;69(2):233–42.

53. Vinson EN, Major NM, Helms CA. The posterolateral corner of the knee. AJR Am J Roentgenol 2008;190(2):449–58.

54. Brown TR, Quinn SF, Wensel JP, et al. Diagnosis of popliteus injuries with MR imaging. Skeletal Radiol 1995;24(7):511–4.

55. Gruel JB. Isolated avulsion of the popliteus tendon. Arthroscopy 1990;6(2):94–5.

56. Burstein DB, Fischer DA. Isolated rupture of the popliteus tendon in a professional athlete. Arthroscopy 1990;6(3):238–41.

57. Geissler WB, Corso SR, Caspari RB. Isolated rupture of the popliteus with posterior tibial nerve palsy. J Bone Joint Surg Br 1992;74(6):811–3.

58. Guha AR, Gorgees KA, Walker DI. Popliteus tendon rupture: a case report and review of the literature. Br J Sports Med 2003;37(4):358–60.

59. Conroy J, King D, Gibbon A. Isolated rupture of the popliteus tendon in a professional soccer player. Knee 2004;11(1):67–9.

60. Quinlan JF, Webb S, McDonald K, et al. Isolated popliteus rupture at the musculo-tendinous junction. J Knee Surg 2011;24(2):137–40.

61. Winge S, Phadke P. Isolated popliteus muscle rupture in polo players. Knee Surg Sports Traumatol Arthrosc 1996;4(2):89–91.

62. Bencardino JT, Rosenberg ZS, Brown RR, et al. Traumatic musculotendinous injuries of the knee: diagnosis with MR imaging. Radiographics 2000; 20(Spec No):S103–20.

63. Yu JS, Salonen DC, Hodler J, et al. Posterolateral aspect of the knee: improved MR imaging with a coronal oblique technique. Radiology 1996; 198(1):199–204.

64. Rajeswaran G, Lee JC, Healy JC. MRI of the popliteofibular ligament: isotropic 3D WE-DESS versus coronal oblique fat-suppressed T2W MRI. Skeletal Radiol 2007;36(12):1141–6.

65. Zhang H, Feng H, Hong L, et al. Popliteofibular ligament reconstruction for posterolateral external rotation instability of the knee. Knee Surg Sports Traumatol Arthrosc 2009;17(9):1070–7.

66. De Maeseneer M, Shahabpour M, Vanderdood K, et al. Medial meniscocapsular separation: MR imaging criteria and diagnostic pitfalls. Eur J Radiol 2002;41(3):242–52.

67. Ross G, Chapman AW, Newberg AR, et al. Magnetic resonance imaging for the evaluation of acute posterolateral complex injuries of the knee. Am J Sports Med 1997;25(4):444–8.

68. Baker CL Jr, Norwood LA, Hughston JC. Acute combined posterior cruciate and posterolateral instability of the knee. Am J Sports Med 1984; 12(3):204–8.

69. LaPrade RF, Ly TV, Wentorf FA, et al. The posterolateral attachments of the knee: a qualitative and quantitative morphologic analysis of the fibular collateral ligament, popliteus tendon, popliteofibular ligament, and lateral gastrocnemius tendon. Am J Sports Med 2003;31(6):854–60.

70. Delgado GJ, Chung CB, Lektrakul N, et al. Tennis leg: clinical US study of 141 patients and anatomic investigation of four cadavers with MR imaging and US. Radiology 2002;224(1):112–9.

71. Juhng SK, Lee JK, Choi SS, et al. MR evaluation of the "arcuate" sign of posterolateral knee instability. AJR Am J Roentgenol 2002;178(3):583–8.

72. Huang GS, Yu JS, Munshi M, et al. Avulsion fracture of the head of the fibula (the "arcuate" sign): MR imaging findings predictive of injuries to the posterolateral ligaments and posterior cruciate ligament. AJR Am J Roentgenol 2003;180(2): 381–7.

73. Segond P. Recherches cliniques et expérimentales sur les épanchements sanguins du genou par entorse. 1879.

74. Woods GW, Stanley RF, Tullos HS. Lateral capsular sign: x-ray clue to a significant knee instability. Am J Sports Med 1979;7(1):27–33.

75. Weber WN, Neumann CH, Barakos JA, et al. Lateral tibial rim (Segond) fractures: MR imaging characteristics. Radiology 1991;180(3):731–4.

76. Dietz GW, Wilcox DM, Montgomery JB. Segond tibial condyle fracture: lateral capsular ligament avulsion. Radiology 1986;159(2):467–9.

77. Goldman AB, Pavlov H, Rubenstein D. The Segond fracture of the proximal tibia: a small avulsion that reflects major ligamentous damage. AJR Am J Roentgenol 1988;151(6):1163–7.

78. Campos JC, Chung CB, Lektrakul N, et al. Pathogenesis of the Segond fracture: anatomic and MR

imaging evidence of an iliotibial tract or anterior oblique band avulsion. Radiology 2001;219(2):381–6.

79. Hayes CW, Brigido MK, Jamadar DA, et al. Mechanism-based pattern approach to classification of complex injuries of the knee depicted at MR imaging. Radiographics 2000;20(Spec No):S121–34.

80. Gottsegen CJ, Eyer BA, White EA, et al. Avulsion fractures of the knee: imaging findings and clinical significance. Radiographics 2008;28(6):1755–70.

81. Sferopoulos NK, Rafailidis D, Traios S, et al. Avulsion fractures of the lateral tibial condyle in children. Injury 2006;37(1):57–60.

82. Bennett DL, George MJ, El-Khoury GY, et al. Anterior rim tibial plateau fractures and posterolateral corner knee injury. Emerg Radiol 2003;10(2):76–83.

83. Daniel DM, Pedowitz RA, O'Connorr JJ, et al. Daniel's Knee Injuries: Ligament and Cartilage Structure, Function, Injury, and Repair. 2nd ed. Philadelphia: Lippincott Williams & Wilkin; 2003.

84. Ruiz ME, Erickson SJ. Medial and lateral supporting structures of the knee. Normal MR imaging anatomy and pathologic findings. Magn Reson Imaging Clin N Am 1994;2(3):381–99.

85. Loredo R, Hodler J, Pedowitz R, et al. Posteromedial corner of the knee: MR imaging with gross anatomic correlation. Skeletal Radiol 1999;28(6):305–11.

86. LaPrade RF, Engebretsen AH, Ly TV, et al. The anatomy of the medial part of the knee. J Bone Joint Surg Am 2007;89(9):2000–10.

87. Indelicato P. Injury to the medial capsuloligamentous complex. In: Feagin JA, editor. The crucial ligaments: diagnosis and treatment of ligamentous injuries about the knee. New York: Churchill Livingstone; 1994. p. 197–206.

88. Irizarry JM, Recht MP. MR imaging of the knee ligaments and the postoperative knee. Radiol Clin North Am 1997;35(1):45–76.

89. Hughston JC, Eilers AF. The role of the posterior oblique ligament in repairs of acute medial (collateral) ligament tears of the knee. J Bone Joint Surg Am 1973;55(5):923–40.

90. Sims WF, Jacobson KE. The posteromedial corner of the knee: medial-sided injury patterns revisited. Am J Sports Med 2004;32(2):337–45.

91. House CV, Connell DA, Saifuddin A. Posteromedial corner injuries of the knee. Clin Radiol 2007;62(6):539–46.

92. Beltran J, Matityahu A, Hwang K, et al. The distal semimembranosus complex: normal MR anatomy, variants, biomechanics and pathology. Skeletal Radiol 2003;32(8):435–45.

93. Kim YC, Yoo WK, Chung IH, et al. Tendinous insertion of semimembranosus muscle into the lateral meniscus. Surg Radiol Anat 1997;19(6):365–9.

94. Flandry F, Perry CC. The anatomy and biomechanics of the posteromedial aspect of the knee. In: Fanelli GC, editor. Posterior cruciate ligament injuries. Heidelberg (Germany): Springer; 2000. 47.

95. O'Donoghue DH. The unhappy triad: etiology, diagnosis and treatment. Am J Orthop 1964;6:242–7. PASSIM.

96. Shelbourne KD, Carr DR. Combined anterior and posterior cruciate and medial collateral ligament injury: nonsurgical and delayed surgical treatment. Instr Course Lect 2003;52:413–8.

97. Harner CD, Waltrip RL, Bennett CH, et al. Surgical management of knee dislocations. J Bone Joint Surg Am 2004;86(2):262–73.

98. Kaeding CC, Pedroza AD, Parker RD, et al. Intra-articular findings in the reconstructed multiligament-injured knee. Arthroscopy 2005;21(4):424–30.

99. Halinen J, Lindahl J, Hirvensalo E, et al. Operative and nonoperative treatments of medial collateral ligament rupture with early anterior cruciate ligament reconstruction: a prospective randomized study. Am J Sports Med 2006;34(7):1134–40.

100. Chan KK, Resnick D, Goodwin D, et al. Posteromedial tibial plateau injury including avulsion fracture of the semimembranous tendon insertion site: ancillary sign of anterior cruciate ligament tear at MR imaging. Radiology 1999;211(3):754–8.

101. Wijdicks CA, Griffith CJ, LaPrade RF, et al. Medial knee injury: part 2, load sharing between the posterior oblique ligament and superficial medial collateral ligament. Am J Sports Med 2009;37(9):1771–6.

102. Petersen W, Loerch S, Schanz S, et al. The role of the posterior oblique ligament in controlling posterior tibial translation in the posterior cruciate ligament-deficient knee. Am J Sports Med 2008;36(3):495–501.

103. Escobedo EM, Mills WJ, Hunter JC. The "reverse Segond" fracture: association with a tear of the posterior cruciate ligament and medial meniscus. AJR Am J Roentgenol 2002;178(4):979–83.

104. Morgan PM, LaPrade RF, Wentorf FA, et al. The role of the oblique popliteal ligament and other structures in preventing knee hyperextension. Am J Sports Med 2010;38(3):550–7.

Magnetic Resonance Imaging of the Extensor Mechanism

Corrie M. Yablon, MD*, Deepa Pai, MD, Qian Dong, MD, Jon A. Jacobson, MD

KEYWORDS

- Magnetic resonance imaging • Extensor mechanism • Quadriceps • Patellar tendon
- Patellofemoral instability

KEY POINTS

- Magnetic resonance (MR) imaging shows high diagnostic accuracy in the characterization of extensor mechanism disorders, especially when the clinical diagnosis is unclear.
- Knowledge of characteristic patterns of injury on MR imaging increases detection of injury.
- Radiologists must be aware of common anatomic variants and imaging pitfalls of the extensor mechanism as seen on MR imaging.

INTRODUCTION

Anterior knee pain, a common clinical complaint, is one of the most frequent referrals for magnetic resonance (MR) imaging of the lower extremity.[1] Types of quadriceps and patellar tendon injury include acute traumatic rupture, chronic repetitive/overuse injury, and tendon degeneration. Patellofemoral instability, patellar dislocation, and tracking abnormalities are common disorders.

Although radiography is the first-line imaging modality in the acute traumatic setting, and ultrasonography is used in the diagnosis of soft tissue injury, MR imaging shows high diagnostic accuracy in the evaluation of anterior knee pain when the physical examination is limited, when the clinical presentation is unclear, or when injury that is occult on radiography is suspected. MR imaging is particularly well suited to imaging the soft tissues because of its high soft tissue contrast and resolution. However, it is important to be aware of common MR imaging pitfalls when evaluating disorders of the extensor mechanism.

NORMAL ANATOMY

The extensor mechanism is composed of the quadriceps femoris tendon and muscles, the patella and patellofemoral joint, and the patellar tendon. The quadriceps tendon is a trilaminar structure formed by the coalescence of the 4 quadriceps tendons, inserting on the superior pole of the patella. The rectus femoris forms the most anterior layer of the quadriceps tendon. The vastus medialis and lateralis together form the intermediate layer, and the vastus intermedius forms the deepest layer. There is ongoing debate in the literature as to the anatomy of the vastus medialis muscle. Two sets of muscle fibers have been described: the vastus medialis longus proximally, and the vastus medialis obliquus, which extends distally to insert on the medial patella. There is no consensus in the literature as to whether these two components are separate muscles, or whether they reflect different directional fibers of the same muscle.[2,3] On MR imaging, the normal appearance of the trilaminar quadriceps

The authors have nothing to disclose.
Department of Radiology, University of Michigan, 1500 East Medical Center Drive, Ann Arbor, MI 48109, USA
* Corresponding author.
E-mail address: cyablon@umich.edu

Magn Reson Imaging Clin N Am 22 (2014) 601–620
http://dx.doi.org/10.1016/j.mric.2014.07.004
1064-9689/14/$ – see front matter © 2014 Elsevier Inc. All rights reserved.

tendon manifests as low-signal tendon fibers with interdigitating fat (**Fig. 1**).[4]

The patella is the largest sesamoid in the body and lies between the quadriceps and patellar tendons. Superficial quadriceps fibers extend over the patella to insert on the tibial tuberosity as part of the patellar tendon, termed the pre-patellar quadriceps continuation.[5–7] The patella plays an important role in extensor mechanism function. The patella protects the distal femoral articular cartilage, links the quadriceps and patellar tendons, and provides increased mechanical leverage of the quadriceps muscles during extension by elevating the extensor tendons from the axis of rotation of the knee, increasing the angle over which the quadriceps tendon can act.[7,8]

The patella has a large, shallow lateral facet and a steeper, shorter medial facet separated by a vertically oriented median ridge. Many patellae also show a medially located odd facet in the medial facet (**Fig. 2**).[9] When the knee is in extension, the patella articulates with the shallow portion of the proximal femoral trochlea; it is in this position that the patella is most prone to

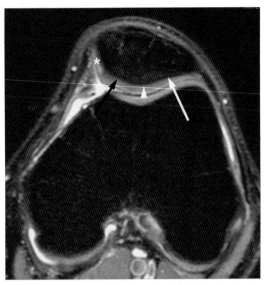

Fig. 2. Normal patellar anatomy. The lateral patellar facet (*white arrow*) is shallower and longer than the medial patellar facet (*black arrow*), which is shorter and steeper. The median ridge (*arrowhead*) lies between the lateral and medial facets. The odd facet (*asterisk*) is a normal anatomic variant at the medial facet.

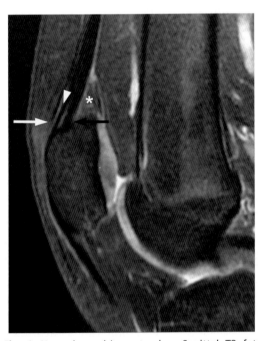

Fig. 1. Normal quadriceps tendon. Sagittal T2 fat-saturated (T2FS) image shows the normal trilaminar appearance of the quadriceps tendon. The anterior layer (*white arrow*) corresponds with the rectus femoris tendon, the middle layer (*arrowhead*) corresponds with the vastus medialis and lateralis, and the deepest layer (*black arrow*) corresponds with the vastus intermedius tendon. Note the normal quadriceps fat pad (*asterisk*).

subluxation or dislocation. When the knee is flexed, the patella is fully engaged within the femoral trochlea. The normal patella shows marrow and cortical signal on all pulse sequences.

The patella is stabilized by the medial and lateral patellar retinacula. The medial patellar retinaculum has been variously described as having 2 or 3 layers; these layers can be difficult to distinguish on MR imaging in normal patients. The most important medial patellar stabilizer is the medial patellofemoral ligament (MPFL), which extends from the medial patella to the medial epicondyle of the distal femur.[10] The lateral retinaculum stabilizes the lateral patella. The normal retinacula show low signal on all pulse sequences (**Fig. 3**).

The patellar tendon is a thick, bandlike structure that extends from the inferior pole of the patella and fans out to insert on the anterior tibial tubercle. The normal patellar tendon is oriented along the axis of the proximal tibia. The normal patellar tendon shows homogeneous low signal intensity on all pulse sequences with the exception of normal, mildly increased signal at the posterior margins of the origin and insertion sites of the tendon.[7]

The quadriceps fat pad lies deep to the quadriceps tendon insertion on the patella, and anterior to the suprapatellar recess. The normal quadriceps fat pad is triangular in shape and

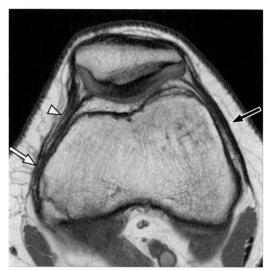

Fig. 3. Normal patellar retinacula. Axial T2FS MR imaging shows the medial patellar retinaculum (*white arrow*) and the MPFL (*arrowhead*), and the lateral patellar retinaculum (*black arrow*).

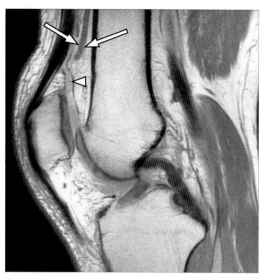

Fig. 4. Articular muscle of the knee. A 43-year-old man underwent MR imaging for a meniscal tear. Note the articular muscle of the knee (*arrows*) arising from the distal femur and inserting on the posterior margin of the suprapatellar recess (*arrowhead*).

demonstrates fat signal on all pulse sequences. The extrasynovial, intracapsular, infrapatellar fat pad (IPFP), or fat pad of Hoffa, lies between the patellar tendon and the anterior knee joint. It is thought that the IPFP may serve to facilitate knee function, increase lubrication of the joint, and may even play a role in inflammation and degeneration of the knee joint. The normal IPFP shows fat signal.[11,12]

Three bursae are present within the anterior knee. The prepatellar bursa lies in the subcutaneous tissues superficial to the patella. The superficial infrapatellar bursa lies anterior to the patellar tendon insertion on the tibia, and the deep infrapatellar bursa lies between the distal patellar tendon and its insertion on the anterior tibial tubercle.

The suprapatellar recess extends cranially from the knee joint, posterior to the quadriceps fat pad and anterior to the prefemoral fat pad. The suprapatellar recess extends medially and laterally over the medial and lateral femoral condyles, and communicates with the medial and lateral recesses beneath each retinaculum. The suprapatellar recess and the joint capsule are stabilized while in extension by the articular muscle of the knee, also known as the musculus articularis genus. This muscle originates from the distal femur and can be seen in most patients on sagittal MR imaging (**Fig. 4**).[13,14]

The extensor mechanism does not have a paratenon.[7] The genicular arteries provide blood supply to the patella and secondarily to the quadriceps and patellar tendons.[15] The relative avascularity of the quadriceps and patellar tendons at their osseous insertions may explain why the quadriceps and patellar tendons tear so frequently in this location.[7,15] The extensor mechanism is supplied additionally by the IPFP, anterior subcutaneous tissues, and the joint capsule.[7,15]

QUADRICEPS INJURY
Quadriceps Rupture and Partial Tear

Acute quadriceps rupture occurs in the setting of sports injury or in the context of chronic quadriceps degeneration or previous trauma. Rupture occurs most frequently in men more than 40 years of age, and is also associated with underlying systemic disease or medications, such as renal failure, diabetes, gout, hyperparathyroidism, rheumatoid arthritis, systemic lupus erythematosus, obesity, and steroid and fluoroquinolone use.[16–21] Bilateral spontaneous ruptures have been reported in patients with gout, diabetes, and steroid use.[20] Ruptures occur most frequently at the insertion of the quadriceps on the patella. Complete quadriceps ruptures are much less common than partial quadriceps tears. MR imaging has been shown to be of higher specificity than ultrasonography for determining whether the quadriceps tear is complete or partial, and thus MR imaging is important for presurgical planning.[16,22]

MR imaging findings of complete quadriceps rupture show fluid signal within a torn and retracted quadriceps tendon; no fibers are identified inserting on the patella. The quadriceps stump retracts cranially and the patella retracts caudally, often associated with a wavy appearance of the patellar tendon. There is frequently a large joint effusion with hematoma at the rupture site (**Fig. 5**). Avulsion fragments may be identified at the quadriceps stump. MR imaging of partial quadriceps tear shows discontinuity of any of the layers of the quadriceps tendon but without complete tendon disruption (**Fig. 6**). The anteriormost rectus femoris is most frequently torn.[7] Injury may also involve the prepatellar quadriceps continuation, which should not be mistaken for prepatellar bursitis (**Fig. 7**).

It is important to differentiate between complete quadriceps ruptures and partial tears, because the treatments are substantially different. Acute quadriceps full-thickness rupture is treated surgically by tunneling the quadriceps tendon into the patella. If the rupture is chronic, or occurs in the setting of a total knee arthroplasty, then the repair may require a tendon graft.[23] If the tear is partial, treatment is conservative.[20]

Quadriceps Tendinosis

Tendinosis of the quadriceps is less common than patellar tendinosis, and occurs most frequently in the setting of chronic underlying systemic disease and/or drug use, as discussed earlier. Calcific tendinosis of the quadriceps tendon has been described.[24] In addition, repetitive microtrauma such as that seen in jumping sports is associated with tendinosis. MR findings show a thickened, abnormal tendon with increased intermediate signal in the tendon fibers (**Fig. 8**).

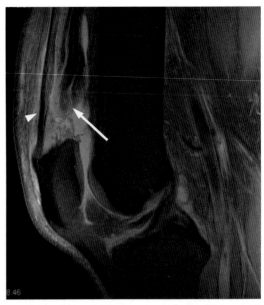

Fig. 6. Quadriceps partial tear. A 32-year-old man with pain after high jumping. Sagittal T2FS MR imaging shows intact anterior rectus femoris fibers (*arrowhead*). The intermediate and deep fibers of the quadriceps are torn and retracted (*arrow*). In partial tears the rectus femoris is usually torn, but that was not so in this case.

PATELLAR TENDON INJURY
Overuse Injuries

Patellar tendinosis is the most commonly encountered disorder of the patellar tendon. Also known as jumper's knee, it typically is seen in a young active population and is commonly associated

A   B

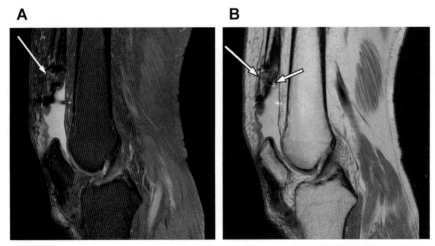

Fig. 5. Quadriceps complete rupture. A 68-year-old man with previous history of quadriceps repair who presented with retear. Sagittal T2FS (*A*) and proton density (PD) (*B*) MR imaging show susceptibility artifact from the previous repair at the quadriceps stump (*arrows*). There is a large joint effusion.

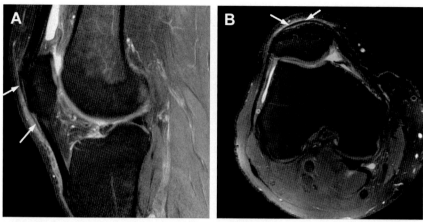

Fig. 7. A 58-year-old man presenting with chronic anterior knee pain. Sagittal PD fat-saturated (PDFS) (*A*) and axial PDFS (*B*) MR imaging show abnormal signal in the quadriceps continuation into the patella (*arrows*). Also note the prepatellar edema.

with running and jumping. This diagnosis can be confirmed with MR imaging, with sagittal and axial fluid-sensitive sequences being the most useful; thickening and increased signal of the tendon proximally at its attachment to the inferior patellar pole are the most common findings in acute cases (**Fig. 9**).[25] Bone marrow edema in the inferior patellar pole can also be seen in severe cases. Chronic cases of patellar tendinosis may show thickening and abnormal signal involving the entire tendon with abnormal signal intensity on both T1-weighted and T2-weighted sequences.[1,26,27] Other described chronic imaging findings include periosteal reaction along the anterior margin of the patella, calcification within the patellar tendon, and elongation of the inferior patellar pole.[25]

Osgood-Schlatter Disease

Repetitive stress or overuse injuries of the patellar tendon such as Osgood-Schlatter disease is caused by chronic traction of the patellar tendon at the level of the tibial tubercle. The apophyseal cartilage of the tibial tuberosity is weak compared with the tensile forces of the extensor mechanism, resulting in fragmentation of the bone and cartilage.[28] This diagnosis is often made clinically with additional imaging usually obtained to exclude other causes of anterior knee pain. When MR imaging is obtained, typical findings include fragmentation and edema of the tibial tubercle with surrounding soft tissue edema. The patellar tendon is also thickened with increased signal distally at the level of the tibial tubercle on

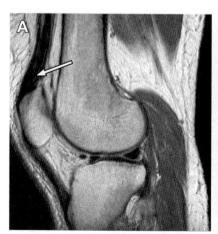
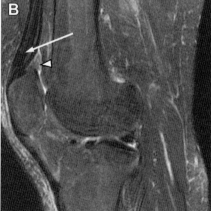

Fig. 8. Fluoroquinolone-induced quadriceps tendinosis. A 24-year-old woman on antibiotics presented with new anterior knee pain after taking fluoroquinolones. Sagittal PD (*A*) and T2FS (*B*) MR imaging show thickening and blurring of the fat planes of the quadriceps insertion on the patella (*arrows*). Note the mild edema in the quadriceps fat pad (*arrowhead*).

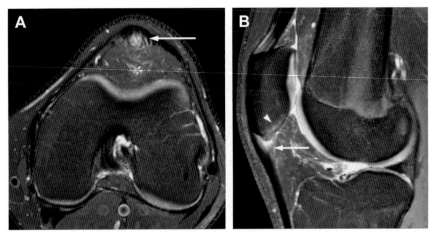

Fig. 9. A 17-year-old basketball player with knee pain. Axial (*A*) and sagittal (*B*) PD-weighted fat-saturated MR image of the knee shows abnormal hyperintense signal and thickening of the patellar tendon (*arrows*) consistent with tendinosis. Bone marrow edema is also present in the inferior patellar pole (*arrowhead*).

the fluid-sensitive sequences (**Fig. 10**). Irregularity of the tibial tubercle often persists into adulthood even when no longer symptomatic.

Sinding-Larsen-Johansson Syndrome

Sinding-Larsen-Johansson syndrome is overuse injury of the proximal patellar tendon at the level of the inferior patellar pole. The inferior patellar pole can appear fragmented and show abnormal hyperintense signal changes on the fluid-sensitive MR sequences depending on the degree

of stress injury (**Fig. 11**). MR imaging is also useful in distinguishing this overuse injury from patellar sleeve fractures.

Patellar Sleeve Fracture

Patellar sleeve fractures are fractures of the inferior pole of the patella with involvement of the unossified patellar cartilage (**Fig. 12**). MR imaging is important to show the full extent of unossified patellar cartilage involvement, which is significantly underestimated on radiography.[29,30] Acute

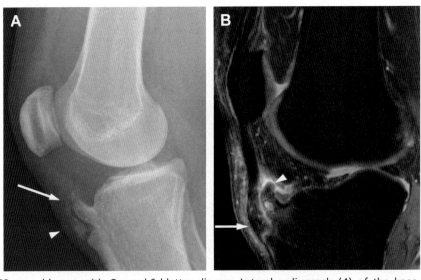

Fig. 10. A 32-year-old man with Osgood-Schlatter disease. Lateral radiograph (*A*) of the knee shows fragmentation of the tibial tubercle (*arrow*) with overlying soft tissue swelling (*arrowhead*). Sagittal PD-weighted fat-saturated MR image of the knee (*B*) shows edema of the tibial tubercle (*arrowhead*) with cystic change and thickening and abnormal signal of the distal patellar tendon (*arrow*). Surrounding soft tissue edema is present.

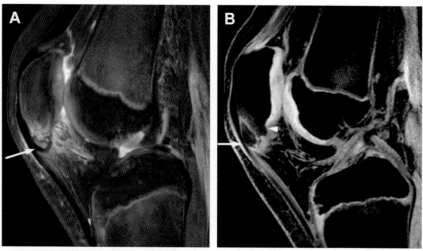

Fig. 11. A 15-year-old boy with anterior knee pain and Sinding-Larsen-Johansson syndrome. (*A*) Sagittal PD-weighted fat-saturated and (*B*) sagittal cartilage-sensitive (water selective) MR images of the knee show fragmentation of the inferior patellar pole (*arrows*) with edema within the fragment and adjacent patella. Small joint effusion and edema of the Hoffa fat pad are present. Note that the cartilage (the inferior margin of which is denoted by the *arrowhead*) is not disrupted.

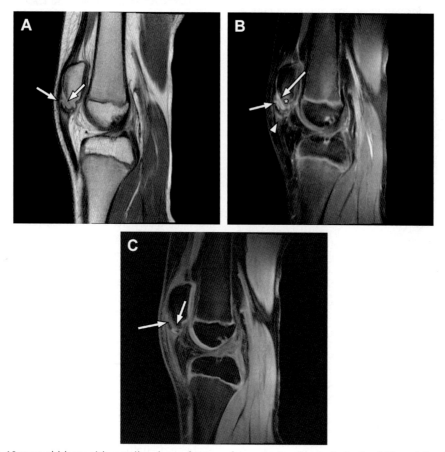

Fig. 12. A 10-year-old boy with patellar sleeve fracture from playing football. Sagittal PD-weighted non–fat-saturated MR image of the knee (*A*) shows linear hypointense signal of the inferior patellar pole extending through unossified cartilage compatible with a sleeve fracture (*arrows*). Sagittal PD-weighted fat-saturated MR image (*B*) of the same patient shows thickening and abnormal signal of the proximal patellar tendon (*arrowhead*) and bone marrow edema of the inferior patellar pole (*asterisk*). Sagittal cartilage-sensitive sequence (water selective) (*C*) shows the fracture line extending through the unossified cartilage (*arrows*).

tensile forces on the extensor mechanism can also lead to avulsion fractures of the distal patellar tendon (**Fig. 13**).

Patellar Tendon Tear

Overuse injuries can progress to focal tears of the patellar tendon. Tearing can also occur in the acute setting. Fluid-sensitive MR sequences show focal cleftlike high-intensity signal within the tendon (**Fig. 14**). Ruptures of the patellar tendon occur but are uncommon. When encountered, patients typically have concomitant systemic disease that predisposes them to such an injury. Patellar tendon ruptures have also been described in certain athletes who receive a substantial direct impact to their anterior knee, such as football players.[31] With MR imaging, there is discontinuity of the patellar tendon with acute tears showing extensive edema of the surrounding soft tissues (**Fig. 15**). Acute patellar tendon ruptures are managed surgically with transpatellar bone tunnels formed when the rupture occurs at the level of the inferior patellar pole.[23]

Patella baja, or low-lying patella with a shortened patellar tendon, can be seen in patients

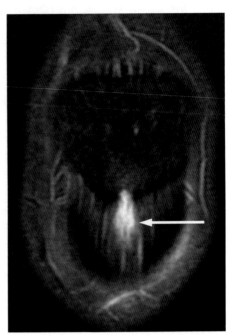

Fig. 14. A 19-year-old basketball player with anterior knee pain. Coronal PD-weighted fat-saturated image through the patellar tendon shows focal, linear, hyperintense signal (*arrow*) within the patellar tendon consistent with a partial tear.

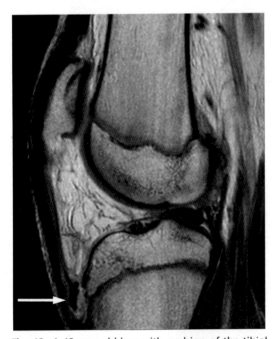

Fig. 13. A 12-year-old boy with avulsion of the tibial tubercle after a fall on ice. Sagittal PD-weighted image of the knee shows separation/fracture of the tibial tubercle (*arrow*) from the adjacent tibia. In pediatric patients, the apophysis is a point of weakness and is usually overcome by the tensile forces of the patellar tendon in the setting of a forceful contraction rather than primary injury of the tendon itself.

who have had prior knee trauma or surgery, especially patellar tendon harvest for anterior cruciate ligament reconstruction.[32,33]

PATELLOFEMORAL INSTABILITY

Patellofemoral instability encompasses a wide spectrum of disease ranging from patellofemoral tracking disorders to frank patellar dislocation. These entities share a common clinical presentation of anterior knee pain. Patellar stability is maintained by a combination of static and dynamic stabilizers. The static stabilizers comprise the patellar retinacula and MPFL. The dynamic stabilizers are the quadriceps tendon and muscles, the patellar tendon, and the joint capsule.

Acute Patellar Dislocation

Patellar dislocation occurs most frequently in women in the second decade of life. Sixty-one percent of acute patellar dislocations occur during a sports activity.[34] The most common mechanism is a twisting injury in which the medial patellar stabilizers rupture, allowing the medial patellar facet to impact on the lateral femoral condyle. At the time of injury, the patient may not be aware that the patella has dislocated, because in most cases the patellar dislocation is transient, with

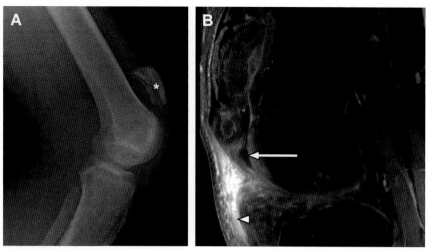

Fig. 15. A 23-year-old man presents with complete patellar tendon rupture after jumping. Lateral radiograph of the knee (*A*) shows abnormal superior positioning of the patella (*asterisk*). Sagittal PD-weighted fat-saturated MR image (*B*) of the same patient shows proximally retracted torn patellar tendon stump (*arrow*) and nonvisualization of any patellar tendon in its expected location (*arrowhead*).

spontaneous relocation. Thus, the patellar dislocation may not be suspected when the patient presents for treatment. MR imaging is usually the first line of imaging.[35] Although radiographs are frequently the first images obtained in the workup, they are frequently unrevealing, with the exception of a joint effusion, although an osteochondral fracture (termed the sliver sign) may be seen.[36] MR imaging has become the imaging modality of choice because it allows assessment of the medial supporting structures and associated soft tissue and osseous injuries that may be occult on radiography.

MR imaging findings include rupture or sprain of the medial patellar retinaculum and MPFL, with fluid signal within and about the ligaments. The MPFL most often tears from its femoral attachment, and in one study MPFL injury was seen in 96% of acute patellar dislocations.[37] Additional findings include bone contusions or subchondral impaction fractures at the lateral femoral condyle and medial patellar facet.[38,39] The patella may be positioned lateral to the femoral trochlea at the time of imaging. There may also be associated cartilage shearing injury, and displaced osteochondral fragments within the suprapatellar recess or medial and lateral recesses. This injury predisposes to the future development of patellofemoral osteoarthritis. There is frequently a large joint effusion with or without lipohemarthrosis. Edema and partial tearing of the vastus medialis muscle are also frequently seen in the acute setting (**Fig. 16**). MR imaging also enables assessment for underlying morphologic abnormalities of the

patellofemoral joint that may predispose to future dislocation.

The initial patellar dislocation and associated medial soft tissue injuries predispose to recurrent

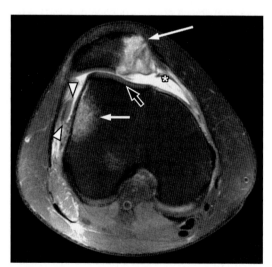

Fig. 16. A 21-year-old woman with transient patellar dislocation caused by a soccer injury. Axial T2FS image shows a contusion of the lateral femoral condyle and a nondisplaced medial patellar fracture with bone marrow edema (*white arrows*). The MPFL is torn at the patellar attachment site (*asterisk*). In addition, there is an osteochondral fragment in the lateral recess (*white arrowheads*). There is lateral subluxation of the patella with respect to the femoral trochlea. Note the shallow lateral trochlear articular surface (*black arrow*). There is a joint effusion.

patellar dislocation. Once the medial retinaculum and the MPFL have been torn, medial restraint to lateral patellar subluxation is compromised, especially when the knee is in flexion. Tearing of the MPFL most frequently occurs at the femoral attachment but can also occur at the patellar attachment. If abnormal signal is identified either at the femoral or patellar attachments of the medial retinaculum on MR imaging, then MPFL injury should be suspected.

There is controversy as to how to treat the initial acute patellar dislocation. Some investigators advocate conservative management, whereas others advocate repair or reconstruction of the MPFL and repair of cartilage or osteochondral injury if present.[40,41] One study showed that, over a minimum 2-year follow-up, 17% of patients with acute dislocation had a subsequent dislocation. Of patients with a history of multiple dislocations, 49% had a subsequent dislocation.[34]

Chronic Patellofemoral Instability

Patients who have recurrent patellofemoral instability often have underlying anatomic variants, such as an abnormally shallow lateral femoral trochlea (trochlear dysplasia), patella alta (high-riding patella), or a lateral location of the anterior tibial tubercle with respect to the trochlear groove (abnormal tibial tubercle–trochlear groove [TT-TG] distance), femoral anteversion, and ligamentous laxity.[35,42]

Trochlear dysplasia is considered a developmental abnormality and can occur bilaterally. This condition manifests as a shallow lateral femoral trochlea and is best estimated using the lateral trochlear inclination angle. When the lateral inclination level is less than 11°, the patella is prone to lateral dislocation from the trochlear notch (**Fig. 17**).[43] Trochlear dysplasia is seen in 85% of patients with patellar dislocation.[44]

Patella alta, or high-riding patella, occurs when the patellar tendon is too long and the patella is positioned high with respect to the trochlear fossa.[35,45] Although this may be considered an asymptomatic normal anatomic variant, it has been reported that 25% of patients with acute patellar dislocation have patella alta on MR imaging and 50% have patella alta on radiography.[32,35,38] On radiography this relationship has been described using the Insall-Salvati ratio.[46] More recently, measurements of the relationship of patellar height to patellar tendon length have been validated on MR imaging and are now considered to be more accurate than radiographic measurements.[32,47,48] A normal ratio is 1.1. Patella alta is a ratio of more than 1.3 (**Fig. 18**).[32]

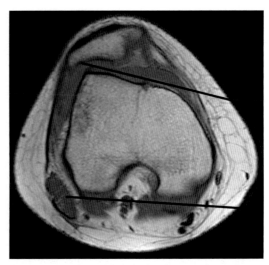

Fig. 17. Lateral trochlear inclination angle. Measurements are made on an axial T1 fat-saturated or fluid-weighted image. A line is drawn along the posterior margins of the femoral condyles. A second line is drawn along the lateral facet of the trochlea. The angle between these two lines is the inclination angle. This patient with recent patellar dislocation has an abnormal trochlear inclination angle of 4°.

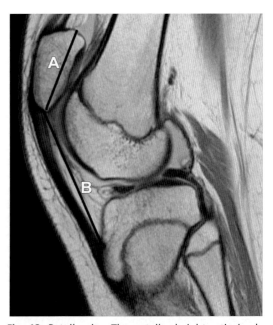

Fig. 18. Patella alta. The patellar height ratio is obtained from a sagittal MR image by measuring the length of the posterior margin of the patellar tendon (line A) and dividing that number by the longest patellar diameter measured superior to inferior (line B). In this patient, the patellar height ratio is 1.7. A normal patellar height ratio is 1.1. Patella alta is defined as a ratio greater than 1.3.

Abnormal TT-TG distance is associated with patellar dislocation.[35,49–51] In a normal patient, the tibial tubercle is vertically aligned with the trochlear groove. Patellar instability and abnormal patellar tracking are frequently seen when the tibial tubercle is located more than 2 cm lateral to the femoral trochlear groove.[44] Note that the original articles described measurement of TT-TG distance on computed tomography (CT); a recent article showed that TT-TG distance on MR imaging was slightly underestimated compared with CT.[52] Treatment of chronic patellar instability is multifactorial and usually involves a combination of MPFL reconstruction and correction of the underlying morphologic abnormality (ie, trochleoplasty, or tibial tubercle osteotomy [Elmslie-Trillat procedure]).[53,54]

Patellofemoral Pain Syndrome

Patellofemoral pain syndrome accounts for 25% of injuries to runners. The same factors that predispose to patellar dislocation are also seen as causes of patellofemoral pain syndrome, including patella alta, trochlear dysplasia, laterally displaced tibial tubercle, and femoral anteversion. Another important factor that is associated with patellofemoral pain syndrome is muscular imbalance between the medial and lateral quadriceps muscles. When the vastus medialis obliquus is weak, its dynamic stabilization of the patella is overridden by the lateral stabilizing factors of the vastus lateralis and iliotibial tract.[55] Tightness of the iliotibial tract can cause lateral patellar tilt and can cause increased pressure on the lateral patella.[42,56] MR imaging findings include abnormally increased fluid signal, thinning, fissuring, full-thickness defects of the lateral patellar facet cartilage, patellofemoral bone marrow edema and subchondral cystic changes, and abnormal lateral patellar tilt or subluxation.

PATELLAR FRACTURE

Patellar fractures account for 0.5% to 1.5% of all reported fractures.[8,57] Most patellar fractures occur as a result of a direct blow or fall and are most commonly transverse in orientation, although vertical and comminuted fractures are seen. Patellar fractures can occur in patients after total knee arthroplasty.[58] Displaced transverse fractures are usually easily identified on radiographs and require surgical intervention. When patellar fractures are vertically oriented and nondisplaced, they may be occult on radiography. MR imaging can be helpful to establish the diagnosis (**Fig. 19**). In addition, MR imaging can evaluate associated findings such as avulsion fragments, osteochondral injuries, and displaced intra-articular osseous or cartilaginous fragments. Displaced patellar fractures are managed surgically, whereas nondisplaced fractures are managed conservatively. In skeletally immature patients, patellar sleeve fractures may occur at the inferior patellar pole, where unossified cartilage is avulsed from the inferior pole of the patella (see **Fig. 12**).[59]

PATELLOFEMORAL OSTEOARTHRITIS

Patellofemoral osteoarthritis is a frequent cause of chronic anterior knee pain in the older patient population.[60] Although osteoarthritis more frequently affects older patients, young patients may also present with osteoarthritis in the setting of prior trauma, participation in high-impact sports, or previous patellar dislocation. MR findings manifest as

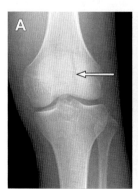 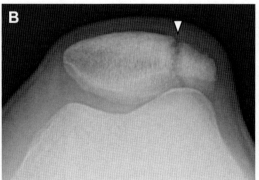 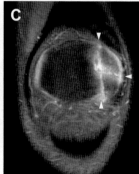

Fig. 19. An 18-year-old man with patellar fracture after a fall. Frontal radiograph of the knee (*A*) shows an irregularly marginated vertically oriented lucency (*arrow*) within the lateral aspect of the patella compatible with a fracture. Merchant view of the knee (*B*) in the same patient shows fracture lucency (*arrowhead*) extending to the articular surface. Coronal PD-weighted fat-saturated MR image of the same patient shows the fracture fragments laterally (*arrowheads*) with associated marrow edema (*C*).

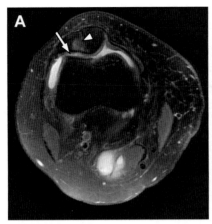
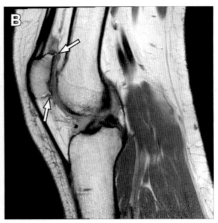

Fig. 20. Patellofemoral osteoarthritis in a 40-year-old woman with chronic knee pain. Axial PDFS image (*A*) shows narrowing of the lateral patellofemoral joint, focal cartilage loss at the lateral patellar facet (*arrow*) and subchondral marrow edema (*arrowhead*). Sagittal PD image (*B*) shows osteophytes at the patella and femoral trochlea.

cartilage thinning, fraying or fissuring, subchondral bone marrow edema, and cystic change (**Fig. 20**).

DISORDERS OF THE FAT PADS
Quadriceps Fat Pad

Quadriceps fat pad edema is of unclear cause and has been reported in 4% to 12% of knee MR imaging examinations.[61,62] Quadriceps fat pad mass effect on the suprapatellar recess has been associated with anterior knee pain. On MR imaging, the quadriceps fat pad appears enlarged and shows intermediate or fluid signal intensity (**Fig. 21**). These findings may be analogous to IPFP edema or Hoffa disease.

IPFP of Hoffa

The IPFP is innervated by nociceptive nerve fibers that may be responsible for the generation of anterior knee pain. Inflammation of the fat pad may play a role in the development of anterior knee pain.[63] Hoffa disease, or impingement of the IPFP, has been described in the setting of patellar trauma or dislocation, anterior cruciate ligament rupture, meniscal tears, and repetitive microtrauma, which lead to hemorrhage and inflammation.[11,12] MR imaging can show enlargement of the fat pad, with abnormal signal and edema, as well as fluid-filled clefts (**Fig. 22**).[12] Scarring in the fat pad is manifested by linear, low signal

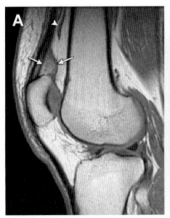
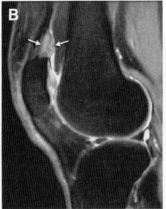
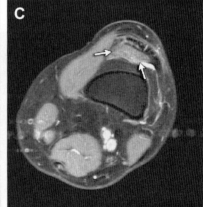

Fig. 21. A 41-year-old woman presenting with anterior knee pain with quadriceps fat pad edema. Sagittal PD (*A*), PDFS (*B*), and axial PDFS (*C*) images show an enlarged quadriceps fat pad (*arrows*) with abnormal signal and convex posterior border. Incidental note is made of an articular muscle (*arrowhead* in *A*). (*From* Roth C, Jacobson J, Jamadar D, et al. Quadriceps fat pad signal intensity and enlargement on MRI: prevalence and associated findings. AJR Am J Roentgenol 2004;182(6):1383–7.)

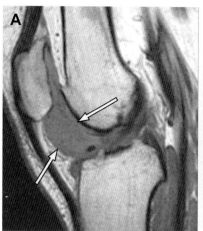
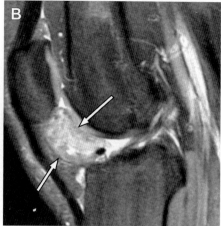

Fig. 22. Hoffa disease. Sagittal PD (*A*) and PDFS (*B*) images of the knee show an enlarged IPFP (*arrows*) with abnormal signal consistent with edema.

intensity and can be seen after arthroscopy and trauma. Recent studies have shown that the IPFP releases cytokines and may play a role in the development of osteoarthritis.[64]

Patellar Maltracking and Impingement on the Superolateral IPFP

Patellar maltracking is a common cause of anterior knee pain, occurring in adolescents and young women. Localized edema in the superolateral IPFP has been described in the setting of lateral patellofemoral friction syndrome, or patellar maltracking, termed patellar tendon–lateral femoral condyle friction syndrome.[65,66] The mechanism is thought to relate to impingement of the superolateral aspect of the fat pad between the lateral femoral condyle and the patellar tendon.[67] MR findings show abnormal signal consistent with edema in the superolateral IPFP, as well as

an association with a high-riding patella, increased TT-TG distance, and diminished patellar tendon–trochlea distance. Abnormal signal in the proximal patellar tendon consistent with tendinosis has also been described (**Fig. 23**).[65] Young patients are most prone to superolateral Hoffa fat pad edema and such edema may be asymptomatic.[68] Anterolateral pain has also been found most often to be associated with tendinosis of the lateral patellar tendon in the setting of superolateral IPFP impingement.

BURSAL DISORDERS
Prepatellar Bursitis

Prepatellar bursitis is associated with many causes such as infection, gout, sarcoid, or CREST (calcinosis, Raynaud syndrome, esophageal dysmotility, sclerodactyly, telangiectasia) syndrome,

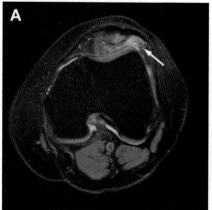
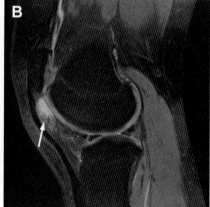

Fig. 23. A 25-year-old woman with lateral patellar friction syndrome and anterior knee pain. Axial (*A*) and sagittal (*B*) T2FS MR images show localized edema in the superolateral aspect of the IPFP (*arrows*).

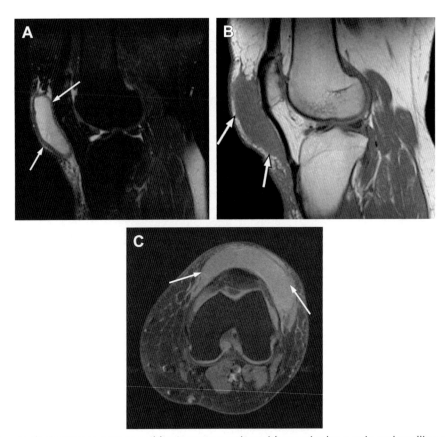

Fig. 24. Prepatellar bursitis in a 45-year-old woman presenting with anterior knee pain and swelling after a fall. Sagittal T2FS (*A*), PD (*B*), and axial T2FS (*C*) images of the knee show a well-defined, crescentic fluid collection (*arrows*) confined to the prepatellar soft tissues, without cranial, medial, or lateral extension into the thigh.

and immunocompromise. Repetitive microtrauma, such as kneeling, is a common cause. Infectious prepatellar bursitis is caused by direct inoculation with an infectious agent, most frequently *Staphylococcus aureus*. The patient presents with a fluctuant soft tissue mass anterior to the patella, with warmth, redness, and pain.[69] Differentiation of septic from aseptic bursitis is made by aspiration. Imaging is seldom required unless there is concern of injury to underlying structures. The usual MR imaging appearance is that of a circumscribed fluid collection anterior to the patella. The collection may show heterogeneous signal if there is hemorrhage or infection present (**Fig. 24**). Management ranges from oral antibiotics to surgical excision.[69]

Morel-Lavallée Lesion of the Knee

More recently, the Morel-Lavallée lesion of the knee has been described in professional football players, as an entity distinct from prepatellar bursitis. It is an internal degloving injury of the prepatellar soft tissues resulting from shearing trauma

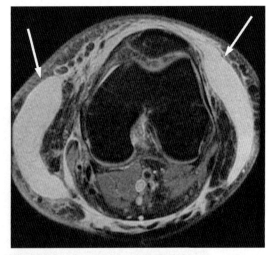

Fig. 25. Morel-Lavallée lesion of the knee in a 52-year-old woman run over by a truck. Axial PDFS image shows lobulated fluid collections in the medial and lateral subcutaneous tissues of the knee (*arrows*) as a result of shearing injury. The fluid collections are contiguous with the prepatellar soft tissues and extend cranially along the distal thigh.

when the knee strikes the ground, in which the skin and subcutaneous tissues are separated from the underlying fascia, with disruption of the perforating vessels.[70] It manifests as an enlarging, fluctuant soft tissue mass extending from the suprapatellar region, medially, laterally, and cranially to the midthigh, beyond the expected margin of the prepatellar bursa (**Fig. 25**). Treatment involves aspiration and compressive wrapping.[70]

Superficial and Deep Infrapatellar Bursa

Superficial and deep infrapatellar bursal fluid can be seen in the setting of direct trauma or patellar tendon disorders. A small amount of asymptomatic fluid is commonly seen in the deep infrapatellar bursa.

NORMAL ANATOMIC VARIANTS AND IMAGING PITFALLS
Dorsal Defect of the Patella

Dorsal defect of the patella (DDP) is usually an incidental finding on MR imaging. A normal anatomic variant, it has an estimated incidence of 0.3% to 1.0 % of the population and presents most frequently in young patients in the second decade of life.[71,72] DDP can be bilateral. On radiography, DDP appears as a lucent lesion with well-defined sclerotic borders at the superolateral aspect of the patella, at the dorsal articular surface. A mature lesion may appear sclerotic and well circumscribed. On MR imaging, DDP appears as a well-defined lesion at the superolateral aspect of the dorsal patella, with sclerotic

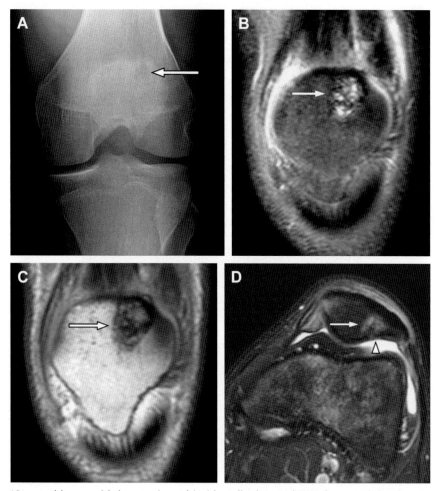

Fig. 26. An 18-year-old man with knee pain and incidentally detected DDP (a normal developmental variant). Frontal radiograph of the knee (*A*) shows a nonspecific lucency with sclerotic borders (*arrow*) within the superolateral patella. Coronal PD-weighted fat-saturated (*B*) and non–fat-saturated (*C*) images of the same patient show focal heterogeneous hyperintense and hypointense signal respectively (*arrow*) in the superolateral patella; a characteristic location for DDP. Axial PDFS MR image of the knee (*D*) shows the typical subchondral marrow signal changes (*arrow*) and preservation of the underlying cartilage (*arrowhead*).

margins with heterogeneous internal signal (iso-intense to hyperintense to cartilage) and with intact overlying cartilage (**Fig. 26**). It should not be mistaken for an osteochondral injury.[73]

Bipartite or Multipartite Patella

Bipartite or multipartite patella is a normal developmental variant with a prevalence of 2% to 3% of the population. It is frequently bilateral and often asymptomatic.[74,75] This entity develops secondary to failure of the secondary ossification center(s) to fuse with the patella. The bipartite fragment most typically arises at the superolateral margin of the patella; the fragment should show normal marrow signal, and the synchondrosis should be smooth and show normal cartilage signal. Osseous and fibrous union can be seen. A bipartite or multipartite patella may be mistaken for fracture in a patient who obtains MR imaging for anterior knee pain. If this anatomic variant is present with normal signal, then additional sources of the disorder should be sought.

The bipartite patella may be the source of anterior knee pain if there is abnormal motion or instability at the synchondrosis. In this case, the most common MR imaging finding is edema in the bipartite fragment. Other findings include fluid signal at the synchondrosis, consistent with a pseudarthrosis. In more chronic cases, cystic subchondral marrow changes are seen at the synchondrosis (**Fig. 27**). Fluid signal may

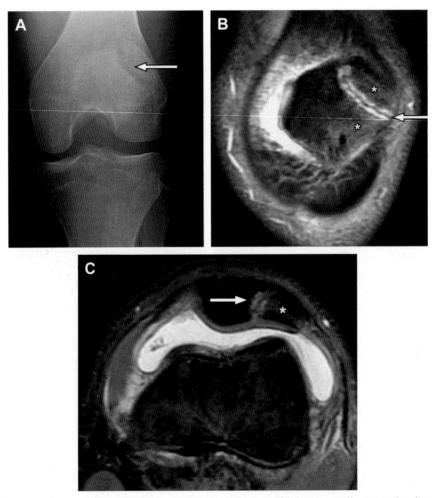

Fig. 27. A 19-year-old man with meniscal tear and incidentally noted bipartite patella. Frontal radiograph of the knee (*A*) shows a lucency in the superolateral quadrant of the patella (*arrow*), a characteristic location and appearance of a bipartite patella, which is a normal developmental variant. Coronal (*B*) and axial (*C*) PD-weighted fat-saturated MR images of the knee of the same patient show the hyperintense linear signal within the patella (*arrows*) consistent with the synchondrosis. Hyperintense signal (edema) is seen in the bone alongside the synchondrosis (*asterisks*), which can be painful.

even be seen between the fragment and the patella.[74]

Magic Angle Artifact

Magic angle artifact is encountered in pulse sequences with a low echo time (TE), in tightly bound collagen structures (such as ligaments or tendons) that course at 55° relative to the main magnetic field, B_0. The patellar tendon is particularly prone to magic angle artifact when low-TE sequences such as T1, proton density (PD), and three-dimensional gradient echo T1-weighted sequences are used.[76] Because of the oblique cranial caudal course of the patellar tendon, magic angle artifact in the form of mildly increased signal is frequently seen at the dorsal margin of the patellar tendon origin from the inferior pole of the patella and at its insertion on the tibial tubercle on low-TE sequences. This finding is normal and should not be misconstrued as a disorder. The critical TE value to eliminate magic angle is 40 milliseconds for conventional spin echo, 70 milliseconds for fast spin echo, and 30 milliseconds for gradient echo; therefore, the TE value should be set higher than these critical values.[77] Correlation with a true T2-weighted sequence helps to differentiate between artifact and disorder (**Fig. 28**).

Trilaminar Structure of the Quadriceps

The normal trilaminar structure of the quadriceps tendon should not be confused with a partial tear of the tendon. The normal layers of fat interdigitating between the tendon fibers show intermediate signal on MR imaging.

SUMMARY

Anterior knee pain is associated with many different causes. The clinical diagnosis may be unclear when the patient presents for treatment. MR imaging is a valuable modality with high diagnostic accuracy in the evaluation of extensor mechanism disorders. MR imaging is highly accurate in differentiating full-thickness from partial-thickness tears of the quadriceps tendon, and in differentiating among the many different causes of patellar tendon disorder. MR imaging is particularly useful in the evaluation of patellar dislocation and the underlying morphologic abnormalities that may predispose to dislocation.

REFERENCES

1. Skiadas V, Perdikakis E, Plotas A, et al. MR imaging of anterior knee pain: a pictorial essay. Knee Surg Sports Traumatol Arthrosc 2013;21(2):294–304.
2. Smith TO, Nichols R, Harle D, et al. Do the vastus medialis obliquus and vastus medialis longus really exist? A systematic review. Clin Anat 2009;22(2):183–99.
3. Roberts VI, Mereddy PK, Donnachie NJ, et al. Anatomical variations in vastus medialis obliquus and its implications in minimally-invasive total knee replacement. An MRI study. J Bone Joint Surg Br 2007;89(11):1462–5.
4. Zeiss J, Saddemi SR, Ebraheim NA. MR imaging of the quadriceps tendon: normal layered configuration and its importance in cases of tendon rupture. AJR Am J Roentgenol 1992;159(5):1031–4.
5. Jacobson J. Fundamentals of musculoskeletal ultrasound. Philadelphia: Saunders Elsevier; 2007. p. 345.
6. Wangwinyuvirat M, Dirim B, Pastore D, et al. Prepatellar quadriceps continuation: MRI of cadavers with gross anatomic and histologic correlation. AJR Am J Roentgenol 2009;192(3):W111–6.
7. Yu JS, Petersilge C, Sartoris DJ, et al. MR imaging of injuries of the extensor mechanism of the knee. Radiographics 1994;14(3):541–51.
8. Lotke PA, Ecker ML. Transverse fractures of the patella. Clin Orthop Relat Res 1981;(158):180–4.
9. Kwak SD, Colman WW, Ateshian GA, et al. Anatomy of the human patellofemoral joint articular cartilage: surface curvature analysis. J Orthop Res 1997;15(3):468–72.
10. Starok M, Lenchik L, Trudell D, et al. Normal patellar retinaculum: MR and sonographic imaging

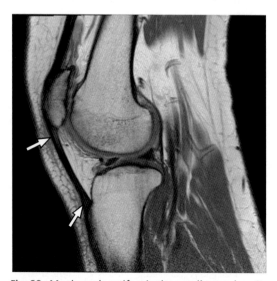

Fig. 28. Magic angle artifact in the patellar tendon. On this PD-weighted sagittal image (TE = 17), the proximal and distal patellar tendon show mildly increased signal caused by magic angle artifact (*arrows*). The tendon otherwise shows normal thickness and morphology.

with cadaveric correlation. AJR Am J Roentgenol 1997;168(6):1493–9.

11. Jacobson JA, Lenchik L, Ruhoy MK, et al. MR imaging of the infrapatellar fat pad of Hoffa. Radiographics 1997;17(3):675–91.

12. Saddik D, McNally EG, Richardson M. MRI of Hoffa's fat pad. Skeletal Radiol 2004;33(8):433–44.

13. Puig S, Dupuy DE, Sarmiento A, et al. Articular muscle of the knee: a muscle seldom recognized on MR imaging. AJR Am J Roentgenol 1996; 166(5):1057–60.

14. Kimura K, Takahashi Y. M. articularis genus. Observations on arrangement and consideration of function. Surg Radiol Anat 1987;9(3):231–9.

15. Scapinelli R. Studies on the vasculature of the human knee joint. Acta Anat (Basel) 1968;70(3): 305–31.

16. Perfitt JS, Petrie MJ, Blundell CM, et al. Acute quadriceps tendon rupture: a pragmatic approach to diagnostic imaging. Eur J Orthop Surg Traumatol 2013. [Epub ahead of print].

17. Stinner DJ, Orr JD, Hsu JR. Fluoroquinolone-associated bilateral patellar tendon rupture: a case report and review of the literature. Mil Med 2010;175(6):457–9.

18. Kayali C, Agus H, Turgut A, et al. Simultaneous bilateral quadriceps tendon rupture in a patient on chronic haemodialysis. (Short-term results of treatment with transpatellar sutures augmented with a quadriceps tendon flap). Ortop Traumatol Rehabil 2008;10(3):286–91.

19. Potasman I, Bassan HM. Multiple tendon rupture in systemic lupus erythematosus: case report and review of the literature. Ann Rheum Dis 1984; 43(2):347–9.

20. Ilan DI, Tejwani N, Keschner M, et al. Quadriceps tendon rupture. J Am Acad Orthop Surg 2003; 11(3):192–200.

21. Kramer J, White LM, Recht MP. MR imaging of the extensor mechanism. Semin Musculoskelet Radiol 2009;13(4):384–401.

22. Swamy GN, Nanjayan SK, Yallappa S, et al. Is ultrasound diagnosis reliable in acute extensor tendon injuries of the knee? Acta Orthop Belg 2012; 78(6):764–70.

23. Lee D, Stinner D, Mir H. Quadriceps and patellar tendon ruptures. J Knee Surg 2013;26(5):301–8.

24. Macurak RB, Goldman JA, Hirsh E, et al. Acute calcific quadriceps tendinitis. South Med J 1980; 73(3):322–5.

25. Johnson DP, Wakeley CJ, Watt I. Magnetic resonance imaging of patellar tendonitis. J Bone Joint Surg Br 1996;78(3):452–7.

26. O'Keeffe SA, Hogan BA, Eustace SJ, et al. Overuse injuries of the knee. Magn Reson Imaging Clin N Am 2009;17(4):725–39, vii.

27. Peace KA, Lee JC, Healy J. Imaging the infrapatellar tendon in the elite athlete. Clin Radiol 2006;61(7):570–8.

28. Hirano A, Fukubayashi T, Ishii T, et al. Magnetic resonance imaging of Osgood-Schlatter disease: the course of the disease. Skeletal Radiol 2002; 31(6):334–42.

29. Bates DG, Hresko MT, Jaramillo D. Patellar sleeve fracture: demonstration with MR imaging. Radiology 1994;193(3):825–7.

30. Gottsegen CJ, Ever BA, White EA, et al. Avulsion fractures of the knee: imaging findings and clinical significance. Radiographics 2008;28(6):1755–70.

31. Boublik M, Schlegel T, Koonce R, et al. Patellar tendon ruptures in National Football League players. Am J Sports Med 2011;39(11):2436–40.

32. Miller TT, Staron RB, Feldman F. Patellar height on sagittal MR imaging of the knee. AJR Am J Roentgenol 1996;167(2):339–41.

33. Tria AJ Jr, Alicea JA, Cody RP. Patella baja in anterior cruciate ligament reconstruction of the knee. Clin Orthop Relat Res 1994;(299):229–34.

34. Fithian DC, Paxton EW, Stone ML, et al. Epidemiology and natural history of acute patellar dislocation. Am J Sports Med 2004;32(5):1114–21.

35. Diederichs G, Issever AS, Scheffler S. MR imaging of patellar instability: injury patterns and assessment of risk factors. Radiographics 2010;30(4): 961–81.

36. Haas JP, Collins MS, Stuart MJ. The "sliver sign": a specific radiographic sign of acute lateral patellar dislocation. Skeletal Radiol 2012;41(5): 595–601.

37. Nomura E, Horiuchi Y, Inoue M. Correlation of MR imaging findings and open exploration of medial patellofemoral ligament injuries in acute patellar dislocations. Knee 2002;9(2):139–43.

38. Elias DA, White LM, Fithian DC. Acute lateral patellar dislocation at MR imaging: injury patterns of medial patellar soft-tissue restraints and osteochondral injuries of the inferomedial patella. Radiology 2002;225(3):736–43.

39. Zaidi A, Babyn P, Astori I, et al. MRI of traumatic patellar dislocation in children. Pediatr Radiol 2006;36(11):1163–70.

40. Panni AS, Vasso M, Cerciello S. Acute patellar dislocation. What to do? Knee Surg Sports Traumatol Arthrosc 2013;21(2):275–8.

41. Sillanpaa PJ, Maenpaa HM. First-time patellar dislocation: surgery or conservative treatment? Sports Med Arthrosc 2012;20(3):128–35.

42. Fredericson M, Powers CM. Practical management of patellofemoral pain. Clin J Sport Med 2002; 12(1):36–8.

43. Carrillon Y, Abidi H, Dejour D, et al. Patellar instability: assessment on MR images by measuring

the lateral trochlear inclination-initial experience. Radiology 2000;216(2):582–5.

44. Dejour H, Walch G, Nove-Josserand L, et al. Factors of patellar instability: an anatomic radiographic study. Knee Surg Sports Traumatol Arthrosc 1994; 2(1):19–26.

45. Neyret P, Robinson AHN, Le Coultre B, et al. Patellar tendon length–the factor in patellar instability? Knee 2002;9(1):3–6.

46. Insall J, Salvati E. Patella position in the normal knee joint. Radiology 1971;101(1):101–4.

47. Ward SR, Terk MR, Powers CM. Patella alta: association with patellofemoral alignment and changes in contact area during weight-bearing. J Bone Joint Surg Am 2007;89(8):1749–55.

48. Shabshin N, Schweitzer ME, Morrison WB, et al. MRI criteria for patella alta and baja. Skeletal Radiol 2004;33(8):445–50.

49. Schoettle PB, Zanetti M, Seifert B, et al. The tibial tuberosity-trochlear groove distance; a comparative study between CT and MRI scanning. Knee 2006;13(1):26–31.

50. Balcarek P, Jung K, Frosch KH, et al. Value of the tibial tuberosity-trochlear groove distance in patellar instability in the young athlete. Am J Sports Med 2011; 39(8):1756–61.

51. Balcarek P, Oberthur S, Hopfensitz S, et al. Which patellae are likely to redislocate? Knee Surg Sports Traumatol Arthrosc 2013. [Epub ahead of print].

52. Camp CL, Stuart MJ, Krych AJ, et al. CT and MRI measurements of tibial tubercle-trochlear groove distances are not equivalent in patients with patellar instability. Am J Sports Med 2013;41(8): 1835–40.

53. Naveed MA, Ackroyd CE, Porteous AJ. Long-term (ten- to 15-year) outcome of arthroscopically assisted Elmslie-Trillat tibial tubercle osteotomy. Bone Joint J 2013;95-B(4):478–85.

54. Banke IJ, Kohn LM, Meidinger G, et al. Combined trochleoplasty and MPFL reconstruction for treatment of chronic patellofemoral instability: a prospective minimum 2-year follow-up study. Knee Surg Sports Traumatol Arthrosc 2013. [Epub ahead of print].

55. Van Tiggelen D, Cowan S, Coorevits P, et al. Delayed vastus medialis obliquus to vastus lateralis onset timing contributes to the development of patellofemoral pain in previously healthy men: a prospective study. Am J Sports Med 2009;37(6): 1099–105.

56. Collado H, Fredericson M. Patellofemoral pain syndrome. Clin Sports Med 2010;29(3):379–98.

57. Mao N, Ni H, Ding W, et al. Surgical treatment of transverse patella fractures by the cable pin system with a minimally invasive technique. J Trauma Acute Care Surg 2012;72(4):1056–61.

58. Chun KA, Ohashi K, Bennett DL, et al. Patellar fractures after total knee replacement. AJR Am J Roentgenol 2005;185(3):655–60.

59. Ostlere S. The extensor mechanism of the knee. Radiol Clin North Am 2013;51(3):393–411.

60. Hinman RS, Lentzos J, Vicenzino B, et al. Patellofemoral osteoarthritis is common in middle-aged people with chronic patellofemoral pain. Arthritis Care Res (Hoboken) 2013. [Epub ahead of print].

61. Roth C, Jacobson J, Jamadar D, et al. Quadriceps fat pad signal intensity and enlargement on MRI: prevalence and associated findings. AJR Am J Roentgenol 2004;182(6):1383–7.

62. Shabshin N, Schweitzer ME, Morrison WB. Quadriceps fat pad edema: significance on magnetic resonance images of the knee. Skeletal Radiol 2006;35(5):269–74.

63. Clockaerts S, Bastiaansen-Jenniskens YM, Runhaar J, et al. The infrapatellar fat pad should be considered as an active osteoarthritic joint tissue: a narrative review. Osteoarthritis Cartilage 2010;18(7):876–82.

64. Clockaerts S, Bastiaansen-Jenniskens YM, Feijt C, et al. Cytokine production by infrapatellar fat pad can be stimulated by interleukin 1beta and inhibited by peroxisome proliferator activated receptor alpha agonist. Ann Rheum Dis 2012;71(6):1012–8.

65. Campagna R, Pessis E, Biau DJ, et al. Is superolateral Hoffa fat pad edema a consequence of impingement between lateral femoral condyle and patellar ligament? Radiology 2012;263(2):469–74.

66. Subhawong TK, Eng J, Carrino JA, et al. Superolateral Hoffa's fat pad edema: association with patellofemoral maltracking and impingement. AJR Am J Roentgenol 2010;195(6):1367–73.

67. Chung CB, Skaf A, Roger B, et al. Patellar tendon-lateral femoral condyle friction syndrome: MR imaging in 42 patients. Skeletal Radiol 2001;30(12): 694–7.

68. De Smet AA, Davis KW, Dahab KS, et al. Is there an association between superolateral Hoffa fat pad edema on MRI and clinical evidence of fat pad impingement? AJR Am J Roentgenol 2012;199(5): 1099–104.

69. Aaron DL, Patel A, Kayiaros S, et al. Four common types of bursitis: diagnosis and management. J Am Acad Orthop Surg 2011;19(6):359–67.

70. Tejwani SG, Cohen SB, Bradley JP. Management of Morel-Lavallee lesion of the knee: twenty-seven cases in the national football league. Am J Sports Med 2007;35(7):1162–7.

71. Johnson JF, Brogdon BG. Dorsal effect of the patella: incidence and distribution. AJR Am J Roentgenol 1982;139(2):339–40.

72. van Holsbeeck M, Vandamme B, Marchal G, et al. Dorsal defect of the patella: concept of its origin

and relationship with bipartite and multipartite patella. Skeletal Radiol 1987;16(4):304–11.

73. Ho VB, Kransdorf MJ, Jelinek JS, et al. Dorsal defect of the patella: MR features. J Comput Assist Tomogr 1991;15(3):474–6.

74. Kavanagh EC, Zoga A, Omar I, et al. MRI findings in bipartite patella. Skeletal Radiol 2007; 36(3):209–14.

75. Ogden JA, McCarthy SM, Jokl P. The painful bipartite patella. J Pediatr Orthop 1982;2(3):263–9.

76. Karantanas AH, Zibis AH, Papanikolaou N. Increased signal intensity on fat-suppressed three-dimensional T1-weighted pulse sequences in patellar tendon: magic angle effect? Skeletal Radiol 2001;30(2):67–71.

77. Li T, Mirowitz SA. Manifestation of magic angle phenomenon: comparative study on effects of varying echo time and tendon orientation among various MR sequences. Magn Reson Imaging 2003;21(7):741–4.

A Biomechanical Approach to Interpreting Magnetic Resonance Imaging of Knee Injuries

Scott E. Sheehan, MD, MS[a],*, Bharti Khurana, MD[b],
Glenn Gaviola, MD[c], Kirkland W. Davis, MD[a]

KEYWORDS

- Knee • Injury • Biomechanics • Mechanism • Instability • MR imaging • Imaging

KEY POINTS

- An understanding of the functional anatomy of the knee aids in recognizing common injury mechanisms of knee trauma at magnetic resonance (MR) imaging and resulting clinical instability.
- The presence of specific osseous and soft-tissue injuries can help elucidate the mechanism of injury and provide a targeted approach to MR imaging evaluation of the knee following trauma.
- Injuries of the knee can be categorized as occurring in hyperextension, in physiologic extension, and in flexion with varying degrees of angulation and rotation, and result in characteristic osteochondral, ligamentous, meniscal, and musculotendinous lesions.
- Recognition by the radiologist of these key injury patterns and clinical instability may aid in the detection of occult and subtle injuries that may require early surgical treatment to prevent subsequent treatment failure.

INTRODUCTION

Magnetic resonance (MR) imaging of knee injuries enables identification of soft-tissue and radiographically occult bone injuries, and facilitates analysis and reporting of injury constellations in the context of functional knee instability. Previous works have described the stabilizing structures of the knee, common destabilizing injury patterns, and the MR imaging appearance of common knee injuries. The purpose of this review is to discuss the normal functional anatomy of key soft-tissue stabilizers of the knee, summarize the currently known etiology and types of posttraumatic knee instability, present the most common

resultant MR imaging injury patterns, and synthesize a unified model for use as a targeted reporting checklist during MR image interpretation. By illustrating the biomechanical mechanism and clinical relevance of potentially destabilizing injuries, an improved understanding will allow the radiologist to better identify significant, subtle, and potentially occult injuries, and thus provide more clinically relevant interpretations.

NORMAL FUNCTIONAL ANATOMY

Normal knee motion involves flexion and extension in the sagittal plane, translation in 3 planes (anterior-posterior, medial-lateral, and proximal-distal),

Disclosures: The authors have no relationships to disclose.
[a] Department of Musculoskeletal Radiology, University of Wisconsin School of Medicine and Public Health, 600 Highland Avenue, Madison, WI 53792, USA; [b] Department of Emergency Radiology, Brigham and Women's Hospital, 75 Francis Street, Boston, MA 02115, USA; [c] Department of Musculoskeletal Radiology, Brigham and Women's Hospital, 75 Francis Street, Boston, MA 02115, USA
* Corresponding author.
E-mail address: sheehan.scott.e@gmail.com

and both internal and external rotation of the femur relative to the tibia.[1] In full extension, the femur is slightly internally rotated, with the lateral femoral condylar rotation locking the knee in place. As a result there is minimal abduction, adduction, or rotational laxity to the fully extended knee. With flexion, the femur rotates externally and unlocks the knee. Moderate passive rotation and mild laxity in lateral motion are normally demonstrated with the knee in 90° of flexion.[2] Destabilizing knee injuries commonly produce clinically detectable increases in rotational or lateral knee laxity than would otherwise be expected for a given state of knee flexion.

Knee instability has been classified according to the Committee on Research and Education of the American Orthopedic Society for Sports Medicine as: (1) 1-plane or straight, (2) rotatory, or (3) combined instability.[2] The osseous structures of the knee provide minimal inherent stability. Rather, the soft-tissue structures that span the joint provide the dynamic stabilizing action. The cruciate and collateral ligaments, the joint capsule, and the musculotendinous units play a crucial role in providing knee stability (**Fig. 1**). The cruciate ligaments are intra-articular but extrasynovial structures that primarily resist anteroposterior displacement of the tibia relative to the femur to stabilize the knee joint. The vertical axis of flexion and rotation of the knee, termed the central pivot, normally lies close to the attachment sites of the posterior cruciate ligament (PCL).[3–5] Destabilizing knee injuries result in the shift of this central pivot away from the injured structures (**Fig. 2**).

The cruciate and collateral ligaments serve complementary roles in stabilizing the knee during rotation. During tibial internal rotation the cruciate ligaments coil and effectively shorten about the central pivot. In particular, the PCL becomes increasingly taut, thus providing proportionally greater stabilization than the anterior cruciate ligament (ACL), with a concomitant increase with knee flexion.[2,6] However, the collateral ligaments straighten during internal rotation, become relatively lax, and provide less stability. Conversely, during tibial external rotation the collateral ligaments shorten, assume more static tension, and provide increased stability. The cruciate ligaments uncoil and effectively lengthen during external rotation, thus diminishing their stabilizing function. With neutral rotation, the cruciate and collateral ligaments are not under any specific tension and provide less overall resistance to motion (**Fig. 3**).[2]

The ACL comprises 2 distinct bundles. The anteromedial bundle primarily resists anterior tibial translation with the knee in flexion, and the posterolateral bundle resists anterior tibial translation and rotation with the knee in extension.[7] The ACL is the primary constraint against anterior tibial translation; straight anterior instability implies complete disruption of the ACL, often accompanied by medial and lateral capsular ligament injury (see later discussion).[2,8,9] The presence of a concomitant complete PCL disruption further exacerbates this instability.[2,3]

The PCL is the primary stabilizer against posterior translation of the tibia, although the posterior

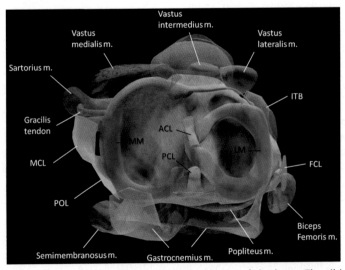

Fig. 1. Computer-generated image showing key anatomic structures of the knee. The tibial articular surface is viewed en face from a superior perspective, and the femoral condyles are transparent. ACL, anterior cruciate ligament; FCL, fibular collateral ligament; ITB, iliotibial band; LM, lateral meniscus; MCL, medial collateral ligament; MM, medial meniscus; PCL, posterior cruciate ligament; POL, posterior oblique ligament.

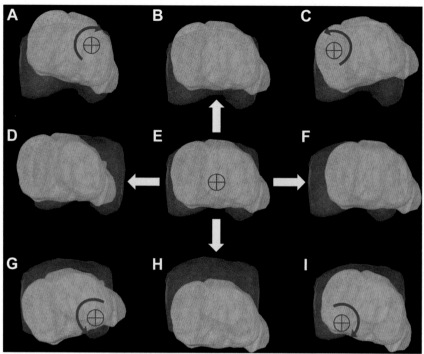

Fig. 2. Computer-generated image showing displacement of the central axis of rotation of the knee (*red crosshairs*) following a destabilizing injury, and the direction of resulting instability. The tibial articular surface is viewed en face from a superior perspective, and the femoral condyles are partially transparent for improved visualization. In the normal anatomic configuration (*E*), the central pivot is defined by the axis of the posterior cruciate ligament (PCL). Rotatory instability generally involves pivot displacement away from, and tibial rotation toward (*curved red arrows*) the injured restraining structures. Simple rotatory instability patterns include anteromedial (*A*), anterolateral (*C*), posteromedial (*G*), and posterolateral (*I*). Disruption of the anterior cruciate ligament (ACL) can produce straight or "1-plane" anterior instability (*B*), which is exacerbated by concomitant PCL injury. Disruption of the PCL results in the most functionally significant straight instability, as indicated by the loss of the rotatory axis in straight anterior (*B*), medial (*D*), lateral (*F*), and posterior (*H*) instability. Combined instability will occur when multiple directions of rotatory instability are present.

oblique ligament (POL), the fibular collateral ligament (FCL), the posterolateral corner structures, and the posterior joint capsule all provide key secondary roles.[3,8,10–12] The PCL has been described as the primary stabilizing ligament of the knee owing in part to its function in determining straight versus rotatory instability.[3,8] True rotatory instability requires that the cruciate ligaments are not completely compromised.

Lateral stabilization of the knee is provided by several structures with the FCL, or lateral collateral ligament, being the primary constraint to lateral joint opening.[13] The anterolateral corner is stabilized primarily by the lateral capsular ligament, a focal thickening of the middle one-third of the lateral joint capsule, and to a lesser extent by the iliotibial band (ITB).[5,13] The ITB represents the distal extension of the fascia lata of the lateral thigh, and helps reinforce the lateral capsular ligament.[13] The ACL and FCL play critical supplementary roles in anterolateral stability.[8,13,14] The

posterolateral corner is primarily stabilized by the arcuate complex, which consists of the FCL, the arcuate ligament, the posterior one-third of the lateral joint capsule, the popliteofibular ligament, and fabellofibular ligament. Additional posterolateral stabilizing structures include the biceps femoris tendon, popliteus muscle and popliteomeniscal ligament, and the lateral head of the gastrocnemius.[5,13,15] These posterolateral corner structures, along with the PCL, help to maintain posterolateral stability and to counter tibial external rotation forces.[6]

Primary constraints against medial joint opening include the superficial medial collateral ligament (MCL) and the POL, a ligament in continuity with the posteromedial joint capsule. The ACL provides supplementary support while the medial head of the gastrocnemius aids in dynamic stabilization.[16,17] The MCL and the POL also provide supplementary and reciprocal support to counter internal and external rotation, depending on the

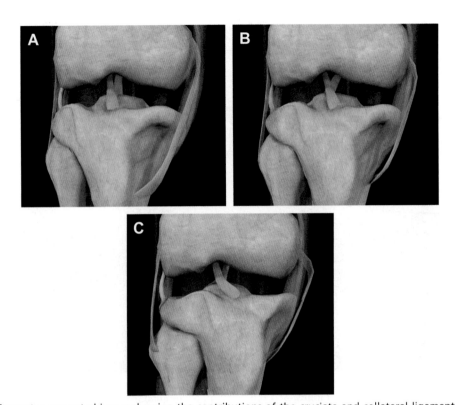

Fig. 3. Computer-generated image showing the contributions of the cruciate and collateral ligaments to knee stabilization during tibial rotation. With tibial external rotation (*A*), the cruciate ligaments uncoil and lengthen while the collateral ligaments shorten and provide more stabilization. In neutral position (*B*), the collateral and cruciate ligaments provide more complementary contributions to knee stabilization, as neither is under specific asymmetric tension. With tibial internal rotation (*C*), the cruciate ligaments coil and effectively shorten and provide increased stability, while the collateral ligaments become relatively lax.

degree of knee flexion.[18] The deep fibers of the medial collateral ligament, the meniscotibial and meniscofemoral ligaments, merge with an area of focal thickening of the middle one-third of the joint capsule termed the medial capsular ligament. These fibers provide a small but significant contribution to constraint against medial joint opening and external rotation.[18] However, the anterior one-third of the medial joint capsule contributes little to medial knee stability and is infrequently torn.[3] The semitendinosus and semimembranosus muscles play complementary but minor roles in medial stabilization; the semitendinosus counteracts valgus forces while the semimembranosus acts as a dynamic stabilizer of the posteromedial corner via its attachment with the POL and posterior capsule.[2,19]

The patella is a sesamoid bone that articulates with the medial and lateral femoral condyles at the intercondylar groove, and serves to magnify the moment arm of knee extension via anterior displacement of the quadriceps myotendinous unit.[20] The quadriceps and patellar tendons merge with the superior and inferior poles of the patella, respectively, and contribute to vertical stability. The normal 15° to 20° angle of the quadriceps insertion relative to the patellar tendon insertion produces a resting valgus orientation of the extensor mechanism during full extension. This situation results in a lateral resting position of the patella in the intercondylar groove on extension, and medial movement of the patella to the intercondylar midline with increasing flexion (**Fig. 4**). Medialization of the patella on flexion increases the surface area of articular contact, thus increasing patellar stability.[20] The patella is stabilized medially by the medial patellofemoral ligament (MPFL) and medial patellar retinaculum, with dynamic stabilization provided by the oblique head of the vastus medialis muscle.[21] The lateral retinaculum merges with both the vastus lateralis muscle and ITB, providing lateral patellar stability.

The angle of the quadriceps tendon relative to the patellar tendon insertion also secondarily determines the magnitude of anterior tibial shear force produced during quadriceps contraction.

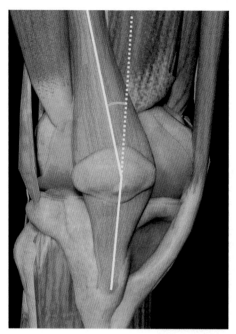

Fig. 4. Computer-generated image of the anterior surface of the knee, showing the normal quadriceps-patella tendon angle of 15° to 20° (*orange arc*), which generates a small lateral force vector component on knee extension and quadriceps contraction, resulting in a lateral position of the patella in the intercondylar groove.

Higher quadriceps-patella tendon angles in extension produce more anterior shear force and result in greater anterior tibial translation than would otherwise occur with knee flexion.[22] This anterior shear force is countered primarily by the ACL, followed by the PCL and medial and lateral capsular ligaments, while the hamstring muscles provide dynamic stabilization.[2,3,8,22,23]

An understanding of the functional anatomy and normal stabilizing role of the soft-tissue structures of the knee can provide an informed and more directed search for specific destabilizing injuries, in the context of the known clinical knee instability according to specific type and subtypes. In particular, the presence of straight instability should specifically raise suspicion for cruciate ligament injury, whereas rotatory instability is suggestive of at least partial PCL integrity (**Table 1**).

IMAGING FINDINGS OF ACUTE INJURY

Traumatic knee injuries often demonstrate characteristic osseous and soft-tissue injury patterns that can reveal the underlying injury mechanism, and the subsequent risk and type of potential instability. Keeping in mind the normal functional anatomy just discussed, the approach to evaluation using MR imaging should begin with an assessment for osseous and osteochondral injuries, as these often best illustrate the primary force vector of the trauma in addition to any secondary contrecoup or contralateral distraction or avulsion components.[24] With this inferred force vector, the stabilizing ligaments at greatest risk for injury should then be evaluated, as ligament injury patterns can suggest the type of resulting instability. Attention should next be directed to the relevant myotendinous units, as these provide secondary stabilization; underlying disruption can suggest the magnitude or severity of the overall injury and subsequent instability. Finally, the menisci should be scrutinized in the setting of specific injury patterns, as unrecognized and inappropriately treated injury can result in chronic disability. The following sections provide general guidance on the assessment and grading of these injuries, although a thorough discussion is beyond the scope of this review.

Osseous and Osteochondral Lesions

Findings of acute knee trauma commonly include bone contusions, isolated or pure chondral injuries, subchondral or osteochondral fractures, or cortical extra-articular fractures. Multiple classification systems of acute traumatic osteochondral lesions have been proposed,[25–27] although commonalities exist between these systems. Bone contusions likely represent microtrabecular fractures with superimposed marrow edema and hemorrhage, without overt cortical bone disruption or an identifiable cortical fracture line.[28] Contusions can appear as ill-defined regions of hypointensity on T1-weighted and proton density (PD)-weighted sequences, with corresponding hyperintensity on short-tau inversion recovery (STIR) or T2-weighted sequences with fat suppression (FS) that often exceeds the area of T1 abnormality.[25] Subchondral fractures are distinguished from contusions by the presence of a hypointense fracture line most often immediately beneath the subchondral lamella on T1-weighted imaging sequences, lying within a larger region of bone edema (**Fig. 5**).[25] These injuries are termed osteochondral fractures if they extend through the articular cartilage into the underlying cortex. Isolated or pure chondral injuries can also be seen, ranging in appearance and severity from signal heterogeneity, fissuring, chondral flap or delamination, chondral depression into an underlying impaction fracture, or osteochondral indentation or flake fractures (**Fig. 6**).[25] Multiple classification systems of osteochondral injury and morphologies on MR imaging have been described, although no single

Table 1
Simplified classification system for the major types of knee instability resulting from ligament injury, proposed by the Committee on Research and Education of the American Orthopedic Society for Sports Medicine, and the key corresponding primary and secondary stabilizing structures that prevent each type of instability

Instability Type	Subtype	Primary Stabilizers	Secondary Stabilizers
One-plane (straight) instability	Anterior	ACL	Medial and lateral capsular ligaments
	Posterior	PCL	Arcuate complex, POL, posterior capsule
	Medial[a]	MCL, POL, medial capsular ligament	PCL[a]
	Lateral[a]	FCL and arcuate complex, lateral capsular ligament	PCL[a], biceps femoris tendon, ITB, ACL
Rotatory instability	Anterolateral	Lateral capsular ligament, FCL and arcuate complex	ACL, ITB
	Anteromedial	MCL, POL, medial capsular ligament	ACL
	Posterolateral	FCL and arcuate complex, lateral capsular ligament	PCL (incomplete injury), popliteus tendon
	Posteromedial	MCL, POL, medial capsular ligament[b]	PCL[b]
Combined rotatory instability	Combinations of the above primary types of rotatory instability	Details are beyond the scope of this review	

The presentation and severity of knee instability can vary depending on the degree of knee flexion, and injuries to the listed primary and secondary structures may not be symptomatic at all tested states of knee flexion.
Abbreviations: ACL, anterior cruciate ligament; FCL, fibular collateral ligament; ITB, iliotibial band; MCL, medial collateral ligament; PCL, posterior cruciate ligament; POL, posterior oblique ligament.
[a] Straight medial and lateral clinical instability require high-grade injury to the PCL, or will alternatively present with rotatory instability.
[b] Posteromedial rotatory instability is controversial, and unlikely in the presence of a high-grade PCL injury.

system has gained universal acceptance. In general, injuries without chondral disruption will more likely undergo conservative nonsurgical treatment, whereas surgical fixation will often be used for chondral and osteochondral fractures, often after a trial of conservative therapy for smaller lesions.[2,25]

Contusion edema patterns occur commonly as a result of impaction or distraction, whereby the incident force vector causes direct impact of 2 or more bones on one side of the knee, with accompanying distraction on the contralateral side. For example, a severe valgus-inducing force may generate lateral knee compression and medial knee distraction. Lateral bony impaction results in bony contusion and/or osteochondral injury, whereas medial knee distraction results in tension on the collateral ligaments and subsequent sprain, tear, or avulsion types of injury (**Fig. 7**). Avulsion fractures are commonly seen on the side of distraction, but cause relatively less bone marrow edema in comparison with impaction injuries

(**Fig. 8**).[29] Avulsion fractures can be subtle on MR imaging, with only mild donor-site bone marrow edema and an often indistinct, small avulsed cortical fragment. Distraction without true avulsion fracture can also manifest as focal or linear edema at the associated ligamentous or tendinous attachment site, similar to a focal contusion.[30]

MR imaging findings of contusions can develop in as little as 1 hour following trauma and can routinely persist for more than 40 weeks.[31,32] Although the overall prognosis of contusion without initial overlying cartilage injury is generally good, late development of chronic overlying chondral or subchondral defects can occur if not appropriately treated.[27,33–35]

Ligamentous Lesions

Grading of collateral ligament injuries, as grade I, II, or III, is based on clinical assessment rather than by strict imaging criteria alone, by assessing the degree of ligament injury and presence of

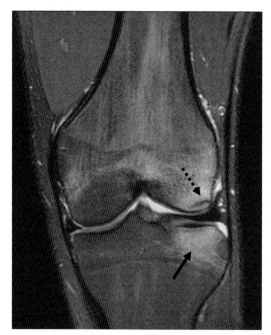

Fig. 5. Coronal proton density–weighted (PD) MR image of the knee with fat suppression (FS) showing axial impaction injury of the lateral femoral condyle and lateral tibial plateau. Hyperintensity within the lateral tibial plateau is consistent with contusion (*black arrow*). Similar hyperintensity within the lateral femoral condyle is noted, although the presence of a superimposed transverse hypointense line indicates a subchondral fracture (*dotted black arrow*).

clinical instability through provocative maneuvers during physical examination.[36] Significant clinical MCL instability qualifies as a grade III injury, and can be further subclassified by the severity of medial joint opening with a valgus-inducing

stress.[19,36] MR imaging grading of collateral ligament injuries categorized as imaging grades I, II, and III describe findings of ligamentous or periligamentous edema, ligament thickening and signal abnormality, and frank ligament discontinuity, respectively, with associated osseous edema at the ligament attachment points (**Fig. 9**).[37,38] However, MR imaging grades have shown inconsistent correlation with clinical findings.[39,40] Isolated MCL injuries are unlikely to cause significant functional instability, leading some clinicians to advocate that suspected MCL injuries should be imaged only if classified as grade III clinically, to evaluate for an associated destabilizing injury to the posteromedial corner structures such as the POL, posterior capsule, semimembranosus tendon, or cruciate ligaments.[19] In contradistinction, FCL and posterolateral corner ligament injuries are less common but pose a higher risk of instability.[13] Whereas isolated grade III MCL injuries often respond well to conservative nonsurgical therapy, grade III FCL injuries or fracture equivalents most often undergo primary surgical repair to restore stability.[5,13,41]

ACL injuries can be identified on MR imaging by the presence of primary and secondary signs or a combination thereof, and are often best evaluated on T2-weighted or PD-weighted imaging.[42] Primary MR imaging signs of ACL injury include abnormal signal within the ligament, abnormal contour and configuration, or frank fiber disruption, the presence of which yield a high degree of diagnostic accuracy (see **Fig. 9**).[43] Secondary signs include anterior translation of the tibia greater than 7 mm, characteristic bony contusions of the lateral femoral condyle and lateral tibial plateau, anterior tibial spine avulsion, or

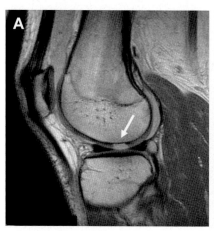
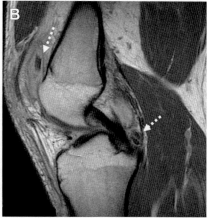

Fig. 6. Sagittal PD MR images of the knee at the level of the lateral compartment (*A*) and the intercondylar notch (*B*) showing a full-thickness cartilage defect of the weight-bearing lateral femoral condyle (*solid white arrow*), with an osteochondral fragment in the joint space (*dotted white arrows*).

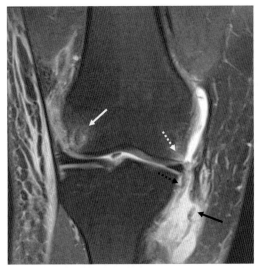

Fig. 7. Coronal PD FS MR image of the knee obtained following traumatic valgus knee injury. Impact on the lateral aspect of the knee causes valgus angulation with axial compression lateral to the central pivot, and concomitant axial distraction medial to the central pivot. A contusion of the lateral femoral condyle (*white arrow*) is likely due to a combination of direct impact and compressive injury, with a corresponding distraction related high-grade tear of the distal medial collateral ligament (MCL) (*black arrow*) and underlying meniscotibial ligament (*dotted black arrow*). A small contusion of the medial femoral condyle likely reflects contrecoup injury (*dotted white arrow*).

buckling of the PCL, among others.[42–46] Partial-thickness ACL injuries are often difficult to accurately diagnose on imaging, likely owing to the nonspecific nature of increased instrasubstance

signal that can be seen to an extent in an intact ACL, and in all grades of ACL injury.[42,47] As partial-thickness injuries are commonly managed nonsurgically, MR imaging is useful to evaluate for full-thickness ACL injury or other associated soft-tissue abnormalities that would lead to progression of instability.[48]

PCL injuries are less common than ACL injuries and most often occur in the setting of multiple injuries, which is thought to contribute in part to its underdiagnosis.[49] Full-thickness PCL tears can be diagnosed on MR imaging if there is increased signal intensity on PD-, T1-, or T2-weighted sequences in the expected location of intact PCL fibers, visualization of frank fiber disruption or retraction, or failure to identify the PCL. Focal PCL thickening greater than 7 mm or increased intrasubstance signal may reflect a partial-thickness tear.[49,50] PCL injuries are commonly associated with ACL, MCL, and posterolateral corner injuries (see later discussion).[42,51,52]

Musculotendinous Lesions

Musculotendinous structures of the knee provide dynamic stabilization across the normal range of knee motion. The myotendinous junction of the musculotendinous unit is usually the weakest structural component and the most common site of injury.[5,53–55] Injuries are most common in muscles that cross 2 joints and demonstrate eccentric contraction (contraction while lengthening), including the semimembranosus, rectus femoris, biceps femoris, and medial head of the gastrocnemius.[5,38,53,55,56] Musculotendinous injuries can be categorized as muscular contusion, tendon

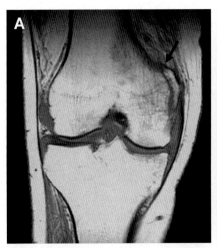 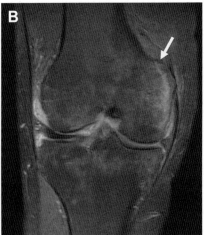

Fig. 8. (*A*) Coronal PD and (*B*) coronal PD FS MR images of the knee showing an avulsion fracture of the proximal attachment of the MCL. An oblique hypointense line with cortical disruption indicates a minimally displaced avulsion fracture at the site of the proximal MCL attachment (*black arrow*) with relatively mild bone marrow edema (*white arrow*).

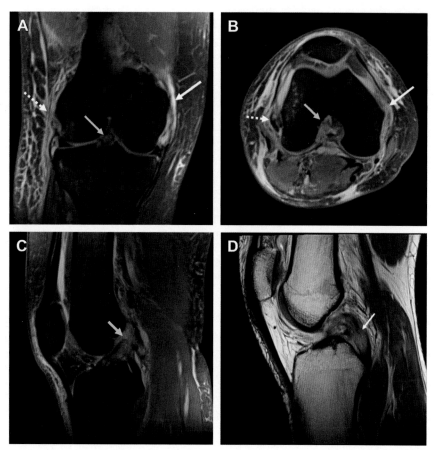

Fig. 9. Multiplanar MR images of the knee showing examples of ligament injuries. (*A*) Coronal T2-weighted MR image of the knee with fat suppression (T2 FS) showing an imaging grade III injury with tear of the proximal MCL in a patient with clinical medial joint-line instability. There is thickening and a wavy contour of the proximal MCL and apparent fiber disruption (*solid white arrow*), with surrounding edema. Edema is noted within the lateral joint space (*dotted white arrow*) surrounding the FCL with thickening and intermediate signal of its proximal attachment. (*B*) Corresponding axial T2 FS image again shows grade III MCL injury (*solid white arrow*), and peril-igamentous edema with mild signal abnormality within the proximal fibular collateral ligament (FCL) (*dotted white arrow*), reflecting sprain and grade II FCL injury. Increased signal within the ACL is partially imaged on coronal and axial images, suggesting underlying injury (*orange arrows*). (*C*) Sagittal T2 FS image at the level of the intercondylar notch confirms increased signal and apparent thickening of the ACL with frank fiber disruption, consistent with high-grade injury and complete tear from its proximal femoral attachment (*orange arrow*). (*D*) Sagittal PD MR image of a different patient following knee trauma shows increased signal in the thickened PCL with discontinuity of fibers (*white arrow*), indicating high-grade injury.

avulsion, or myotendinous strain. Increased fluid within the injured soft tissue is common to all grades of musculotendinous injury in the acute setting, and is best visualized with STIR or T2-weighted FS sequences oriented in the short and long axes of the imaged muscle.[5] T1-weighted sequences are also useful to evaluate for architectural abnormality, associated hematoma, or fatty infiltration and atrophy.[56]

Although multiple classification systems of strain injuries have been proposed,[38,55,57] they are most commonly graded according to combined clinical and MR imaging findings. Low- to moderate-grade injuries usually show a "feathery" pattern of increased signal within the muscle, with small areas of frank fluid signal representing partial tears of muscle fibers on MR imaging (**Fig. 10**). High-grade injuries generally show near full-thickness to complete rupture of the myotendinous unit with a hematoma or fluid-filled gap in the myotendinous unit and varying degrees of tendon retraction on MR imaging, and clinically present with near complete loss of muscle function.[38] Most musculotendinous injuries are treated conservatively, depending on the involved muscle and degree of clinical dysfunction.[53,56] However,

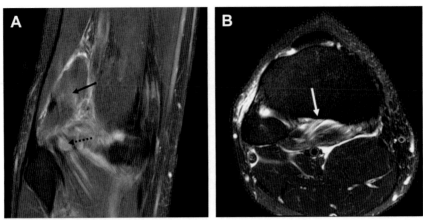

Fig. 10. (*A*) Coronal short-tau inversion recovery and (*B*) axial T2 FS MR images of the knee show a moderate strain of the popliteus muscle (*white arrow*), with focal fluid signal indicating partial-thickness tearing of fibers at the myotendinous junction (*dotted black arrow*). Edema in the lateral head of the gastrocnemius is also noted (*solid black arrow*), consistent with associated mild strain.

myotendinous injuries should be distinguished from avulsion fractures of the adjacent osseous attachment, as avulsion injuries are often best treated with early surgical repair if displaced more than 2 to 3 cm.[38]

Meniscal Lesions

The menisci are fibrocartilaginous structures that distribute axial load-bearing forces across the articular surface and increase the surface area for femoral condylar motion, ultimately improving joint stability.[38] Thus meniscal injuries can contribute to knee instability and predispose patients to knee pain, locking, joint maltracking, and early degeneration. The medial meniscus is attached along its peripheral circumference to the joint capsule, closely approximated with the deep fibers of the MCL, rendering the medial meniscus vulnerable to damage with associated MCL injury.[1,38] The lateral meniscus is more loosely approximated with the lateral capsule and has no direct attachment to the FCL, but is dynamically posteriorly displaced with initiation of knee flexion because of its attachment to the popliteus tendon.[38]

The normal menisci are uniformly hypointense structures on virtually all MR imaging sequences, with a characteristic morphology.[58] Increased signal within the abnormal meniscus in an adult patient is best seen on T1-weighted, PD-weighted, or gradient-echo sequences, and can reflect mucoid degeneration if the signal is punctate, amorphous, or linear in morphology but confined within the substance of the meniscus.[59] Meniscal tears are diagnosed if the signal abnormality

extends through the meniscus and comes into contact with the adjacent articular surface, or if the meniscus is morphologically abnormal.[58,59] Secondary signs of meniscal injury include an underlying bone contusion or osteochondral lesion, presence of parameniscal cysts, peripheral meniscal extrusion, soft-tissue edema, or adjacent effusion.[58,60]

Traumatic meniscal tears most commonly occur with femoral rotation against a fixed tibia during flexion or extension, with the resulting shear force applied to the meniscal surface, most often producing a vertical longitudinal tear morphology.[2,38,61,62] Longitudinal tears usually occur in the peripheral one-third of the meniscus, begin in the posterior horn and propagate anteriorly, and are often associated with ACL tears.[38,58] Traumatic vertical longitudinal tears can often displace or flip and can take on a bucket-handle configuration if extensive, occurring more commonly in the medial meniscus.[60] In the case of ACL disruption attention should be directed to the posterior root of the lateral meniscus, which can sustain an associated tear,[63,64] possibly because of traction on the meniscofemoral ligament of Wrisburg during the ACL injury. Traumatic radial meniscal tears can also occur; these are vertical tears arising from the free edge and extending peripherally, with or without combined complex or horizontal tear morphologies.[58] Meniscal root tears and traumatic radial tears should be suspected in the presence of peripheral meniscal extrusion, compromising the ability of the meniscus to counteract stresses from axial loading. Extrusion is thought to predispose the patient to accelerated articular cartilage loss in the affected compartment, although a causal relationship has not been definitively demonstrated.[1,63,65–67] In contradistinction, displaced or flipped longitudinal tears show normal resistance to axial stresses and can demonstrate meniscal intrusion, which is a meniscal fragment displaced toward the intercondylar notch, best identified on coronal MR images (**Fig. 11**).[68]

Meniscocapsular separation is defined as disruption of the meniscotibial or meniscofemoral ligaments that attach the meniscus to the deep joint capsule, more commonly occurring on the posterior and medial margins of the medial meniscus. These injuries can be difficult to identify on MR imaging, but should be suspected in the setting of high-grade MCL injuries or in patients with persistent pain in the absence of frank MCL injury, as they can be associated with peripheral meniscal tears, and can cause meniscal destabilization and chronic knee pain.[38,69] MR Imaging findings may include meniscal displacement, fluid

signal interposed between the meniscus and capsule, irregular peripheral meniscus margin, or disrupted ligament fascicles.[38,69,70]

INJURY MECHANISMS

Multiple classification systems have been proposed to describe the constellation of traumatic knee injuries from the perspective of injury mechanism, most often based on contusion patterns, dominant soft-tissue injuries, and resulting instability.[2,24,61] Injury mechanisms can be intuitively grouped as occurring with the knee in hyperextension, in full physiologic extension, or in flexion with varying degrees of rotation and varus/valgus angulation.[61]

Hyperextension Injuries

Hyperextension injuries commonly occur following a direct impact force to the anterior tibia with the

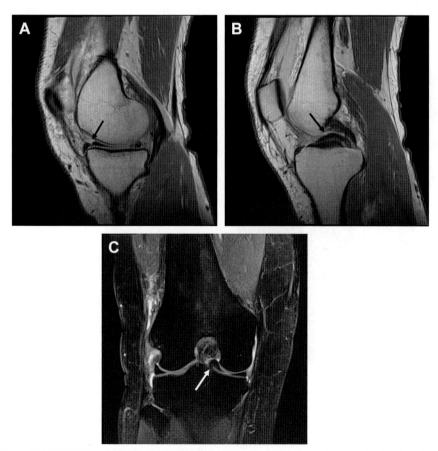

Fig. 11. (*A*) Sagittal PD MR image of the medial compartment of the knee shows a bucket-handle tear of the medial meniscus with a flipped fragment showing a double-delta sign (*black arrow*). (*B*) Additional sagittal PD MR image at the level of the intercondylar notch shows a medially flipped fragment underlying the PCL producing a double-PCL sign (*black arrow*). (*C*) Corresponding coronal PD FS image showing apparent intrusion of the displaced meniscal fragment into the intercondylar notch (*white arrow*).

knee in extension and the foot immobile, or can alternatively be seen with indirect mechanisms such as a forceful kicking motion (**Fig. 12**).[24] The degree of tibial internal or external rotation at the time of injury determines the direction of the hyperextension force vector transmitted through the knee, and can indicate potentially injured structures along the force vector (**Fig. 13**).

Pure hyperextension

A pure hyperextension mechanism will often show broad contusions at the anterior femur and tibia, owing to either impaction of the femoral and tibial margins with anterior joint closure or a direct anterior impact. The soft-tissue structures of the posterocentral knee and both the posteromedial and posterolateral corners may be injured, depending on the severity of hyperextension. Posteromedially, the POL is commonly injured, and the posterolateral structures such as the arcuate complex and popliteus tendon are frequently damaged. Occasionally, avulsion of the proximal fibula styloid process is demonstrated, a finding that has been termed the arcuate sign, as it reflects avulsion injury of the arcuate complex from its

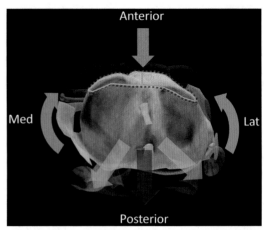

Fig. 13. Computer-generated image demonstrating the effect of internal and external tibial rotation on force vector transmission with hyperextension injuries. A posteriorly directed force vector (*yellow arrow*) on a neutral tibia is transmitted directly through the joint (*red arrow*), potentially causing both medial and lateral tibial and femoral contusions (*dotted red area*). External tibial rotation (*curved green arrow*) translates the force vector to produce a valgus moment, which relatively shortens and unloads the posterolateral corner structures, causing most of the force vector to be absorbed by the lengthened posteromedial corner structures, which are under higher relative tension (*straight green arrow*). The contusion pattern follows the net vector, involving the anterolateral tibia and femur (*green area*). Conversely, hyperextension during internal tibial rotation (*curved blue arrow*) generates a valgus moment that shortens and unloads the posteromedial structures and lengthens the posterolateral corner structures, which absorb most of the injury burden (*straight blue arrow*). The contusion pattern again follows the net vector, usually involving the anteromedial tibia and femur (*blue area*). Lat, lateral; Med, medial.

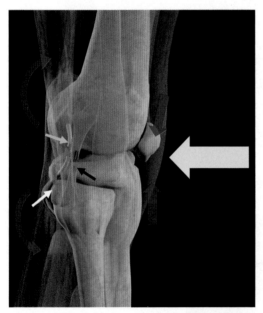

Fig. 12. Computer-generated image of a posteriorly directed impact force vector (*yellow arrow*) on to the anterior knee with the tibia in neutral position, producing closure of the anterior joint space (*straight red arrows*) and opening of the posterior joint space (*curved red arrows*). The vector is transmitted through the posterior knee, causing injury to soft-tissue structures such as the FCL (*black arrow*), the arcuate ligament (*white arrow*), and popliteus tendon (*orange arrow*). The posteromedial corner injuries are not shown.

fibular attachment with implied posterolateral corner instability (**Fig. 14**).[71] Centrally, the posterior capsule and PCL can be damaged if there is severe hyperextension, with concomitant ACL injury sometimes observed.[8,61,72] Extensive soft-tissue edema is commonly seen posteriorly. With disruption of the POL, PCL, and arcuate complex, marked straight posterior instability is likely.[3]

Hyperextension with varus

Impact on the anteromedial knee with the knee extended and the tibia internally rotated produces a hyperextension with varus injury mechanism whereby the force vector is directed through the posterolateral corner, often injuring the cruciate and posterolateral corner ligaments and tendons (**Fig. 15**).[8,24] Contusions commonly occur on the anteromedial tibia and femur, following the force

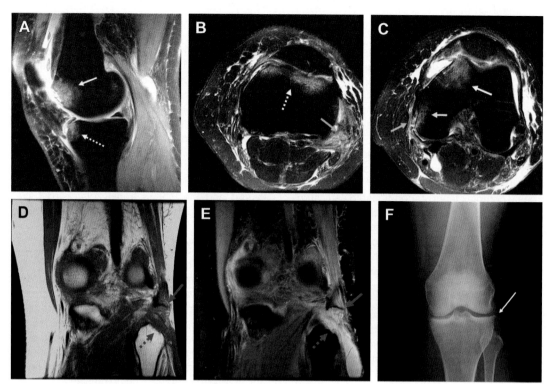

Fig. 14. MR imaging findings of the knee following a severe hyperextension injury during mild internal rotation. (*A*) Sagittal and (*B, C*) axial PD FS images showing contusions of the anterior femoral condyle (*solid white arrows*), and anterior tibial plateau (*dotted white arrows*). The mild internal rotation causes the force vector to be primarily transmitted through the posterolateral corner, with extensive soft-tissue edema surrounding the posterolateral corner suggestive of injury to the FCL and arcuate complex (*blue arrow*). However, as the internal rotation is mild, some of the force is transmitted through the posteromedial corner, with resultant injury to the MCL and posterior oblique ligament (POL) (*orange arrow*) with periligamentous edema and likely underlying traction stress injury of the medial femoral condyle with resulting marrow edema (*yellow arrow*). (*D*) Coronal PD and (*E*) PD FS images show a superiorly displaced avulsion fragment (*red arrow*) and edema surrounding the distal arcuate complex. Cortical irregularity of the proximal fibula avulsion donor site is noted (*dotted red arrow*). (*F*) Anteroposterior radiograph confirms an avulsion fracture of the proximal fibula (*white arrow*), consistent with the arcuate sign.

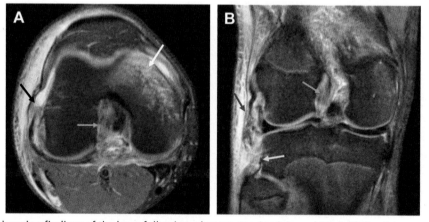

Fig. 15. MR imaging findings of the knee following a hyperextension injury obtained following an anterior knee impact during knee internal rotation. (*A*) Axial and (*B*) coronal PD FS images showing a characteristic contusion to the anterior aspect of the medial femoral condyle (*white arrow*), with small fluid level in the lateral joint recess (*black arrow*) suggestive of hemarthrosis. The force vector is primarily transmitted through the posterolateral corner, with resulting full-thickness tear of the FCL with ligament retraction (*red arrow*), and arcuate ligament injury (*yellow arrow*) best appreciated on the coronal view. Increased signal within the proximal ACL with discontinuity of the hypointense fibers indicates a high-grade tear (*orange arrows*).

vector.[24,73] Cortical fractures of the anteromedial tibial plateau, though uncommon, are highly correlated with posterolateral corner ligamentous injury.[15] Damage to the posterolateral corner structures such as the arcuate complex, popliteus tendon, and lateral capsular ligament can cause significant posterolateral rotatory instability, the severity of which increases with associated PCL injury; however, straight lateral instability results if the PCL is frankly disrupted.[6,8,13] High-grade arcuate complex tears respond best to early surgical intervention, and can ultimately lead to failure of cruciate ligament repair and early osteoarthritis if undetected.[6,72] If a significant rotational component is present in these mechanisms producing posterolateral rotatory instability, injury to the anterior horn of the medial meniscus may result.[8]

Hyperextension with valgus

If the tibia is externally rotated at the time of injury, impact on the anterolateral knee will produce mirror-image injuries to the contralateral medial side via a hyperextension with valgus injury mechanism. This injury often shows characteristic anterolateral femoral and tibial contusions, and injuries to the posteromedial soft-tissue structures (**Fig. 16**). The POL, posteromedial capsule, and sometimes the MCL, PCL, and semimembranosus muscle can be injured.[2,8,24,61] Controversy exists regarding PCL injury and true posteromedial rotatory instability. It has been suggested that

posteromedial rotatory instability can occur with an intact ACL but injured POL, medial capsular ligament, PCL, and medial portion of the posterior capsule.[8] Others have suggested that instability is unlikely in the presence of an intact PCL, because the intact PCL should become taut in internal tibial rotation, essentially precluding posteromedial rotatory instability.[3] This issue remains controversial, but it has been shown that 1-plane medial instability will occur if the medial ligaments are injured and the PCL is frankly disrupted,[3] likely making true posteromedial instability uncommon.

Injuries in Physiologic Extension

As previously discussed, the knee normally demonstrates minimal rotatory motion in full physiologic extension. Impaction forces on the lateral or medial aspects of the extended knee generate predominately valgus or varus stress injury patterns, respectively. Impact on the posterior aspect of the extended knee and nonimpact but high-energy direction change may produce a shear injury mechanism, owing to anterior tibial translation.

Pure valgus injury (clip injury)

Lateral impact to the extended knee is a common occurrence in contact sports such as American football, and has been termed the clip injury.[24] This mechanism produces valgus angulation, which closes the lateral joint space and opens the medial joint space (**Fig. 17**). Contusions of the lateral femoral condyle or the lateral tibial plateau can occur, either from direct lateral impact or from indirect axial impaction of the lateral femoral condyle and tibial plateau on joint-space closure, with a potential resulting osteochondral lesion.[38,74] Opening and widening of the medial joint space can produce an associated traction or avulsion injury at the MCL attachment points.[24] Pure valgus mechanisms commonly injure the MCL, POL, medial capsular ligament, and often the ACL (**Fig. 18**) with resulting anteromedial instability, and possible straight medial instability if the PCL is also disrupted.[3,8] Identification of cruciate ligament injury is critical in valgus injuries with high-grade MCL tear, because associated cruciate ligament damage can cause instability at all ranges of flexion, and may necessitate early surgical intervention.[18,38]

Pure varus injury

Impact on the medial aspect of the extended knee is less common, but can produce a primarily varus injury pattern with imaging findings that mirror those seen with valgus injuries: contusion of the medial femoral condyle or medial tibia, and damage to the lateral stabilizers of the knee (**Fig. 19**).

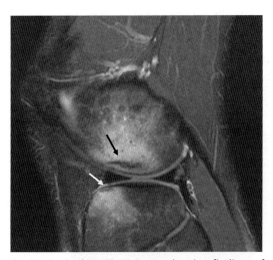

Fig. 16. Sagittal PD FS MR image showing findings of a knee hyperextension injury sustained following an anterior impact during tibial external rotation. Characteristic contusions of the anterolateral femoral (*black arrow*) and tibial (*white arrow*) articular surfaces are present, with underlying subchondral impaction fractures. Low-grade injuries to the MCL and POL were noted (not shown).

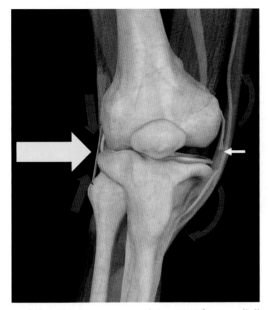

Fig. 17. Computer-generated image of a medially directed impact force vector (*yellow arrow*) on the lateral aspect of the extended knee, causing valgus knee angulation with closing of the lateral joint space (*straight red arrows*), concomitant opening of the medial joint space (*curved red arrows*), and disruption of the MCL (*white arrow*).

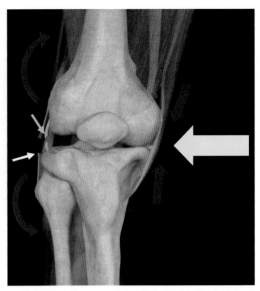

Fig. 19. Computer-generated image of a laterally directed impact force vector (*yellow arrow*) on the medial aspect of the extended knee, causing varus knee angulation with closure of the medial joint space (*straight red arrows*) and concomitant opening of the lateral joint space (*curved red arrows*), with disruption of the FCL (*white arrow*) and popliteus tendon (*orange arrow*).

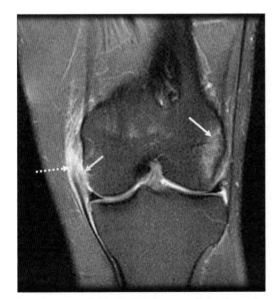

Fig. 18. Coronal PD FS MR image of the knee following pure valgus injury. A direct impact on the lateral femoral condyle causes a characteristic bone contusion (*solid white arrow*), with medial joint opening causing high-grade injury to the proximal MCL (*dotted white arrow*) and underlying meniscofemoral ligament (*yellow arrow*).

Injuries to the FCL and posterolateral corner structures are more destabilizing than medial knee ligament injuries, owing to the relatively higher static tension on the lateral ligaments during normal ambulation,[13] and often require primary surgical repair for acute high-grade injury.[6] Experimental studies suggest that the FCL is likely to fail first under varus loading,[75] with resulting increased varus knee laxity at low levels of flexion and possible posterolateral rotatory instability. Injuries to the lateral capsular ligament, biceps femoris tendon, arcuate ligaments, and popliteus myotendinous unit, and potentially the ITB are also seen (**Fig. 20**). With a posterolateral corner injury, a coexisting ACL injury will exacerbate resultant posterolateral or anterolateral rotatory instability, whereas an associated full-thickness PCL injury will produce marked straight lateral instability.[8,13] As previously mentioned, postoperative graft failure may occur if coexisting cruciate and posterolateral corner injuries are not both addressed surgically.

Anterior tibial translation injury

A direct impact onto the posterior aspect of the fully extended knee can cause anterior tibial

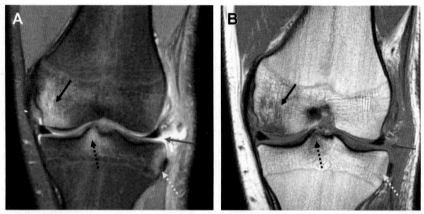

Fig. 20. (*A*) Coronal PD FS and (*B*) coronal PD MR images of the knee following a pure varus knee injury. An impact on the medial aspect of the knee causes varus angulation with medial knee joint closure, and resulting osseous contusion to the medial femoral condyle (*solid black arrows*), which is likely due to a combination of direct medial and axial impaction. There is corresponding opening of the lateral joint space with disruption of the FCL and meniscotibial portion of the lateral capsular ligament (*red arrows*), with fluid noted underneath the lateral meniscus. Bone edema of the lateral tibial plateau (*dotted yellow arrows*) is likely due to traction at the posterior aspect of the iliotibial band (ITB) insertion on the Gerdy tubercle, suggestive of ITB injury. Subcortical edema within the medial tibial eminence and subtle cortical disruption (*dotted black arrows*) indicate an avulsive injury to the ACL tibial attachment.

translation and a resulting contact ACL injury (**Fig. 21**).[4,8,76,77] However, ACL injuries are more commonly indirect noncontact injuries, often resulting from flexion combination injury mechanisms (described next) or excessive axial loading on landing, or, importantly, on rapid change of direction at near full extension or with mild knee

flexion.[76] With sudden direction change during knee extension, a high quadriceps-patella tendon angle ensures a high shear component force from the strong eccentric quadriceps contraction, which overpowers the posterior stabilizing effect of the weaker hamstring muscles, resulting in excessive anterior tibial translation and ACL shear

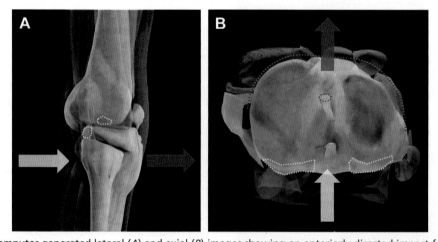

Fig. 21. Computer-generated lateral (*A*) and axial (*B*) images showing an anteriorly directed impact force vector on the posterior aspect of the extended knee (*yellow arrow*), causing anterior translation of the proximal tibia (*red arrows*). The ACL (*dotted red circle*), medial and lateral capsular ligaments, and anterior capsule are at particular risk of injury (*dotted red line*). Characteristic contusions of the medial and lateral femoral condyles and corresponding posterior aspect of the medial and lateral tibial plateaus are often seen (*dashed yellow areas*). This injury pattern can also commonly occur as a result of strong quadriceps contraction in knee extension, overpowering the weaker posterior hamstring muscles and causing anterior tibial translation without a direct posterior impact (*yellow arrow*).

injury.[2,22,23,76] The risk of ACL injury may be exacerbated with increasing tibial internal rotation, owing to the increased static tension of the coiled cruciate ligaments.[2] Contusions of the posterior aspect of the lateral tibial plateau and central or anterior aspect of the lateral femoral condyle, termed kissing contusions, are generally characteristic of ACL injuries, owing to anterior tibial translation and impaction. However, noncontact mechanisms without significant valgus loading also commonly show a similar kissing-contusion pattern of the medial femoral condyle and medial tibial plateau, owing to more symmetric anterior displacement with less of a rotational component (**Fig. 22**).[23] Although isolated ACL injury and mild straight anterior instability may occur with these mechanisms, if marked straight anterior instability or anteromedial/anterolateral rotatory instability is present, it is likely that the ACL and medial and/or lateral capsular ligaments are injured.[2,8]

Flexion Combination Injuries

With increasing flexion, the knee demonstrates less anatomic stability to rotation, abduction, and adduction forces. Injuries during flexion therefore more commonly involve some degree of internal or external rotation, and associated varus or valgus angulation, than do injuries in extension. Meniscal injuries are also more commonly seen during flexion, as increased anatomic rotational knee laxity during flexion can lead to trapping of the meniscus posteriorly during a significant rotational force, and subsequent knee extension can cause shearing of the meniscal surface in a "trap-and-twist" mechanism.[2,61]

Impact onto the lateral aspect of the flexed knee can commonly produce a valgus and external rotation injury pattern, although this can also occur with noncontact mechanisms. A similar injury pattern can occur on the contralateral side of the

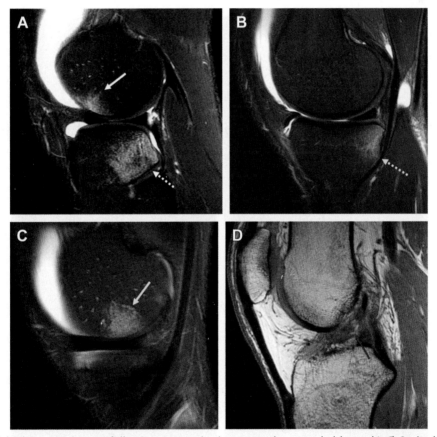

Fig. 22. Multiplanar MR images following a posterior impact to the extended knee. (*A–C*) Sagittal T2 FS and (*D*) sagittal PD images show contusions to the lateral femoral condyle (*solid white arrow*) and posterior aspect of the lateral tibial plateau (*dotted white arrow*), and the posterior aspect of the medial tibial plateau (*dotted yellow arrow*) and medial femoral condyle (*solid yellow arrow*). The contusions are presumed to be due to anterior tibial translation and subsequent impaction, owing to the high-grade tear of the ACL (*red arrow*). which appears wavy with disrupted fibers.

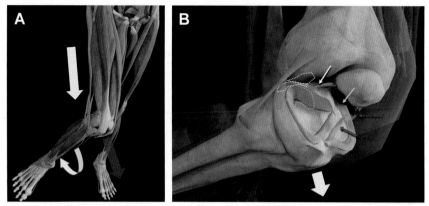

Fig. 23. Computer-generated anterolateral view (*A*) of the knee during a pivot-shift injury. Loading of the knee occurs along the axis of the femur (*straight yellow arrow*) with the foot planted, and the knee flexed and in external tibial rotation (*curved yellow arrow*). The resulting force vector (*red arrow*) causes combined anterior translation, valgus angulation, and exacerbated external rotation of the proximal tibia. Anterolateral view (*B*) following anterior tibial translation (*yellow arrow*) shows disruption of the ACL (*solid red arrow*), and opening of the medial joint space with valgus angulation causing injury to the MCL (*dotted red arrow*), POL, and/or medial capsular ligament. Characteristic contusions of the lateral femoral condyle and the posterior aspect of the lateral tibial plateau are most often seen (*dashed yellow areas*). Meniscal injuries due to shear forces produced during tibial rotation are commonly seen, and attention should be directed to the posterior horn of the medial meniscus, which may be disrupted because of a "trap-and-twist" mechanism with the medial femoral condyle (*orange arrow*) and the posterior horn of the lateral meniscus (*dashed green area*), which may be torn owing to traction on the ligament of Wrisburg (*white arrow*).

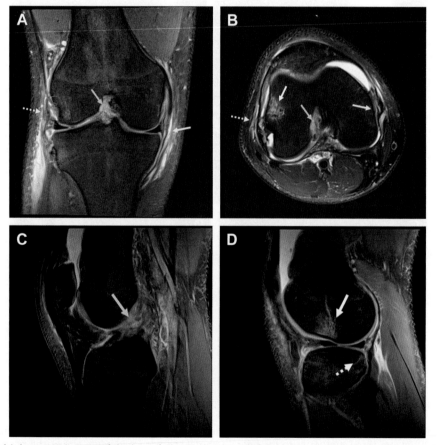

Fig. 24. Multiplanar MR images of the knee following a pivot-shift injury to the knee in flexion and relative tibial external rotation. (*A*) Coronal, (*B*) axial, and (*C*) sagittal PD FS images show hyperintense signal within the disrupted ACL (*orange arrows*), a grade II MCL injury (*solid yellow arrows*), and likely minimal FCL and lateral capsular injury (*dotted yellow arrows*). Note is made of a lateral femoral condyle contusion (*solid white arrow*). (*D*) Sagittal PD FS image of the lateral compartment further shows contusions of the lateral femoral articular surface (*solid white arrow*) and posterior aspect of the lateral tibial plateau (*dotted white arrow*).

knee following a varus and internal rotation injury mechanism, which is less commonly due to a direct medial impact. A direct impact onto the anterior aspect of the flexed knee can produce a translation or shear injury to the structures of the knee. Finally, progressive knee flexion and external rotation during weight bearing can cause lateral patellar dislocation without preceding traumatic impact.

Flexion with valgus and external rotation (pivot shift)

Internal rotation of the femur on a flexed knee with the foot planted produces a combination of valgus knee angulation and, most commonly, external rotation of the tibia, termed the pivot-shift injury (**Fig. 23**).[8,24,61] This mechanism is common in skiers and American football players, owing to simultaneous rapid deceleration and direction

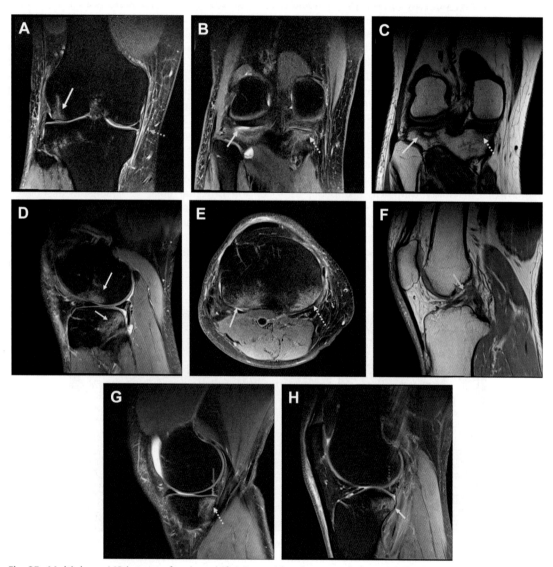

Fig. 25. Multiplanar MR images of a pivot-shift injury with valgus angulation and tibial external rotation components. (*A, B*) Coronal PD FS, (*C*) coronal PD, (*D*) sagittal PD FS, and (*E*) axial PD FS images show a characteristic lateral femoral condyle contusion (*solid white arrows*), and osteochondral impaction injury to the posterolateral tibial plateau (*yellow arrows*). An impaction fracture of the posteromedial tibial plateau is also seen, likely caused by contrecoup impaction (*dotted yellow arrows*). A grade I MCL injury is present (*dotted orange arrow*). (*F*) Sagittal PD image at the level of the intercondylar notch confirms complete disruption of the ACL (*orange arrow*). Additional sagittal PD FS images at the level of the medial (*G*) and lateral (*H*) compartments show a vertical longitudinal tear of the posterior horn of the medial meniscus (*solid red arrow*), and similar complex vertical tear of the posterior horn lateral meniscus (*dotted red arrow*) overlying the medial (*dotted yellow arrow*) and lateral (*solid yellow arrow*) tibial plateau impaction injuries.

change.[24] The ACL and MCL are maximally loaded during flexion and valgus stress, resulting in medial distraction and joint-space opening, with further exacerbation if tibial internal rotation occurs.[74] Disruption of the ACL and MCL allows anterior translation of the tibia about the flexed and abducted knee, producing a characteristic kissing-contusion pattern whereby the lateral femoral condyle impacts the posterior aspect of the lateral tibial plateau (**Fig. 24**).[24] Contusions of the medial tibial plateau can also occur posteriorly, possibly because of contrecoup impaction or semimembranosus tendon avulsion.[24,61] The pivot-shift injury pattern most commonly results in anteromedial rotatory instability, owing to distraction injury to the MCL, medial capsular ligament, ACL, and often also the POL.[8] Injuries to the ACL, MCL, and medial meniscus have been described as the triad of O'Donoghue, although lateral meniscus injuries are more common in the acute setting.[74,78,79] Damage to the posterior horn of the lateral meniscus is also commonly seen in anteromedial instability with ACL disruption, as previously discussed, possibly attributable to traction on the ligament of Wrisburg at the time of ACL injury.[8,63,64,80] Medial meniscus posterior horn and body tears, in addition to bucket-handle tears, are often observed, although the

acuity or chronicity of these injuries remains controversial (**Fig. 25**).[2,38,58,80]

Flexion with varus and internal rotation

A less common variation of flexion combination injuries can occur during external rotation of the femur with the knee in flexion and the foot planted, with resulting varus angulation and relative internal rotation of the tibia producing distraction of the lateral knee and posterolateral corner (**Fig. 26**).[61] This injury can also be seen with sudden cutting maneuvers or rapid deceleration, and is less commonly due to a medial impact. The osseous injury pattern of this mechanism is similar to that of the classic pivot-shift injury, including contusions or osteochondral injury to the lateral femoral condyle and posterolateral tibial plateau, and is again generally seen with ACL disruption.[8,61] Anterolateral rotatory instability may result, owing to potential injury to the ACL, lateral capsular ligament, and arcuate complex.[5,8,13,14] The Segond fracture, an avulsion fracture of the lateral aspect of the proximal tibia, is noticeably associated with these varus and tibial internal rotation mechanisms. This fracture may reflect avulsion of the lateral capsular ligament, anterior oblique band of the FCL, or iliotibial tract, and is strongly associated with ACL injury (**Fig. 27**).[71,81,82] As discussed

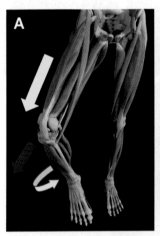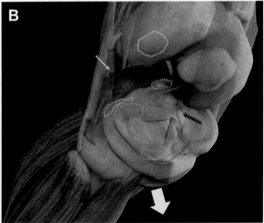

Fig. 26. (*A*) Computer-generated anterior view of the flexed knee during varus and tibial internal rotation injury. Loading of the knee occurs along the axis of the femur (*straight yellow arrow*) with the foot planted, and the knee flexed and in internal tibial rotation (*curved yellow arrow*). The resulting force vector (*red arrow*) causes combined anterior translation, varus angulation, and exacerbated internal rotation of the proximal tibia. (*B*) Anterolateral view following anterior tibial translation (*yellow arrow*) and tibial rotation shows disruption of the ACL (*red arrow*), and opening of the lateral joint space with varus angulation causing injury to the FCL (*dotted red arrow*) and arcuate complex structures, in addition to myotendinous injury to the popliteus muscle (*orange arrow*). Characteristic contusions of the lateral femoral condyle and the posterior aspect of the lateral tibial plateau are most often seen with continued tibial rotation and translation with subsequent impaction (*dashed yellow areas*). Similar to the external rotation pivot-shift injury, injuries to the posterior horn of the medial and lateral menisci can be seen, but characteristic injury to the anterior horn of the lateral meniscus is also often noted (*dashed green areas*).

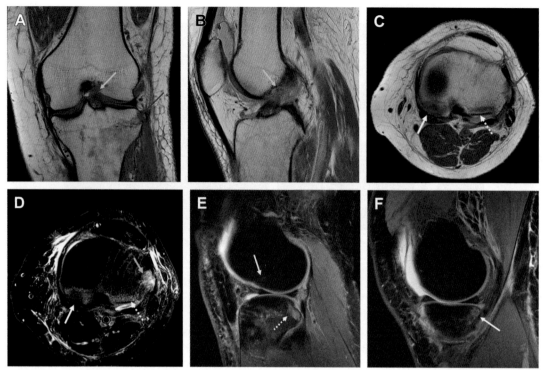

Fig. 27. Multiplanar MR images of the knee showing a knee injury in flexion with varus angulation and internal rotation. (*A*) Coronal and (*B*) sagittal PD MR images show a tiny cortical avulsion fracture of the lateral margin of the proximal tibia (*red arrow*), consistent with a Segond fracture. Increased signal within the ACL with apparent hypointense fiber disruption (*orange arrows*) is consistent with a full-thickness tear. (*C*) Axial PD and (*D*) PD FS images show a small avulsed fragment (*red arrow*) with a relatively small area of associated hyperintense bone marrow edema (*blue arrow*). Impaction fractures of the medial (*solid white arrows*) and lateral (*dotted white arrows*) tibial plateaus are also noted. (*E*) Sagittal PD FS image of the lateral compartment and (*F*) sagittal PD FS image of the medial compartment show a subtle contusion of the lateral femoral condyle (*yellow arrow*), and impaction injuries of the lateral (*dotted white arrow*) and medial (*solid white arrow*) tibial plateaus posteriorly.

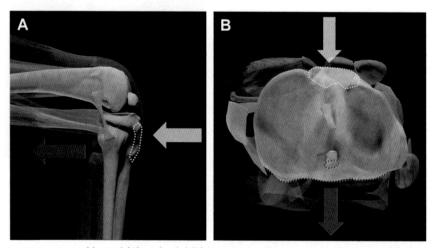

Fig. 28. Computer-generated lateral (*A*) and axial (*B*) images showing a posteriorly directed impact force vector (*yellow arrows*) on the anterior aspect of the proximal tibia with the knee flexed, generating posterior translation of the tibia (*red arrows*). The PCL (*dotted red ellipse*) can be injured in isolation, although the reinforcing posterior capsule is often also disrupted (*dotted red line*). There is occasionally a characteristic contusion to the anterior margin of the proximal tibia or tibial tuberosity (*dotted yellow areas*), although this is inconsistently present. The POL and posterolateral corner are usually not injured with this mechanism, but should be evaluated if significant instability is present.

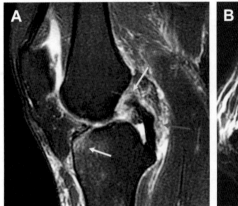
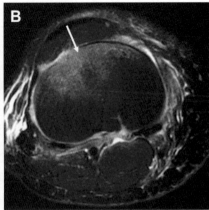

Fig. 29. Multiplanar MR images of the knee obtained following a dashboard-type injury mechanism caused by a fall onto a flexed knee. (*A*) Sagittal and (*B*) axial T2 FS images show a full-thickness tear of the PCL near its femoral attachment (*yellow arrow*). A broad contusion of the anterior margin of the proximal tibia is due to direct impact onto the flexed knee (*white arrows*). Edema is noted within the soft tissues posterior to the knee, with apparent disruption of the posterior capsule (*red arrow*).

earlier, the presence of a fibular head avulsion indicates more severe damage to the arcuate complex of the posterolateral corner. These fractures can be occult, and warrant special attention in the setting of the classic contusion pattern and lateral knee soft-tissue injury, because significant anterolateral or posterolateral rotatory instability may result. Anterolateral rotatory instability is often associated with a characteristic injury to the anterior horn of the lateral meniscus, although posterior horn medial and lateral meniscus injuries are also commonly noted in the setting of associated ACL disruption.[8,13,63,64,80]

Flexion with anterior impact

With increasing knee flexion the collateral ligaments become relatively lax and the ACL is relatively shortened and unloaded, leaving the PCL to provide most of the posterior stabilization of the flexed knee, reinforced by the posterior capsule.[8,12,22] Therefore, in flexion with an anterior impact mechanism, a significant posterior tibial translation force sustained during knee flexion approaching 90° can cause PCL injury with possible capsular injury, resulting in 1-plane posterior instability. These injuries have been termed dashboard injuries because of the commonly observed injury mechanism in automobile accidents of the anterior margin of the proximal tibia impacting the dashboard of a car with the knee flexed. A fall sustained onto a flexed knee may also have a similar injury pattern (**Fig. 28**).[24,61] Contusions of the tibial tuberosity or anterior tibial margin are commonly seen on early MR imaging after direct impact,[24] but may not be present if there is significant delay before imaging is obtained, possibly

because of delayed identification of subtle clinical instability (**Fig. 29**). Although an isolated PCL tear is generally rare, these injuries are often clinically occult in the acute setting. Therefore, attention to

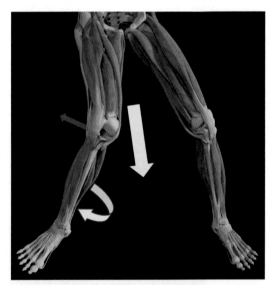

Fig. 30. Computer-generated anterior view of the knee during lateral patellar dislocation. Axial loading of the knee along the axis of the femur (*straight yellow arrow*) during slight knee flexion and significant tibial external rotation (*curved yellow arrow*) with both feet planted causes lateral subluxation of the patella (*red arrow*). On continued flexion, the patella fully dislocates and impacts the lateral femoral condyle, causing characteristic kissing contusions and medial patellar retinaculum and medial patellofemoral ligament injury. Note that the rectus femoris muscle and quadriceps tendon are partially transparent for improved patellar visualization.

the PCL and posterior capsule is warranted on subsequent MR imaging in the setting of predisposing mechanism or characteristic contusion pattern; untreated PCL tears can lead to chronic posterior instability, resulting from progressive stretching and increasing laxity of the overstressed posteromedial and posterolateral ligamentous structures over time.[3,12] If significant posterior instability is present acutely, particularly in extension, considerable posterolateral and posteromedial corner injuries are also likely to be present.[3,8,49] Occasionally PCL avulsion of its femoral attachment or, more commonly, its tibial attachment posteriorly, can be seen.[24,49] Finally, one must bear in mind that posterior displacement of the tibia caused by hyperextension mechanisms can also occur with a characteristic anterior tibial and femoral margin kissing-contusion pattern, a critical distinction to recognize given the more

severe soft-tissue injuries generally seen with hyperextension mechanisms.[49]

Patella dislocation

In knee extension, the patella takes a lateral position in the intercondylar groove and is under slight valgus tension, as discussed earlier. On initiation of flexion, internal rotation of the mildly flexed knee with the foot planted produces relative external tibial rotation. With sufficiently rapid tibial external rotation, the patella may dislocate laterally beyond the intercondylar groove and become wedged on the lateral femoral condyle (**Fig. 30**). Subsequent quadriceps contraction will cause potentially destabilizing injury to the medial patellar retinaculum and MPFL.[24,61] This mechanism can occur with altered weight bearing, with increased loading of the affected side during bending or crouching. This injury mechanism produces

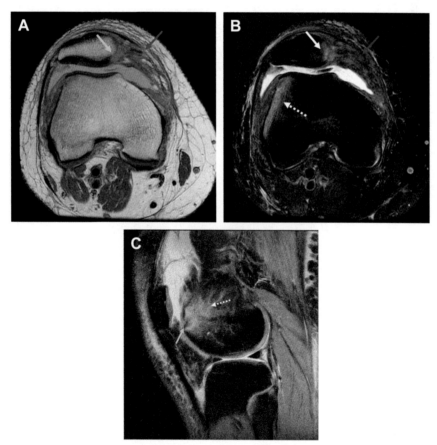

Fig. 31. Multiplanar MR images of the knee following patella dislocation. (*A*) Axial PD and (*B*) axial PD FS images show disruption of the hypointense medial patella retinaculum (*red arrows*), with characteristic kissing contusions of the medial margin of the patella (*solid white arrow*) and lateral femoral condyle (*dotted white arrow*), along with an associated full-thickness chondral defect of the medial patella facet (*orange arrow*). (*C*) Sagittal PD FS image of the same injury again illustrates a lateral femoral condylar contusion (*dotted white arrow*), with a small impaction injury (*orange arrow*).

Table 2
Summary of common injury mechanisms, the most distinguishing imaging findings, associated destabilizing injuries, and the more common resulting instability patterns

	Injury Mechanism	Key Imaging Findings	Destabilizing Injuries	Resulting Instability
Hyperextension	Neutral	Anterior femoral and tibial contusions, posterolateral and posteromedial corner injuries	PCL, POL, arcuate complex, ACL	Straight posterior
	With varus	Anteromedial femoral and tibial contusions, posterolateral corner injuries	Lateral capsular ligament, arcuate complex, ACL, ± PCL	Posterolateral rotatory or straight lateral
	With valgus	Anterolateral femoral and tibial contusions, posteromedial corner injuries	MCL, POL, medial capsular ligament, ACL, ± PCL	Straight medial, ± posteromedial rotatory[a]
Extension	Pure varus	Ipsilateral joint space osseous impact injuries, contralateral joint-space distraction injuries	Lateral capsular ligament, FCL, posterolateral corner, ACL, PCL (rarely)	Anterolateral or posterolateral rotatory, or straight lateral
	Pure valgus		MCL, POL, medial capsular ligament, ACL, PCL (rarely)	Anteromedial rotatory, or straight medial
	Anterior tibial translation	ACL disruption, ± classic mid-femoral and posterior tibial contusions bilaterally	ACL, medial and lateral capsular ligaments	Anteromedial or anterolateral rotatory, or straight anterior
Flexion	Valgus and external tibial rotation	ACL disruption with lateral femoral and tibial contusions, medial distraction injuries	ACL, MCL, medial capsular ligament, POL	Anteromedial rotatory
	Varus and internal tibial rotation	ACL disruption with lateral femoral and tibial contusions	ACL, lateral capsular ligament, arcuate complex	Anterolateral or posterolateral rotatory
	Anterior impact	PCL injury ± anterior tibial contusion	PCL	Straight posterior
	Patella subluxation	Kissing contusions of the medial patella and lateral femoral condyle, medial retinaculum disruption	Medial retinaculum and MPFL	Recurrent patella subluxation

Abbreviation: MPFL, medial patellofemoral ligament.
[a] Posteromedial rotatory instability is controversial, but is unlikely in the presence of an intact PCL, and straight instability is more common if the PCL is disrupted.

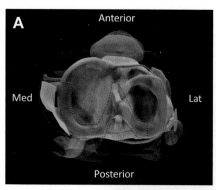
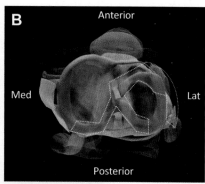
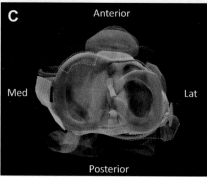

Fig. 32. Computer-generated view of the knee showing locations of common injury constellations seen with different forms of rotatory instability. The tibial articular surface is viewed en face from a superior perspective, and the femoral condyles are partially transparent for improved visualization. Mechanisms that produce (*A*) anteromedial rotatory instability most often demonstrate injury to the medial capsular ligament, the MCL, POL, and ACL, and often show longitudinal tears of the posterior horns of the medial and lateral menisci if the causative mechanism contains a significant rotatory component (*dotted red area*). Mechanisms that produce (*B*) anterolateral rotatory instability most often demonstrate injury to the lateral capsular ligament but also often show injuries to the ITB, ACL, and arcuate complex, and can show characteristic injury to the anterior horn of the lateral meniscus, and the posterior horns of the medial and lateral menisci if the ACL is disrupted (*dotted yellow area*). Mechanisms producing (*C*) posterolateral rotatory instability often demonstrate injuries to the lateral capsular ligament, arcuate complex, popliteus musculotendinous unit, partial PCL tear, and occasional injury to the anterior horn of the medial meniscus (*dotted blue areas*). The presence of full-thickness PCL tear in the setting of these injury patterns suggests more severe straight or 1-plane instability rather than true rotatory instability. Lat, lateral; Med, medial.

characteristic kissing contusions of the medial patellar facet and anterolateral aspect of the lateral femoral condyle (**Fig. 31**). Overlying osteochondral injuries are commonly seen. The patella often returns to the intercondylar groove by the time MR imaging is performed, but usually maintains some degree of excess resting lateralization, and suspicion for dislocation should therefore be raised in the setting of a characteristic contusion pattern or lateralization.[83] Injury to the MPFL and medial retinaculum are most commonly graded under a standard lexicon, with complete disruption seen as discontinuity of the normally hypointense ligaments best seen on axial T2 FS or gradient-echo sequences, often with retracted or wavy fibers and intervening edema.[83] Attention should be directed to identifying the site of ligamentous

injury, as disruption of the MPFL near the femoral attachment or avulsion injury of the MPFL attachment at the adductor tubercle of the femur may necessitate early surgical repair.[84] Surgery is also often pursued in the presence of significant clinical instability or osteochondral injury.[84] Additional signs of dislocation include vastus medialis obliquus (VMO) musculotendinous injury or VMO elevation from the medial femoral condyle, owing to underlying effusion or hemorrhage.[24,83]

SUMMARY

MR imaging evaluation of traumatic osseous and soft-tissue lesion patterns can aid in identification of the mechanism of knee injury, and can suggest the type and degree of resulting knee instability

(Table 2). If clinical instability is present but the cruciate ligaments are intact, rotatory instability should be suspected, with different types and magnitudes of rotatory instability resulting from specific injury patterns (Fig. 32). Complete disruption of the cruciate ligaments, particularly the PCL, will most commonly produce straight or 1-plane instability, which is exacerbated by additional osseous and soft-tissue injuries. Thus, recognition of the likely injury mechanism can better direct the radiologist's attention to potentially occult associated lesions, and can aid in the identification or evaluation of clinical knee instability.

REFERENCES

1. Scott WN. Anatomy. In: Scott WN, Insall JN, editors. Insall & Scott surgery of the knee. 5th edition. Philadelphia: Elsevier/Churchill Livingstone; 2012. p. 2–45.

2. Miller RH, Azar FM. Knee injuries. In: Campbell WC, Canale ST, Beaty JH, editors. Campbell's operative orthopaedics. 11th edition. Philadelphia: Mosby/Elsevier; 2008. p. 2395–600.

3. Hughston JC, Andrews JR, Cross MJ, et al. Classification of knee ligament instabilities. Part I. The medial compartment and cruciate ligaments. J Bone Joint Surg Am 1976;58(2):159–72.

4. Nicholas JA. The five-one reconstruction for anteromedial instability of the knee. Indications, technique, and the results in fifty-two patients. J Bone Joint Surg Am 1973;55(5):899–922.

5. Recondo JA, Salvador E, Villanua JA, et al. Lateral stabilizing structures of the knee: functional anatomy and injuries assessed with MR imaging. Radiographics 2000;20(Spec No):S91–102.

6. Covey DC. Injuries of the posterolateral corner of the knee. J Bone Joint Surg Am 2001;83-A(1):106–18.

7. Zantop T, Herbort M, Raschke MJ, et al. The role of the anteromedial and posterolateral bundles of the anterior cruciate ligament in anterior tibial translation and internal rotation. Am J Sports Med 2007; 35(2):223–7.

8. Chung CB, Lektrakul N, Resnick D. Straight and rotational instability patterns of the knee: concepts and magnetic resonance imaging. Radiol Clin North Am 2002;40(2):203–16.

9. Lerat JL, Moyen BL, Cladiere F, et al. Knee instability after injury to the anterior cruciate ligament. Quantification of the Lachman test. J Bone Joint Surg Br 2000;82(1):42–7.

10. Butler DL, Noyes FR, Grood ES. Ligamentous restraints to anterior-posterior drawer in the human knee. A biomechanical study. J Bone Joint Surg Am 1980;62(2):259–70.

11. Gollehon DL, Torzilli PA, Warren RF. The role of the posterolateral and cruciate ligaments in the stability of the human knee. A biomechanical study. J Bone Joint Surg Am 1987;69(2):233–42.

12. Scott WN. Decision making and surgical treatment of posterior cruciate ligament ruptures. In: Scott WN, Insall JN, editors. Insall & Scott surgery of the knee. 5th edition. Philadelphia: Elsevier/Churchill Livingstone; 2012. p. 494–538.

13. Hughston JC, Andrews JR, Cross MJ, et al. Classification of knee ligament instabilities. Part II. The lateral compartment. J Bone Joint Surg Am 1976; 58(2):173–9.

14. Zantop T, Schumacher T, Diermann N, et al. Anterolateral rotational knee instability: role of posterolateral structures. Winner of the AGA-DonJoy Award 2006. Arch Orthop Trauma Surg 2007; 127(9):743–52.

15. Vinson EN, Major NM, Helms CA. The posterolateral corner of the knee. AJR Am J Roentgenol 2008;190(2):449–58.

16. Grood ES, Noyes FR, Butler DL, et al. Ligamentous and capsular restraints preventing straight medial and lateral laxity in intact human cadaver knees. J Bone Joint Surg Am 1981;63(8):1257–69.

17. Scott WN. Classification of knee ligament injuries. In: Scott WN, Insall JN, editors. Insall & Scott surgery of the knee. 5th edition. Philadelphia: Elsevier/Churchill Livingstone; 2012. p. 318–38.

18. Wijdicks CA, Griffith CJ, Johansen S, et al. Injuries to the medial collateral ligament and associated medial structures of the knee. J Bone Joint Surg Am 2010;92(5):1266–80.

19. Phisitkul P, James SL, Wolf BR, et al. MCL injuries of the knee: current concepts review. Iowa Orthop J 2006;26:77–90.

20. Scott WN. Disorders of the patellofemoral joint. In: Scott WN, Insall JN, editors. Insall & Scott surgery of the knee. 5th edition. Philadelphia: Elsevier/Churchill Livingstone; 2012. p. 592–623.

21. Phillips BB. Recurrent dislocations. In: Campbell WC, Canale ST, Beaty JH, editors. Campbell's operative orthopaedics. 11th edition. Philadelphia: Mosby/Elsevier; 2008. p. 2655–735.

22. Yu B, Garrett WE. Mechanisms of non-contact ACL injuries. Br J Sports Med 2007;41(Suppl 1):i47–51.

23. Viskontas DG, Giuffre BM, Duggal N, et al. Bone bruises associated with ACL rupture: correlation with injury mechanism. Am J Sports Med 2008; 36(5):927–33.

24. Sanders TG, Medynski MA, Feller JF, et al. Bone contusion patterns of the knee at MR imaging: footprint of the mechanism of injury. Radiographics 2000;20(Spec No):S135–151.

25. Bohndorf K. Imaging of acute injuries of the articular surfaces (chondral, osteochondral and subchondral fractures). Skeletal Radiol 1999;28(10):545–60.

26. Mink JH, Deutsch AL. Occult cartilage and bone injuries of the knee: detection, classification, and

assessment with MR imaging. Radiology 1989; 170(3 Pt 1):823–9.

27. Vellet AD, Marks PH, Fowler PJ, et al. Occult posttraumatic osteochondral lesions of the knee: prevalence, classification, and short-term sequelae evaluated with MR imaging. Radiology 1991; 178(1):271–6.

28. Rangger C, Kathrein A, Freund MC, et al. Bone bruise of the knee: histology and cryosections in 5 cases. Acta Orthop Scand 1998;69(3):291–4.

29. Palmer WE, Levine SM, Dupuy DE. Knee and shoulder fractures: association of fracture detection and marrow edema on MR images with mechanism of injury. Radiology 1997;204(2):395–401.

30. Eustace S, Keogh C, Blake M, et al. MR imaging of bone oedema: mechanisms and interpretation. Clin Radiol 2001;56(1):4–12.

31. Blankenbaker DG, De Smet AA, Vanderby R, et al. MRI of acute bone bruises: timing of the appearance of findings in a swine model. AJR Am J Roentgenol 2008;190(1):W1–7.

32. Boks SS, Vroegindeweij D, Koes BW, et al. MRI follow-up of posttraumatic bone bruises of the knee in general practice. AJR Am J Roentgenol 2007;189(3):556–62.

33. Boks SS, Vroegindeweij D, Koes BW, et al. Follow-up of occult bone lesions detected at MR imaging: systematic review. Radiology 2006;238(3):853–62.

34. Nakamae A, Engebretsen L, Bahr R, et al. Natural history of bone bruises after acute knee injury: clinical outcome and histopathological findings. Knee Surg Sports Traumatol Arthrosc 2006;14(12): 1252–8.

35. Roemer FW, Bohndorf K. Long-term osseous sequelae after acute trauma of the knee joint evaluated by MRI. Skeletal Radiol 2002;31(11): 615–23.

36. Hughston JC. The importance of the posterior oblique ligament in repairs of acute tears of the medial ligaments in knees with and without an associated rupture of the anterior cruciate ligament. Results of long-term follow-up. J Bone Joint Surg Am 1994; 76(9):1328–44.

37. Kaplan P. Musculoskeletal MRI. 1st edition. Philadelphia: Saunders; 2001.

38. Stoller DW. The knee. In: Stoller DW, editor. Magnetic resonance imaging in orthopaedics and sports medicine. 3rd edition. Philadelphia: Lippincott Williams & Wilkins; 2007. p. 553–77.

39. Schweitzer ME, Tran D, Deely DM, et al. Medial collateral ligament injuries: evaluation of multiple signs, prevalence and location of associated bone bruises, and assessment with MR imaging. Radiology 1995;194(3):825–9.

40. Yao L, Dungan D, Seeger LL. MR imaging of tibial collateral ligament injury: comparison with clinical examination. Skeletal Radiol 1994;23(7):521–4.

41. Haims AH, Medvecky MJ, Pavlovich R Jr, et al. MR imaging of the anatomy of and injuries to the lateral and posterolateral aspects of the knee. AJR Am J Roentgenol 2003;180(3):647–53.

42. Sanders TG, Miller MD. A systematic approach to magnetic resonance imaging interpretation of sports medicine injuries of the knee. Am J Sports Med 2005;33(1):131–48.

43. Brandser EA, Riley MA, Berbaum KS, et al. MR imaging of anterior cruciate ligament injury: independent value of primary and secondary signs. AJR Am J Roentgenol 1996;167(1):121–6.

44. Cobby MJ, Schweitzer ME, Resnick D. The deep lateral femoral notch: an indirect sign of a torn anterior cruciate ligament. Radiology 1992; 184(3):855–8.

45. Graf BK, Cook DA, De Smet AA, et al. "Bone bruises" on magnetic resonance imaging evaluation of anterior cruciate ligament injuries. Am J Sports Med 1993;21(2):220–3.

46. Vahey TN, Hunt JE, Shelbourne KD. Anterior translocation of the tibia at MR imaging: a secondary sign of anterior cruciate ligament tear. Radiology 1993;187(3):817–9.

47. Umans H, Wimpfheimer O, Haramati N, et al. Diagnosis of partial tears of the anterior cruciate ligament of the knee: value of MR imaging. AJR Am J Roentgenol 1995;165(4):893–7.

48. DeFranco MJ, Bach BR Jr. A comprehensive review of partial anterior cruciate ligament tears. J Bone Joint Surg Am 2009;91(1):198–208.

49. Sonin AH, Fitzgerald SW, Friedman H, et al. Posterior cruciate ligament injury: MR imaging diagnosis and patterns of injury. Radiology 1994; 190(2):455–8.

50. Rodriguez W Jr, Vinson EN, Helms CA, et al. MRI appearance of posterior cruciate ligament tears. AJR Am J Roentgenol 2008;191(4):1031.

51. Huang GS, Yu JS, Munshi M, et al. Avulsion fracture of the head of the fibula (the "arcuate" sign): MR imaging findings predictive of injuries to the posterolateral ligaments and posterior cruciate ligament. AJR Am J Roentgenol 2003;180(2): 381–7.

52. Scott WN. Internal derangements: ligaments and tendons. In: Scott WN, Insall JN, editors. Insall & Scott surgery of the knee. 5th edition. Philadelphia: Elsevier/Churchill Livingstone; 2012. p. 87–105.

53. Azar FM. Traumatic disorders. In: Campbell WC, Canale ST, Beaty JH, editors. Campbell's operative orthopaedics. 11th edition. Philadelphia: Mosby/Elsevier; 2008. p. 2737–88.

54. Noonan TJ, Garrett WE Jr. Injuries at the myotendinous junction. Clin Sports Med 1992;11(4):783–806.

55. Palmer WE, Kuong SJ, Elmadbouh HM. MR imaging of myotendinous strain. AJR Am J Roentgenol 1999;173(3):703–9.

56. Noonan TJ, Garrett WE Jr. Muscle strain injury: diagnosis and treatment. J Am Acad Orthop Surg 1999;7(4):262–9.

57. Mueller-Wohlfahrt HW, Haensel L, Mithoefer K, et al. Terminology and classification of muscle injuries in sport: the Munich consensus statement. Br J Sports Med 2012;47(6):342–50.

58. De Smet AA. How I diagnose meniscal tears on knee MRI. AJR Am J Roentgenol 2012;199(3):481–99.

59. Stoller DW, Martin C, Crues JV 3rd, et al. Meniscal tears: pathologic correlation with MR imaging. Radiology 1987;163(3):731–5.

60. Scott WN. Internal derangements: menisci and cartilage. In: Scott WN, Insall JN, editors. Insall & Scott surgery of the knee. 5th edition. Philadelphia: Elsevier/Churchill Livingstone; 2012. p. 106–23.

61. Hayes CW, Brigido MK, Jamadar DA, et al. Mechanism-based pattern approach to classification of complex injuries of the knee depicted at MR imaging. Radiographics 2000;20(Spec No):S121–134.

62. Smillie IS. The current pattern of internal derangements of the knee joint relative to the menisci. Clin Orthop Relat Res 1967;51:117–22.

63. Brody JM, Lin HM, Hulstyn MJ, et al. Lateral meniscus root tear and meniscus extrusion with anterior cruciate ligament tear. Radiology 2006; 239(3):805–10.

64. De Smet AA, Blankenbaker DG, Kijowski R, et al. MR diagnosis of posterior root tears of the lateral meniscus using arthroscopy as the reference standard. AJR Am J Roentgenol 2009;192(2):480–6.

65. Lerer DB, Umans HR, Hu MX, et al. The role of meniscal root pathology and radial meniscal tear in medial meniscal extrusion. Skeletal Radiol 2004;33(10):569–74.

66. Pula DA, Femia RE, Marzo JM, et al. Are root avulsions of the lateral meniscus associated with extrusion at the time of acute anterior cruciate ligament injury?: a case control study. Am J Sports Med 2013;42(1):173–6.

67. Sharma L, Eckstein F, Song J, et al. Relationship of meniscal damage, meniscal extrusion, malalignment, and joint laxity to subsequent cartilage loss in osteoarthritic knees. Arthritis Rheum 2008; 58(6):1716–26.

68. Schlossberg S, Umans H, Flusser G, et al. Bucket handle tears of the medial meniscus: meniscal intrusion rather than meniscal extrusion. Skeletal Radiol 2007;36(1):29–34.

69. Barber BR, McNally EG. Meniscal injuries and imaging the postoperative meniscus. Radiol Clin North Am 2013;51(3):371–91.

70. Rubin DA, Britton CA, Towers JD, et al. Are MR imaging signs of meniscocapsular separation valid? Radiology 1996;201(3):829–36.

71. Gottsegen CJ, Eyer BA, White EA, et al. Avulsion fractures of the knee: imaging findings and clinical significance. Radiographics 2008;28(6):1755–70.

72. Fornalski S, McGarry MH, Csintalan RP, et al. Biomechanical and anatomical assessment after knee hyperextension injury. Am J Sports Med 2008;36(1):80–4.

73. Scott WN. Imaging of osseous knee trauma. In: Scott WN, Insall JN, editors. Insall & Scott surgery of the knee. 5th edition. Philadelphia: Elsevier/Churchill Livingstone; 2012. p. e49–64.

74. MacMahon PJ, Palmer WE. A biomechanical approach to MRI of acute knee injuries. AJR Am J Roentgenol 2011;197(3):568–77.

75. Maynard MJ, Deng X, Wickiewicz TL, et al. The popliteofibular ligament. Rediscovery of a key element in posterolateral stability. Am J Sports Med 1996;24(3):311–6.

76. Boden BP, Dean GS, Feagin JA Jr, et al. Mechanisms of anterior cruciate ligament injury. Orthopedics 2000;23(6):573–8.

77. Kennedy JC, Fowler PJ. Medial and anterior instability of the knee. An anatomical and clinical study using stress machines. J Bone Joint Surg Am 1971; 53(7):1257–70.

78. Shelbourne KD, Nitz PA. The O'Donoghue triad revisited. Combined knee injuries involving anterior cruciate and medial collateral ligament tears. Am J Sports Med 1991;19(5):474–7.

79. Yoon KH, Yoo JH, Kim KI. Bone contusion and associated meniscal and medial collateral ligament injury in patients with anterior cruciate ligament rupture. J Bone Joint Surg Am 2011;93(16): 1510–8.

80. Cipolla M, Scala A, Gianni E, et al. Different patterns of meniscal tears in acute anterior cruciate ligament (ACL) ruptures and in chronic ACL-deficient knees. Classification, staging and timing of treatment. Knee Surg Sports Traumatol Arthrosc 1995;3(3):130–4.

81. Campos JC, Chung CB, Lektrakul N, et al. Pathogenesis of the Segond fracture: anatomic and MR imaging evidence of an iliotibial tract or anterior oblique band avulsion. Radiology 2001;219(2):381–6.

82. Goldman AB, Pavlov H, Rubenstein D. The Segond fracture of the proximal tibia: a small avulsion that reflects major ligamentous damage. AJR Am J Roentgenol 1988;151(6):1163–7.

83. Diederichs G, Issever AS, Scheffler S. MR imaging of patellar instability: injury patterns and assessment of risk factors. Radiographics 2010;30(4): 961–81.

84. Sillanpaa PJ, Maenpaa HM. First-time patellar dislocation: surgery or conservative treatment? Sports Med Arthrosc 2012;20(3):128–35.

Quantitative Magnetic Resonance Imaging of the Articular Cartilage of the Knee Joint

Richard Kijowski, MD*, Rajeev Chaudhary, BS

KEYWORDS

- Cartilage • Magnetic resonance imaging • Quantitative • Proteoglycan • Collagen • Review

KEY POINTS

- Quantitative magnetic resonance imaging can be used to noninvasively assess the composition and ultrastructure of articular cartilage.
- Quantitative magnetic resonance imaging can be used in clinical practice to detect early cartilage degeneration.
- Quantitative magnetic resonance imaging can be used in osteoarthritis research studies to monitor disease-related and treatment-related changes in articular cartilage over time.

INTRODUCTION

Osteoarthritis is one of the most common chronic medical conditions and is second only to cardiovascular disease as the leading cause of disability in the United States.[1–5] Osteoarthritis may be caused by idiopathic or posttraumatic degeneration of articular cartilage. Characteristic changes in articular cartilage occur during the disease process including a decrease in the proteoglycan content and disruption of the highly organized collagen fiber network.[6–11] Identifying the sequence of events that occur during cartilage degeneration is essential for better understanding of the pathogenesis of osteoarthritis and developing improved treatment options. Quantitative magnetic resonance (MR) imaging provides a noninvasive method to assess cartilage composition and ultrastructure. This article reviews the role of quantitative MR imaging for evaluating the articular cartilage of the knee joint, which is one of the joints most commonly affected by osteoarthritis.

CARTILAGE COMPOSITION AND FUNCTION

Articular cartilage is composed of chondrocytes, which compose approximately 4% of the net weight of the tissue, and an abundant extracellular matrix. The extracellular matrix of cartilage consists primarily of water, composing between 65% and 85% of its net weight, and lower concentrations of proteoglycan and type II collagen.[12,13] Proteoglycan composes 3% to 10% of the net weight of cartilage and allows the tissue to withstand high compressive forces during joint loading. Collagen composes 15% to 20% of the net weight of cartilage and is responsible for the tensile strength of the tissue.[12,13] Articular cartilage is devoid of lymphatics, blood vessels, and

The authors have no disclosures regarding subject matter or materials discussed in the article.

Department of Radiology, University of Wisconsin School of Medicine and Public Health, 600 Highland Avenue, Madison, WI 53792-3252, USA

* Corresponding author. Department of Radiology, University of Wisconsin School of Medicine and Public Health, Clinical Science Center - E3/311, 600 Highland Avenue, Madison, WI 53792-3252.

E-mail address: rkijowski@uwhealth.org

Magn Reson Imaging Clin N Am 22 (2014) 649–669
http://dx.doi.org/10.1016/j.mric.2014.07.005
1064-9689/14/$ – see front matter © 2014 Elsevier Inc. All rights reserved.

nerves, limiting its potential for healing and repair.[13] Thus, preservation of the cartilage macromolecular matrix is vital to joint health.

The macromolecular matrix of articular cartilage is composed of type II collagen organized in a complex 3-dimensional orientation, which provides tensile strength and determines tissue anisotropy.[14] The articular surface is covered by the lamina splendins; dense bundles of collagen fibers lubricated by a proteoglycan called lubricin; and synovial fluid, which allows for low friction load transmission across the joint.[15] The superficial zone of cartilage is composed of collagen fibers and elongated chondrocytes orientated parallel to the articular surface, whereas the middle zone is characterized by a random orientation of collagen fibers intermixed with round chondrocytes. The deep zone of cartilage consists of thick bundles of collagen fibers and elongated chondrocytes oriented perpendicular to the bone-cartilage interface. The radially oriented collagen fibers in

the deeper layer of cartilage pass through the calcified zone to attach to subchondral bone (**Fig. 1**).[13]

The major proteoglycan constituent of articular cartilage is aggrecan, which is composed of a core protein with alternating domains of the negatively charged sulfated glycosaminoglycan side chains keratan sulfate and chondroitin sulfate. Aggrecans are assembled into a macromolecular structure of monomers, which are bound to a hyaluronan backbone through a link protein. The core protein of aggrecan consists of 3 globular domains (G1, G2, and G3) and 3 interglobular domains.[16] The G1 domain resides on the N-terminus and interacts with the link protein to attach aggrecan to the hyaluronan backbone, whereas the G3 domain is located at the C-terminus of the glycoprotein. Located between the G2 and G3 domains are the attachment domains, which link the keratan sulfate and chondroitin sulfate side chains to the core protein (**Fig. 2**).[17]

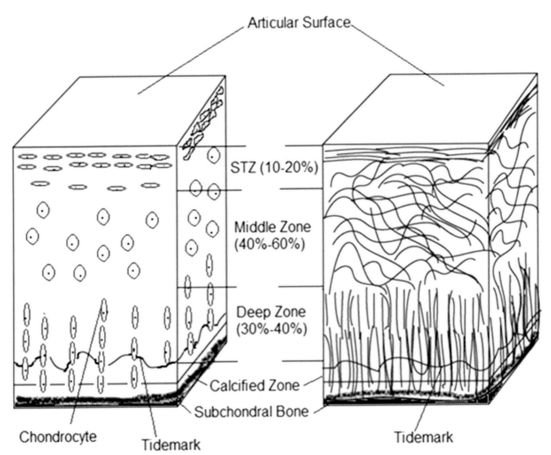

Fig. 1. Articular cartilage divided into its histologic zones. The image depicts the cellular structure and organization as well as the collagen fiber orientation of cartilage from surface to bone. Note the randomness of collagen fibers in the middle zone of cartilage. STZ, superficial zone. (*Adapted from* Xia Y. Averaged and depth-dependent anisotropy of articular cartilage by microscopic imaging. Semin Arthritis Rheum 2008;37(5):317–27.)

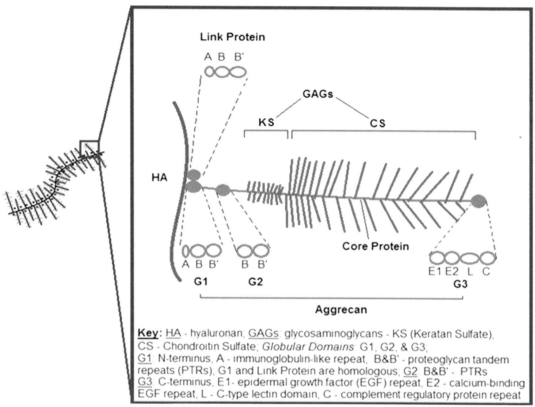

Key: HA - hyaluronan; GAGs: glycosaminoglycans - KS (Keratan Sulfate), CS - Chondroitin Sulfate; *Globular Domains:* G1, G2, & G3; G1: N-terminus, A - immunoglobulin-like repeat, B&B' - proteoglycan tandem repeats (PTRs); G1 and Link Protein are homologous; G2: B&B' - PTRs G3: C-terminus, E1- epidermal growth factor (EGF) repeat, E2 - calcium-binding EGF repeat, L - C-type lectin domain, C - complement regulatory protein repeat

Fig. 2. The macromolecular structure of aggrecan within articular cartilage. (*Adapted from* Aspberg A. The different roles of aggrecan interaction domains. J Histochem Cytochem 2012; 60(12):987–96; with permission.)

The negative charge of the densely packed glycosaminoglycan chains of aggrecan become fixed to the extracellular matrix, called a *fixed charge*; the concentration of this fixed charge is termed the *fixed charge density of articular cartilage*.[16,18] The fixed charge density attracts water and positively charged ions from the synovial fluid. This produces a swelling pressure built up by the electrostatic repulsion between the glycosaminoglycan side chains in the cartilage extracellular matrix, which provides the underlying viscoelastic properties necessary for load distribution.[16,18,19] However, the swelling pressure is constrained by the collagen fiber network, which provides the tensile force opposing the expansion of cartilage. Thus, the complex structure of the cartilage extracellular matrix requires a delicate balance between the compressive forces of aggrecan and the tensile strength of the collagen fiber network for normal function.

SODIUM IMAGING

Sodium imaging can be used to assess the fixed charge density of articular cartilage. Sodium-23 atoms are associated with the negatively charged glycosaminoglycan side chains of proteoglycan macromolecules within cartilage. Decreased proteoglycan concentration within cartilage reduces the fixed charge density, which results in a decreased concentration of sodium ions. Thus, measurement of the sodium signal within cartilage can provide sensitive and specific information regarding the proteoglycan concentration of the tissue. Previous studies have reported strong correlations between the sodium concentration within cartilage measured using sodium imaging and nuclear MR spectroscopy.[20] Furthermore, the concentration of sodium within both native and trypsin degraded ex vivo cartilage samples measured using sodium imaging has been shown to correlate strongly with proteoglycan concentration.[21–23]

Sodium imaging is a promising method for evaluating articular cartilage but is technically challenging. The signal from sodium-23 atoms within cartilage is very low because of its low natural abundance and its reduced gyromagnetic ratio. These factors along with the very short T2 relaxation time of sodium-23 atoms make measuring sodium concentration within cartilage extremely difficult. Two-dimensional and 3-dimensional Cartesian-based sequences have been used for sodium imaging, but scan times are very long even when using high-field-strength 7.0-T scanners.[24–26] Three-dimensional non–Cartesian-based techniques using radial,[27] cone,[28] and twisted projection[29] k-space trajectories have more recently been used to improve the signal-to-noise ratio (SNR) and reduce the scan time for sodium imaging.

Additional limitation of sodium imaging is the need for specialized transmit and receive coils tuned to the resonance frequency of sodium-23 atoms and the difficulty in differentiating the sodium signal arising from articular cartilage and adjacent tissues, such as synovial fluid. Various techniques have been developed to suppress the sodium signal from synovial fluid, including the use of inversion recovery pulses[30,31] and T1-weighted sequences with short repetition times.[32] With the use of more SNR-efficient 3-dimensional non–Cartesian-based imaging techniques and improved methods for suppressing synovial fluid signal, sodium concentration within articular cartilage can be measured with high repeatability and with reasonable scan times.[33,34] Sodium imaging has been used in multiple studies to detect differences in proteoglycan concentration between asymptomatic volunteers and patients with osteoarthritis[32,35] and to monitor changes in the proteoglycan concentration of cartilage repair tissue over time (**Figs. 3 and 4**).[26,36,37]

DELAYED GADOLINIUM-ENHANCED IMAGING

Delayed gadolinium-enhanced imaging (DGEMRIC) measures the T1 relaxation time of articular cartilage in the presence of gadolinium contrast. DGEMRIC can be used to indirectly assess the fixed charge density of cartilage, as the distribution of negatively charged gadolinium contrast within cartilage is in theory indirectly proportional to the concentration of negatively charged glycosaminoglycan side chains of proteoglycan macromolecules. Decreased proteoglycan concentration within cartilage allows accumulation of more gadolinium contrast, which results in more rapid T1 relaxation of adjacent water protons within cartilage.

There is strong evidence to suggest that DGEMRIC can provide a sensitive and specific measure of the proteoglycan concentration of articular cartilage. The T1 relaxation time of both native and enzymatically degraded ex vivo cartilage samples in the presence of gadolinium contrast has been shown to strongly correlate with the proteoglycan concentration of cartilage.[38–44] DGEMRIC measurements have also been found to correlate strongly with the compressive stiffness of cartilage, which is primarily determined by the proteoglycan concentration within the macromolecular matrix.[45–47] Multiple studies have also shown that the T1 relaxation time of cartilage in the presence of gadolinium contrast is higher in the deep than in the superficial layers of cartilage and on the weight-bearing than non–weight-bearing surfaces of the knee joint, which corresponds to the spatial distribution of proteoglycan within cartilage.[42,45,46]

DGEMRIC requires the administration of a double dose of gadolinium contrast followed by a 10-minute exercise period and then a 60- to 120-minute waiting period before T1 relaxation time measurements can be performed.[48,49] The administration of a triple dose of gadolinium contrast has

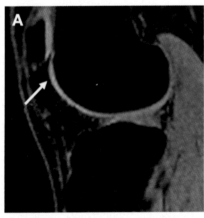
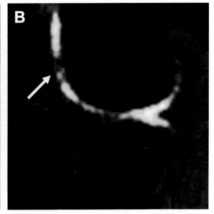

Fig. 3. (*A*) Sagittal fat-suppressed spoiled gradient-echo image in a patient 10 years after anterior cruciate ligament reconstruction surgery shows morphologically normal articular cartilage on the femoral trochlea (*arrow*). (*B*) Corresponding sagittal sodium image shows decreased sodium concentration within the articular cartilage on the femoral trochlea (*arrow*) indicating early proteoglycan loss. (*Courtesy of* Garry Gold, MD, Stanford University, Stanford, CA.)

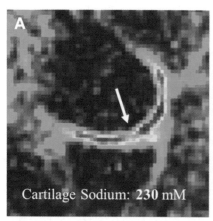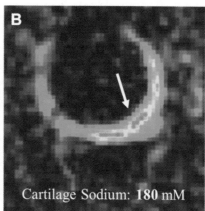

Fig. 4. (A) Sagittal sodium image in an asymptomatic volunteer shows high sodium concentration within the articular cartilage on the medial femoral condyle (arrow). (B) Sagittal sodium image in a patient with Kellgren-Lawrence grade 1 osteoarthritis shows lower sodium concentration within the articular cartilage on the medial femoral condyle (arrow) indicating early proteoglycan loss. (Courtesy of Ravinder Regatte, PhD, New York University, New York, NY.)

been found to improve the sensitivity of the technique for detecting early cartilage degeneration.[49] The disadvantages of DGEMRIC include the long waiting time between contrast administration and MR imaging and the small risk of allergic reactions and even smaller risk of nephrogenic systemic sclerosis with use of ionic gadolinium contrast.[50,51] Initially, T1 relaxation time measurements were performed both before and following the administration of gadolinium contrast; the change in T1 relaxation time was used to assess cartilage composition.[38–44,48,49,52] However, the current DGEMRIC protocols typically measure T1 relaxation time only following gadolinium contrast administration to reduce the scan time, as this measurement has been shown to correlate strongly with both the change in T1 relaxation time[53] and the concentration of proteoglycan within cartilage.[38,40]

T1 relaxation time measurements of articular cartilage in DGEMRIC protocols were originally performed using 2-dimensional inversion recovery fast spin-echo and 3-dimensional inversion recovery spoiled gradient echo sequences with long scan times.[48,49,54] More rapid 3-dimensional techniques for T1 relaxation time measurements including look-locker[55,56] and variable flip-angle[57,58] methods with complementary flip-angle correction have recently been developed. With the use of these new techniques, the T1 relaxation time measurement of articular cartilage following gadolinium contrast administration can be performed with high repeatability and in relatively short scan times.[59–61] However, DGEMRIC measurements within articular cartilage can be influenced by the degree of cartilage loading.[62]

Furthermore, the presence of gadolinium can have deleterious effects on the accuracy of both the T2 relaxation time[63] and the thickness measurements[64] of articular cartilage.

DGEMRIC has been used in multiple studies to detect changes in the proteoglycan concentration of articular cartilage. Animal models of osteoarthritis have shown a decreased T1 relaxation time of cartilage following gadolinium contrast administration, which corresponds to areas of proteoglycan loss on histologic analysis.[65,66] DGEMRIC has been shown to have high sensitivity for detecting surgically and histologically confirmed early cartilage degeneration in human subjects.[52,67] Studies have also found lower T1 relaxation times of cartilage following gadolinium contrast administration in patients with higher radiographic grades of knee osteoarthritis indicating greater proteoglycan loss in individuals with more severe joint degeneration.[68] Decreased T1 relaxation time of articular cartilage after gadolinium contrast administration has been reported in patients following an anterior cruciate ligament tear[69,70] and meniscetomy[71] indicating that DGEMRIC can detect early posttraumatic cartilage degeneration within the knee joint (Fig. 5). DGEMRIC has also been used to monitor changes in the proteoglycan concentration of cartilage following cartilage repair procedures.[37,72–75]

T1-rho MAPPING

T1-rho mapping uses a long-duration and low-power radiofrequency pulse applied to magnetization in the transverse plane which effectively spin-locks the magnetization around the B1 field and prevents T2 relaxation. T1-rho relaxation

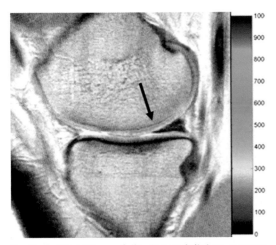

Fig. 5. Sagittal T1 map following gadolinium contrast administration in a patient 3 weeks after anterior cruciate ligament injury shows decreased T1 relaxation time within the articular cartilage on the medial femoral condyle (*arrow*) indicating early proteoglycan loss caused by acute cartilage injury. (*Courtesy of* Carl Tiderius, MD, PhD, Lund, Sweden.)

time is the time constant of the exponential decay of magnetization during application of the spin-lock pulse. T1-rho relaxation time is influenced by low-frequency molecular interactions between water molecules and their local macromolecular environment, with water protons in close proximity to macromolecules having a greater dissipation of energy during the spin-lock pulse than free water protons. T1-rho relaxation time is always longer than T2 relaxation time, as the B1 field attenuates the effects of bipolar interactions, chemical exchange, and static dipolar coupling on signal decay.[76,77]

Initial applications of T1-rho mapping consisted of single-slice acquisitions through articular cartilage.[78,79] Multi-slice T1-rho sequences were later developed based on multi-echo fast spin-echo[80] and spiral[81] imaging methods, but scan times remained long. Various 3-dimensional T1-rho techniques are now available that combine a spin-lock pulse to create T1-rho contrast with gradient-echo acquisition methods that use parallel imaging to reduced scan time.[82,83] The currently used 3-dimensional techniques can measure the T1-rho relaxation time of articular cartilage with high repeatability and in relatively short scan times.[84,85] However, a disadvantage of T1-rho imaging is the relatively large radiofrequency power applied during the spin-lock preparation pulse, which creates problems with the specific absorption rate and tissue heating, especially when using high-field-strength scanners.

T-rho relaxation time is influenced by low-frequency molecular interactions between water

molecules and the cartilage macromolecular matrix.[76] The exchange of protons between water molecules and the hydroxyl and amine groups on the glycosaminoglycan side chains of proteoglycan macromolecules is thought to be the primary mechanism for T1-rho dispersion within cartilage.[77] A strong correlation has been found between the T1-rho relaxation time of cartilage and the fixed charge density measured using sodium imaging.[86] Multiple studies have also shown that the T1-rho relaxation time of both native and enzymatically degraded ex vivo cartilage samples is strongly correlated with the proteoglycan concentration of cartilage.[87–90] However, T1-rho relaxation time is not a specific measure of the proteoglycan concentration of cartilage and is also influenced by other biological changes, which occur during cartilage degeneration,[91,92] the orientation of cartilage relative to the main magnetic field,[93] and the degree of cartilage loading.[94]

T1-rho mapping has been used in multiple studies to detect changes in the macromolecular matrix of articular cartilage in patients with osteoarthritis. The T1-rho relaxation time of cartilage has been found to increase with age[95] and early cartilage degeneration (**Fig. 6**).[96] Studies have shown that T1-rho relaxation time is more sensitive than T2 relaxation time for detecting early cartilage degeneration in both ex vivo specimens[97] and human subjects.[98,99] Texture analysis of the spatial distribution of T1-rho within cartilage has been found to provide even better identification of early cartilage degeneration than global T1-rho relaxation time measurements.[100] Elevated T1-rho within cartilage in patients with osteoarthritis has also been shown to predict the progression of cartilage degeneration over time.[101]

T1-rho mapping also has been used to evaluate posttraumatic and postsurgical changes in articular cartilage. Increased T1-rho relaxation times in areas of acute cartilage injury have been reported in patients with anterior cruciate ligament tears and have been shown to persist at the 1-year follow-up despite the resolution of underlying bone marrow edema.[102–104] Studies have also found significantly higher T1-rho relaxation time within the articular cartilage of the medial compartment of the knee joint in patients with anterior cruciate ligament injury when compared with asymptomatic volunteers at both 1-year and 2-year follow-up periods indicating the presence of early posttraumatic cartilage degeneration (**Fig. 7**).[105,106] T1-rho mapping has also been used to monitor changes in the macromolecular matrix of articular cartilage following cartilage repair procedures (**Fig. 8**).[107,108]

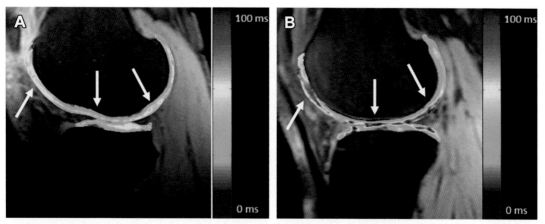

Fig. 6. (*A*) Sagittal T1-rho map in an asymptomatic volunteer shows normal T1-rho relaxation time within the articular cartilage on the femoral trochlea and medial femoral condyle (*arrows*). (*B*) Sagittal T1-rho map in a patient with Kellgren-Lawrence grade 1 osteoarthritis shows increased T1-rho relaxation time within the articular cartilage on the femoral trochlea and medial femoral condyle (*arrows*) indicating early cartilage degeneration. (*Courtesy of* Ravinder Regatte, PhD, New York University, New York, NY.)

T2 MAPPING

T2 mapping measures the spin-spin relaxation time of articular cartilage. When dipoles are aligned in a static magnetic field and a 90° radiofrequency pulse is applied, the dipoles absorb energy. This absorption of energy makes them unstable, and they start to relax back to equilibrium by dispersing energy within the spin system itself or transferring it out of the spin system to the lattice. The T2 relaxation time reflects the time it takes the dipoles to disperse energy following excitation.[109] The T2 relaxation time of cartilage is a complex measurement that is influenced by multiple factors, including water and macromolecular concentration,[110–113] organization of the collagen fiber network,[114–116] cartilage loading,[117–119] and orientation of cartilage relative to the main magnetic field.[120] Thus, changes in the T2 relaxation time of cartilage may be difficult to interpret because of the multiple competing biological and mechanical factors that influence the measurement.

The highly organized macromolecular matrix of articular cartilage restricts the motion of water molecules and enhances dipole-dipole interactions, which shorten the T2 relaxation time of cartilage. These dipole-dipole interactions are dictated by the geometric factor $3\cos^2\theta-1$ of the z-component

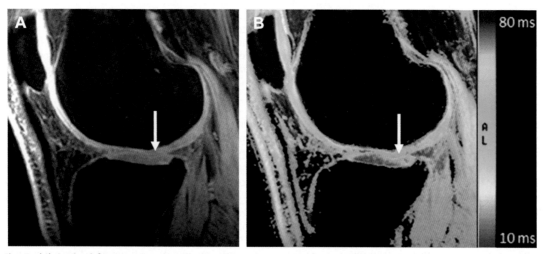

Fig. 7. (*A*) Sagittal fat-suppressed spoiled gradient-echo image in a patient 3 years after anterior cruciate ligament reconstruction surgery shows morphologically normal articular cartilage on the medial tibial plateau (*arrow*). (*B*) Corresponding sagittal T1-rho map shows increased T1-rho relaxation time within the articular cartilage on the medial tibial plateau (*arrow*) indicating early cartilage degeneration.

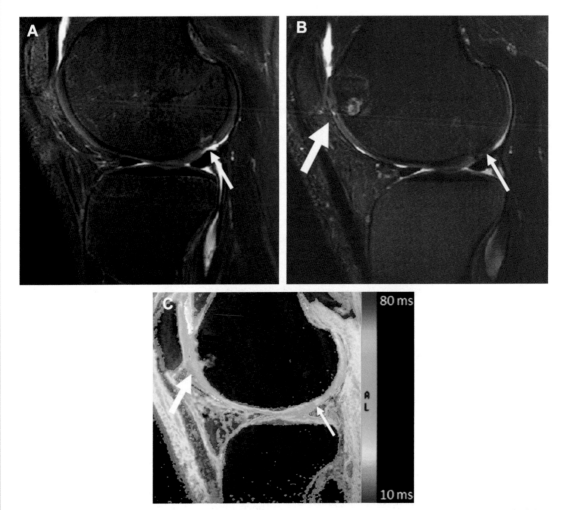

Fig. 8. (*A*) Sagittal fat-suppressed T2-weighted fast spin-echo image in a patient with acute traumatic injury shows a focal cartilage defect on the medial femoral condyle (*arrow*). (*B*) Sagittal fat-suppressed T2-weighted fast spin-echo image in the same patient 1 year following autologous chondrocyte transplantation shows complete fill in of the cartilage defect on the medial femoral condyle (*small arrow*). The patient also underwent abrasion chondroplasty of the donor site defect on the femoral trochlea, which is partially filled in with cartilage (*large arrow*). (*C*) Corresponding sagittal T1-rho map shows normal T1-rho relaxation time within the articular cartilage on the medial femoral condyle (*small arrow*). However, there is increased T1-rho relaxation time within the articular cartilage on the femoral trochlea (*large arrow*) indicating failure to restore normal cartilage composition and ultrastructure following abrasion chondroplasty.

of the electromagnetic field. Consequently, when $\theta = 54.7°$, the interactions go to zero, and an increase in T2 relaxation time is observed, which is referred to as the *magic angle effect*.[120–125] The magic angle effect in cartilage is thought to be caused by the orientation-dependent effect on the T2 relaxation time of water bound to collagen.[114,115,121,126] Thus, the T2 relaxation time of cartilage may provide information regarding collagen fiber orientation and the integrity of the collagen fiber network.[115,116,126–129] However, water bound to collagen has an extremely short T2 relaxation time of approximately 2.2 milliseconds,

which cannot be directly measured using most T2 relaxation time techniques.[130–135] Therefore, the magic angle effect is likely influenced by interactions between collagen-bound water and the other measurable water components, either through water exchange or the influence of collagen fiber orientation on the orientation of other cartilage constituents.[120,129]

The exact relationship between the T2 relaxation time and chemical composition of articular cartilage remains unknown with conflicting reports in the literature. Some enzymatic degradation studies have shown that proteoglycan depletion of ex vivo cartilage samples using trypsin results in increased T2 relaxation time,[112,136] whereas other studies have found no such change in T2 relaxation time with proteoglycan depletion.[22,88,137] Collagenase degradation of ex vivo cartilage samples has been shown to increase T2 relaxation time in one study suggesting that collagen content may also influence the T2 relaxation time of cartilage.[137] Studies comparing the T2 relaxation time of articular cartilage with biochemical measurements of water, proteoglycan, and collagen content have also reported inconsistent findings. Some studies using human cartilage specimen obtained during total knee arthroplasty have found an inverse correlation between the T2 relaxation time and the proteoglycan content of cartilage,[111,113] whereas other studies using similar methodology have found no such relationship.[93] Although increased hydration of articular cartilage should theoretically lead to an increase in T2 relaxation time, not all studies have shown a direct correlation between the T2 relaxation time and the water content of ex vivo cartilage samples.[110,111]

T2 mapping techniques can measures the T2 relaxation time of articular cartilage on a pixel-by-pixel basis by acquiring images at multiple echo times and fitting the signal decay using a nonlinear least squares algorithm.[138] Originally, T2 mapping was performed using single-slice 2-dimensional spin-echo sequences with extremely long scan times.[139] The introduction of fast spin-echo methods have greatly improved the speed of T2 mapping, but the drawback of these techniques is that slice-selective refocusing pulses can lead to stimulated echo signal from the presence of nonrectangular slice select profiles caused by an inhomogeneous B1 field.[140,141] Three-dimensional spoiled gradient-echo techniques have more recently been developed for T2 mapping, which provide thin continuous slices through articular cartilage and eliminate the need for slice-selective refocusing pulses, which reduce the risk of excess signal in and between slices caused by simulated echoes.[142] Currently used techniques can measure the T2 relaxation time of articular cartilage with high repeatability and in relatively short scan times.[84] However, the T2 relaxation time of cartilage is influenced by multiple factors, including the type of sequence, imaging parameters, and radiofrequency coil used to obtain the measurement, which is important to consider when performing longitudinal or multicenter studies.[142–144]

T2 mapping has been extensively used to evaluate the composition and ultrastructure of articular cartilage in patients with osteoarthritis. The T2 relaxation time of cartilage has been shown to increase with age, especially in the superficial layer where senescent changes tend to occur.[145,146] T2 relaxation time has been shown to have high sensitivity for detecting early cartilage degeneration in ex vivo specimens[93] and human subjects (Fig. 9).[147–151] Higher T2 relaxation time of cartilage has also been reported in patients with increasing radiographic grades of osteoarthritis.[147] In addition, higher and more heterogeneous cartilage T2 relaxation time has been noted in subjects with risk factors for osteoarthritis when compared with asymptomatic volunteers despite both groups of individuals having normal

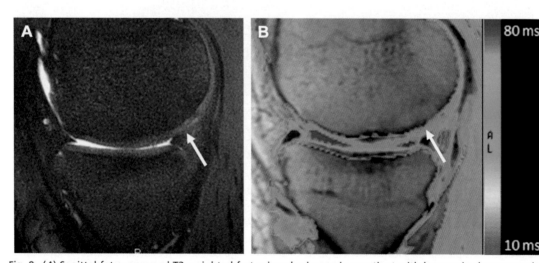

Fig. 9. (A) Sagittal fat-suppressed T2-weighted fast spin-echo image in a patient with knee pain shows morphologically normal articular cartilage on the medial femoral condyle (arrow) in an area where cartilage fibrillation was identified at arthroscopy. (B) Corresponding sagittal T2 map shows increased T2 relaxation time within the articular cartilage on the medial femoral condyle (arrow) indicating early cartilage degeneration.

radiographs.[152,153] Associations between higher cartilage T2 relaxation time and the presence of cartilage lesions,[153] meniscus tears,[154] bone marrow edema lesions,[155] and knee pain[156] have been reported. Higher T2 relaxation time of articular cartilage has also been shown to predict the progression of focal cartilage lesions within the knee joint in longitudinal studies.[157]

T2 mapping has also been used to evaluate post-traumatic and postsurgical changes in articular cartilage. Studies have found elevated T2 relaxation time within the posterior lateral tibial plateau in areas of acute cartilage injury during the early phase after anterior cruciate ligament tear,[102,103] which persisted at both the 1-year[102,105] and 2-year[106] follow-up despite resolution of adjacent bone marrow lesions. Longitudinal follow-up in the same group of patients has demonstrated increased T2 relaxation time within the central medial femoral condyle 2 years after injury with higher T2 values in individuals with associated meniscus tears.[105] Another cross-sectional study using the healthy contralateral knee as a reference to the injured knee has shown elevated cartilage T2 relaxation time within the medial femoral condyle 6 months following anterior cruciate ligament reconstruction surgery.[158] In addition, increased T2 relaxation time within the articular cartilage of the tibial plateau has been reported in patients with meniscus tears.[159] T2 mapping has also been used to monitor changes in the macromolecular matrix of articular cartilage following cartilage repair procedures.[160–164] Restoration of the normal zonal stratification of T2 relaxation time with increasing values from the deep to the superficial layers has been shown to correspond to maturation of the cartilage repair tissue over time (**Fig. 10**).[161]

ULTRASHORT ECHO TIME IMAGING

Ultrashort echo time (UTE) imaging can be used to investigate the short T2 components of articular cartilage. Spin-echo and gradient-echo techniques typically used for cartilage imaging have minimum echo times ranging between 2 milliseconds and 10 milliseconds and, thus, cannot detect signal from water protons in the deep and calcified zones of cartilage where highly organized collagen fibers contribute to very short T2 relaxation times.[165] UTE imaging uses echo times as short as 0.08 milliseconds, which can capture signal from the short T2 components of cartilage. However, UTE imaging assesses effective T2 relaxation time (T2*), which is influenced by tissue susceptibility and magnetic field inhomogeneity along with the T2 relaxation characteristics of cartilage.

Various UTE techniques have been used for evaluating articular cartilage. Most 2-dimensional UTE sequences use a radial k-space trajectory with a half excitation pulse followed by another half excitation pulse with the polarity of the slice selection gradient reversed.[166,167] Three-dimensional UTE sequences typically use a short hard pulse excitation followed by 3-dimensional ramp sampling.[168,169] Conspicuity of the short T2 components on UTE images can be enhanced

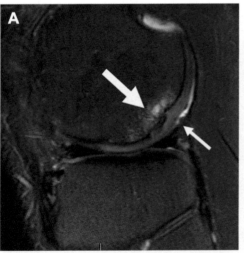
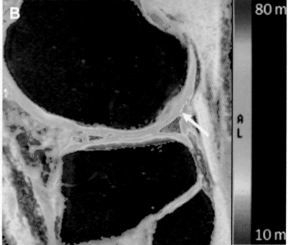

Fig. 10. (A) Sagittal fat-suppressed T2-weighted fast spin-echo image in a patient 1 year following autologous chondrocyte transplantation shows complete fill in of the cartilage defect on the lateral femoral condyle (*small arrow*) with cysts and edema present at the graft-bone interface (*large arrow*). (B) Corresponding sagittal T2 map shows increased T2 relaxation time within the articular cartilage on the lateral femoral condyle (*arrow*) indicating failure to restore normal cartilage composition and ultrastructure following autologous chondrocyte transplantation.

by suppressing signal from fat and long T2 components through the use of saturation or inversion nulling techniques.[168,170,171] Quantitative assessment of articular cartilage using UTE T2* mapping can be performed by acquiring images with multiple echo times, with the lowest being 0.5 milliseconds or less, and fitting the signal decay using a single-component[165,172] or bicomponent model.[173,174]

UTE imaging has identified distinct linear signal intensity at the bone-cartilage interface, which has been shown to correspond to the deepest layer of cartilage and the calcified zone of cartilage on histologic analysis (**Fig. 11**).[175] These deep regions within cartilage, which have a T2* relaxation time of 1.3 milliseconds,[165] may play a role in the pathogenesis and progression of osteoarthritis.[176] UTE T2* relaxation time has been shown to decrease with cartilage degeneration.[172] It has been speculated that the lower UTE T2* relaxation time in degenerative cartilage is caused by loss of water trapped between collagen fibers secondary to collagen denaturation, which results in a greater fraction of short T2 components that contribute to an overall decreased T2* value of cartilage. UTE T2* relaxation time has also been found to have higher sensitivity than T2 relaxation time for distinguishing between healthy and degenerative cartilage because of its ability to assess the short T2 components within the deepest layers of the tissue where cartilage degeneration may occur.[172]

Bicomponent UTE T2* mapping has identified 2 distinct T2* components within articular cartilage, a short component with a T2* relaxation time between 1 millisecond and 6 milliseconds, which corresponds to macromolecular-bound water and a long component with a T2* relaxation time of approximately 22 milliseconds, which corresponds to bulk water.[173,174] Whether the short T2* component corresponds exclusively to collagen-bound water[174] or to water bound to both collagen and proteoglycan remains unknown.[177] Enzymatic degradation of cartilage has been shown to cause a decrease in the short T2* relaxation time with no change in the long T2* relaxation time.[174] However, another study comparing UTE T2* parameters with histology and polarized light microscopy has found that cartilage degeneration has no influence on the short T2* relaxation time but increases the long T2* relaxation time. This study has also shown that the fraction of the short T2 component has the strongest correlation with the degree of cartilage degeneration and disruption of the collagen fiber network.[177] It has been speculated that the higher fraction of the short T2 component in degenerative cartilage is caused by disruption of the collagen fiber network, which results in increased surface area on the collagen fiber for water binding. However, further studies are needed to better understand the mechanisms responsible for changes in UTE T2* parameters at various stages of cartilage degeneration.

MAGNETIZATION TRANSFER IMAGING

Magnetization transfer (MT) imaging can be used to assess the macromolecular matrix of articular cartilage by measuring the magnetization exchange between free water and macromolecular-bound protons. Protons bound to the cartilage macromolecules matrix have a much broader

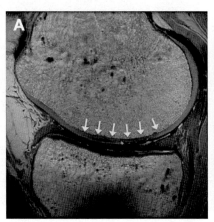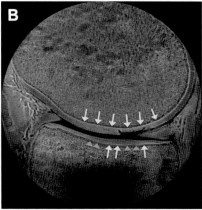

Fig. 11. (*A*) Conventional T1-weighted fast spin-echo image of a cadaver knee joint cannot distinguish between subchondral bone and the deeper layers of articular cartilage (*arrows*). (*B*) Corresponding UTE subtraction image shows a line of high signal intensity (*arrows*) corresponding to the deepest layer of cartilage and the calcified zone of cartilage along with focal areas of diminished signal intensity (*arrowheads*), which suggests abnormality in the deep cartilage region. (*Courtesy of* Christine Chung, MD, University of California at San Diego, San Diego, CA.)

absorption line shapes than free water protons and can be preferentially saturated using an off-resonance radiofrequency pulse. The saturated macromolecular-bound protons undergo magnetization exchange with free water protons through chemical exchange or dipole-dipole interactions, which reduces the longitudinal magnetization of the free water protons available to generate signal during MR imaging.[178]

MT ratio (MTR) measures the change in signal intensity of articular cartilage on MR images acquired with and without an off-resonance radiofrequency pulse. MTR is primarily influenced by the content and molecular structure of collagen within cartilage.[179–181] However, MTR is not a specific measure of collagen within cartilage and is also influenced by other factors, including the T1 relaxation time[182] and proteoglycan content[179] of the tissue. MTR measurements also depend highly on experimental parameters and vary across scanners, transceiver, and scanned objects even when using the same imaging protocol. Studies have shown that MTR is relatively insensitive for detecting early cartilage degeneration in human subjects.[183] However, the technique has been found useful for monitoring changes in the macromolecular matrix of articular cartilage following cartilage repair procedures.[164]

Chemical exchange saturation transfer (CEST) imaging is another technique that investigates the exchange of magnetization between free water and macromolecular-bound protons within articular cartilage. In CEST imaging, the exchangeable proton spins on the hydroxyl groups on the glycosaminoglycan side chains of proteoglycan are selectively saturated with an off-resonance pulse, and the saturation effect is transferred to free water protons through magnetization exchange. The change in the signal measured in the free water pool is directly proportionate to the number of macromolecular-bound protons being saturated and, hence, the concentration of proteoglycan within cartilage.[184] A strong correlation between CEST and sodium values within both healthy cartilage and cartilage repair tissue has been reported, which suggests that CEST imaging can be used to assess the fixed charge density of cartilage.[185]

CEST imaging has been performed at 3.0 T and 7.0 T in reasonable scan times using 3-dimensional gradient-echo sequences.[184–186] The disadvantages of CEST imaging include the need to achieve high-magnetic-field homogeneity and the inadvertent suppression of water signal with the off-resonance pulse, which is especially problematic when using lower-strength 3.0-T scanners.[187] The clinical applications of CEST imaging for evaluating articular cartilage remain largely unknown.

One study has reported a decrease in CEST values of cartilage repair tissue when compared with healthy cartilage (**Fig. 12**).[188] However, little additional work has been performed to correlate CEST measurements with the concentration of proteoglycan within cartilage or to determine the feasibility of using the technique to investigate cartilage degeneration and acute cartilage injury in human patients.

DIFFUSION IMAGING

Diffusion imaging is performed with the use of 2 diffusion-sensitive gradients with the same area but opposite polarity. The paired gradients dephase magnetization from water protons that have undergone diffusion during the time delay between the pulses, resulting in signal attenuation. The degree of signal attenuation is directly proportional to the amount of diffusion of water protons, which is quantified as the apparent diffusion coefficient.[189] Diffusion imaging of articular cartilage was originally performed using 2-dimensional sequences.[189] Three-dimensional steady-state techniques were later developed to provide higher SNR when imaging the short T2 components of cartilage.[190] A 3-dimensional method has recently been developed using 2 modified dual-echo in the steady-state scans acquired with different flip angles and spoiler gradient areas, which can simultaneously measure the T2 relaxation time and apparent diffusion coefficient with the added

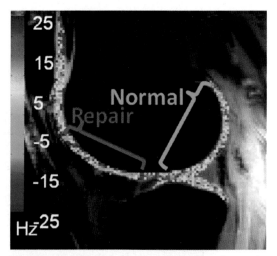

Fig. 12. Sagittal CEST image in a patient 3 months following autologous chondrocyte transplantation shows decreased CEST values of the cartilage repair tissue when compared with healthy cartilage indicating failure to restore normal proteoglycan content immediately following surgery. (*Courtesy of* Ravinder Regatte, PhD, New York University, New York, NY.)

benefit of high-quality source images to assess cartilage morphology (**Fig. 13**).[191] Diffusion tensor imaging can assess the directional components of the diffusion pathway by applying several diffusion-sensitive gradient pairs in different directions and can measure both apparent diffusional coefficient and fractional anisotropy.[192,193] Fractional anisotropy allows determination of the main direction of local diffusion of water protons, which can provide information regarding cartilage ultrastructure.

Diffusion imaging has been used to evaluate the composition and ultrastructure of articular cartilage. Studies using enzymatic degradation of ex vivo cartilage specimens have shown changes in apparent diffusion coefficient with proteoglycan depletion[194–196] and changes in both apparent diffusion coefficient and fractional anisotropy with collagen depletion.[195] Fractional anisotropy has been found to correlate strongly with the orientation of the collagen fiber network assessed using polarized light microscopy and electron scanning microscopy.[194,197,198] Apparent diffusion coefficient and fractional anisotropy have also been shown to be highly sensitive for detecting early cartilage degeneration in both ex vivo[199] and in vivo[200] studies. Diffusor tensor imaging has the unique advantage of simultaneously assessing

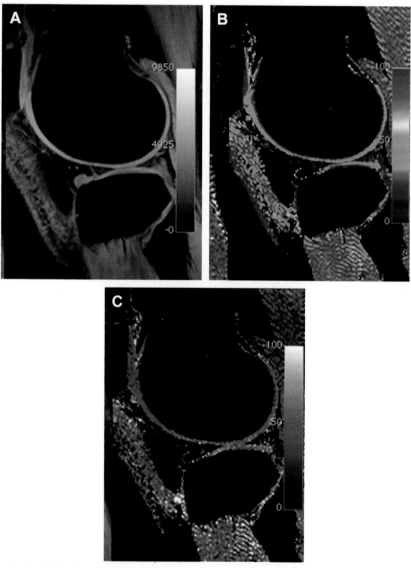

Fig. 13. (*A*) Dual-echo in the steady-state source image, (*B*) T2 map, and (*C*) apparent diffusion coefficient map of the articular cartilage of the knee joint in an asymptomatic volunteer acquired in a single 10-minute scan. (*Courtesy of* Garry Gold, MD, Stanford University, Stanford, CA.)

the proteoglycan and collagen components of articular cartilage in a single scan. However, diffusion tensor imaging is technically challenging to perform on the human knee joint in vivo because of the need for high spatial resolution and thin slices and typically requires the use of high-field-strength scanners and custom-made coils to maximize SNR efficiency.

SUMMARY

Multiple quantitative MR techniques have been developed to noninvasively evaluate the composition and ultrastructure of the articular cartilage of the knee joint. The large number of currently available methods illustrates the inherent limitations of each imaging strategy and the difficulty in providing sensitive and specific information regarding the proteoglycan and collagen components of cartilage. Despite their limitations, quantitative MR techniques have been successfully used in clinical practice to detect early cartilage degeneration and in osteoarthritis research studies to monitor disease-related and treatment-related changes in cartilage over time. However, additional studies using these advanced imaging methods are needed to better understand the sequence of events that occur in the pathogenesis and progression of osteoarthritis.

REFERENCES

1. From the Centers for Disease Control and Prevention. Arthritis prevalence and activity limitations–United States, 1990. JAMA 1994;272(5):346–7.
2. Felson DT. An update on the pathogenesis and epidemiology of osteoarthritis. Radiol Clin North Am 2004;42(1):1–9, v.
3. Felson DT, Zhang Y. An update on the epidemiology of knee and hip osteoarthritis with a view to prevention. Arthritis Rheum 1998;41(8):1343–55.
4. Lawrence RC, Helmick CG, Arnett FC, et al. Estimates of the prevalence of arthritis and selected musculoskeletal disorders in the United States. Arthritis Rheum 1998;41(5):778–99.
5. Oliveria SA, Felson DT, Reed JI, et al. Incidence of symptomatic hand, hip, and knee osteoarthritis among patients in a health maintenance organization. Arthritis Rheum 1995;38(8):1134–41.
6. Squires GR, Okouneff S, Ionescu M, et al. The pathobiology of focal lesion development in aging human articular cartilage and molecular matrix changes characteristic of osteoarthritis. Arthritis Rheum 2003;48(5):1261–70.
7. Poole AR, Kobayashi M, Yasuda T, et al. Type II collagen degradation and its regulation in articular cartilage in osteoarthritis. Ann Rheum Dis 2002; 61(Suppl 2):ii78–81.
8. Wu W, Billinghurst RC, Pidoux I, et al. Sites of collagenase cleavage and denaturation of type II collagen in aging and osteoarthritic articular cartilage and their relationship to the distribution of matrix metalloproteinase 1 and matrix metalloproteinase 13. Arthritis Rheum 2002;46(8):2087–94.
9. Lippiello L, Hall D, Mankin HJ. Collagen synthesis in normal and osteoarthritic human cartilage. J Clin Invest 1977;59(4):593–600.
10. Billinghurst RC, Dahlberg L, Ionescu M, et al. Enhanced cleavage of type II collagen by collagenases in osteoarthritic articular cartilage. J Clin Invest 1997;99(7):1534–45.
11. Hollander AP, Pidoux I, Reiner A, et al. Damage to type II collagen in aging and osteoarthritis starts at the articular surface, originates around chondrocytes, and extends into the cartilage with progressive degeneration. J Clin Invest 1995;96(6):2859–69.
12. Venn M, Maroudas A. Chemical composition and swelling of normal and osteoarthrotic femoral head cartilage. I. Chemical composition. Ann Rheum Dis 1977;36(2):121–9.
13. Pearle AD, Warren RF, Rodeo SA. Basic science of articular cartilage and osteoarthritis. Clin Sports Med 2005;24(1):1–12.
14. Responte DJ, Natoli RM, Athanasiou KA. Collagens of articular cartilage: structure, function, and importance in tissue engineering. Crit Rev Biomed Eng 2007;35(5):363–411.
15. Clark JM. The organisation of collagen fibrils in the superficial zones of articular cartilage. J Anat 1990; 171:117–30.
16. Aspberg A. The different roles of aggrecan interaction domains. J Histochem Cytochem 2012;60(12): 987–96.
17. Knudson CB, Knudson W. Cartilage proteoglycans. Semin Cell Dev Biol 2001;12(2):69–78.
18. Borthakur A, Mellon E, Niyogi S, et al. Sodium and T1rho MRI for molecular and diagnostic imaging of articular cartilage. NMR Biomed 2006;19(7):781–821.
19. Nap RJ, Szleifer I. Structure and interactions of aggrecans: statistical thermodynamic approach. Biophys J 2008;95(10):4570–83.
20. Shapiro EM, Borthakur A, Dandora R, et al. Sodium visibility and quantitation in intact bovine articular cartilage using high field (23)Na MRI and MRS. J Magn Reson 2000;142(1):24–31.
21. Shapiro EM, Borthakur A, Gougoutas A, et al. 23Na MRI accurately measures fixed charge density in articular cartilage. Magn Reson Med 2002;47(2): 284–91.
22. Borthakur A, Shapiro EM, Beers J, et al. Sensitivity of MRI to proteoglycan depletion in cartilage: comparison of sodium and proton MRI. Osteoarthritis Cartilage 2000;8(4):288–93.

23. Insko EK, Kaufman JH, Leigh JS, et al. Sodium NMR evaluation of articular cartilage degradation. Magn Reson Med 1999;41(1):30–4.

24. Reddy R, Insko EK, Noyszewski EA, et al. Sodium MRI of human articular cartilage in vivo. Magn Reson Med 1998;39(5):697–701.

25. Wheaton AJ, Borthakur A, Shapiro EM, et al. Proteoglycan loss in human knee cartilage: quantitation with sodium MR imaging–feasibility study. Radiology 2004;231(3):900–5.

26. Trattnig S, Welsch GH, Juras V, et al. 23Na MR imaging at 7 T after knee matrix-associated autologous chondrocyte transplantation preliminary results. Radiology 2010;257(1):175–84.

27. Wang L, Wu Y, Chang G, et al. Rapid isotropic 3D-sodium MRI of the knee joint in vivo at 7T. J Magn Reson Imaging 2009;30(3):606–14.

28. Staroswiecki E, Bangerter NK, Gurney PT, et al. In vivo sodium imaging of human patellar cartilage with a 3D cones sequence at 3 T and 7 T. J Magn Reson Imaging 2010;32(2):446–51.

29. Borthakur A, Hancu I, Boada FE, et al. In vivo triple quantum filtered twisted projection sodium MRI of human articular cartilage. J Magn Reson 1999; 141(2):286–90.

30. Madelin G, Lee JS, Inati S, et al. Sodium inversion recovery MRI of the knee joint in vivo at 7T. J Magn Reson 2010;207(1):42–52.

31. Feldman RE, Stobbe R, Watts A, et al. Sodium imaging of the human knee using soft inversion recovery fluid attenuation. J Magn Reson 2013;234:197–206.

32. Newbould RD, Miller SR, Upadhyay N, et al. T1-weighted sodium MRI of the articulator cartilage in osteoarthritis: a cross sectional and longitudinal study. PLoS One 2013;8(8):e73067.

33. Madelin G, Babb JS, Xia D, et al. Reproducibility and repeatability of quantitative sodium magnetic resonance imaging in vivo in articular cartilage at 3 T and 7 T. Magn Reson Med 2012;68(3):841–9.

34. Newbould RD, Miller SR, Tielbeek JA, et al. Reproducibility of sodium MRI measures of articular cartilage of the knee in osteoarthritis. Osteoarthritis Cartilage 2012;20(1):29–35.

35. Madelin G, Babb J, Xia D, et al. Articular cartilage: evaluation with fluid-suppressed 7.0-T sodium MR imaging in subjects with and subjects without osteoarthritis. Radiology 2013;268(2):481–91.

36. Zbyn S, Stelzeneder D, Welsch GH, et al. Evaluation of native hyaline cartilage and repair tissue after two cartilage repair surgery techniques with 23Na MR imaging at 7 T: initial experience. Osteoarthritis Cartilage 2012;20(8):837–45.

37. Chang G, Madelin G, Sherman OH, et al. Improved assessment of cartilage repair tissue using fluid-suppressed (2)(3)Na inversion recovery MRI at 7 Tesla: preliminary results. Eur Radiol 2012;22(6): 1341–9.

38. Bashir A, Gray ML, Boutin RD, et al. Glycosaminoglycan in articular cartilage: in vivo assessment with delayed Gd(DTPA)(2-)-enhanced MR imaging. Radiology 1997;205(2):551–8.

39. Bashir A, Gray ML, Burstein D. Gd-DTPA2- as a measure of cartilage degradation. Magn Reson Med 1996;36(5):665–73.

40. Bashir A, Gray ML, Hartke J, et al. Nondestructive imaging of human cartilage glycosaminoglycan concentration by MRI. Magn Reson Med 1999; 41(5):857–65.

41. Trattnig S, Mlynarik V, Breitenseher M, et al. MRI visualization of proteoglycan depletion in articular cartilage via intravenous administration of Gd-DTPA. Magn Reson Imaging 1999;17(4):577–83.

42. Nieminen MT, Rieppo J, Silvennoinen J, et al. Spatial assessment of articular cartilage proteoglycans with Gd-DTPA-enhanced T1 imaging. Magn Reson Med 2002;48(4):640–8.

43. Allen RG, Burstein D, Gray ML. Monitoring glycosaminoglycan replenishment in cartilage explants with gadolinium-enhanced magnetic resonance imaging. J Orthop Res 1999;17(3):430–6.

44. Gillis A, Gray M, Burstein D. Relaxivity and diffusion of gadolinium agents in cartilage. Magn Reson Med 2002;48(6):1068–71.

45. Kurkijarvi JE, Nissi MJ, Kiviranta I, et al. Delayed gadolinium-enhanced MRI of cartilage (dGEMRIC) and T2 characteristics of human knee articular cartilage: topographical variation and relationships to mechanical properties. Magn Reson Med 2004; 52(1):41–6.

46. Nissi MJ, Rieppo J, Toyras J, et al. Estimation of mechanical properties of articular cartilage with MRI - dGEMRIC, T2 and T1 imaging in different species with variable stages of maturation. Osteoarthritis Cartilage 2007;15(10):1141–8.

47. Samosky JT, Burstein D, Eric Grimson W, et al. Spatially-localized correlation of dGEMRIC-measured GAG distribution and mechanical stiffness in the human tibial plateau. J Orthop Res 2005;23(1):93–101.

48. Burstein D, Velyvis J, Scott KT, et al. Protocol issues for delayed Gd(DTPA)(2-)-enhanced MRI (dGEMRIC) for clinical evaluation of articular cartilage. Magn Reson Med 2001;45(1):36–41.

49. Tiderius CJ, Olsson LE, de Verdier H, et al. (Gd-DTPA2)-enhanced MRI of femoral knee cartilage: a dose-response study in healthy volunteers. Magn Reson Med 2001;46(6):1067–71.

50. Bellin MF, Van Der Molen AJ. Extracellular gadolinium-based contrast media: an overview. Eur J Radiol 2008;66(2):160–7.

51. Wiginton CD, Kelly B, Oto A, et al. Gadolinium-based contrast exposure, nephrogenic systemic fibrosis, and gadolinium detection in tissue. AJR Am J Roentgenol 2008;190(4):1060–8.

52. Tiderius CJ, Olsson LE, Leander P, et al. Delayed gadolinium-enhanced MRI of cartilage (dGEMRIC) in early knee osteoarthritis. Magn Reson Med 2003; 49(3):488–92.

53. Williams A, Mikulis B, Krishnan N, et al. Suitability of T(1Gd) as the dGEMRIC index at 1.5T and 3.0T. Magn Reson Med 2007;58(4):830–4.

54. McKenzie CA, Williams A, Prasad PV, et al. Three-dimensional delayed gadolinium-enhanced MRI of cartilage (dGEMRIC) at 1.5T and 3.0T. J Magn Reson Imaging 2006;24(4):928–33.

55. Li W, Scheidegger R, Wu Y, et al. Accuracy of T1 measurement with 3-D Look-Locker technique for dGEMRIC. J Magn Reson Imaging 2008;27(3): 678–82.

56. Siversson C, Tiderius CJ, Dahlberg L, et al. Local flip angle correction for improved volume T1-quantification in three-dimensional dGEMRIC using the Look-Locker technique. J Magn Reson Imaging 2009;30(4):834–41.

57. Andreisek G, White LM, Yang Y, et al. Delayed gadolinium-enhanced MR imaging of articular cartilage: three-dimensional T1 mapping with variable flip angles and B1 correction. Radiology 2009;252(3):865–73.

58. Mamisch TC, Dudda M, Hughes T, et al. Comparison of delayed gadolinium enhanced MRI of cartilage (dGEMRIC) using inversion recovery and fast T1 mapping sequences. Magn Reson Med 2008; 60(4):768–73.

59. Siversson C, Tiderius CJ, Neuman P, et al. Repeatability of T1-quantification in dGEMRIC for three different acquisition techniques: two-dimensional inversion recovery, three-dimensional look locker, and three-dimensional variable flip angle. J Magn Reson Imaging 2010;31(5):1203–9.

60. van Tiel J, Reijman M, Bos PK, et al. Delayed gadolinium-enhanced MRI of cartilage (dGEMRIC) shows no change in cartilage structural composition after viscosupplementation in patients with early-stage knee osteoarthritis. PLoS One 2013; 8(11):e79785.

61. Multanen J, Rauvala E, Lammentausta E, et al. Reproducibility of imaging human knee cartilage by delayed gadolinium-enhanced MRI of cartilage (dGEMRIC) at 1.5 Tesla. Osteoarthritis Cartilage 2009;17(5):559–64.

62. Mayerhoefer ME, Welsch GH, Mamisch TC, et al. The in vivo effects of unloading and compression on T1-Gd (dGEMRIC) relaxation times in healthy articular knee cartilage at 3.0 Tesla. Eur Radiol 2010;20(2):443–9.

63. Nieminen MT, Menezes NM, Williams A, et al. T2 of articular cartilage in the presence of Gd-DTPA2. Magn Reson Med 2004;51(6):1147–52.

64. Eckstein F, Wyman BT, Buck RJ, et al. Longitudinal quantitative MR imaging of cartilage morphology in the presence of gadopentetate dimeglumine (Gd-DTPA). Magn Reson Med 2009;61(4):975–80.

65. Laurent D, O'Byrne E, Wasvary J, et al. In vivo MRI of cartilage pathogenesis in surgical models of osteoarthritis. Skeletal Radiol 2006;35(8):555–64.

66. Laurent D, Wasvary J, O'Byrne E, et al. In vivo qualitative assessments of articular cartilage in the rabbit knee with high-resolution MRI at 3 T. Magn Reson Med 2003;50(3):541–9.

67. Woertler K, Buerger H, Moeller J, et al. Patellar articular cartilage lesions: in vitro MR imaging evaluation after placement in gadopentetate dimeglumine solution. Radiology 2004;230(3):768–73.

68. Williams A, Sharma L, McKenzie CA, et al. Delayed gadolinium-enhanced magnetic resonance imaging of cartilage in knee osteoarthritis: findings at different radiographic stages of disease and relationship to malalignment. Arthritis Rheum 2005; 52(11):3528–35.

69. Tiderius CJ, Olsson LE, Nyquist F, et al. Cartilage glycosaminoglycan loss in the acute phase after an anterior cruciate ligament injury: delayed gadolinium-enhanced magnetic resonance imaging of cartilage and synovial fluid analysis. Arthritis Rheum 2005;52(1):120–7.

70. Fleming BC, Oksendahl HL, Mehan WA, et al. Delayed gadolinium-enhanced MR imaging of cartilage (dGEMRIC) following ACL injury. Osteoarthritis Cartilage 2010;18(5):662–7.

71. Ericsson YB, Tjornstrand J, Tiderius CJ, et al. Relationship between cartilage glycosaminoglycan content (assessed with dGEMRIC) and OA risk factors in meniscectomized patients. Osteoarthritis Cartilage 2009;17(5):565–70.

72. Domayer SE, Welsch GH, Nehrer S, et al. T2 mapping and dGEMRIC after autologous chondrocyte implantation with a fibrin-based scaffold in the knee: preliminary results. Eur J Radiol 2010;73(3):636–42.

73. Gillis A, Bashir A, McKeon B, et al. Magnetic resonance imaging of relative glycosaminoglycan distribution in patients with autologous chondrocyte transplants. Invest Radiol 2001;36(12):743–8.

74. Bekkers JE, Bartels LW, Benink RJ, et al. Delayed gadolinium enhanced MRI of cartilage (dGEMRIC) can be effectively applied for longitudinal cohort evaluation of articular cartilage regeneration. Osteoarthritis Cartilage 2013;21(7):943–9.

75. Watanabe A, Wada Y, Obata T, et al. Delayed gadolinium-enhanced MR to determine glycosaminoglycan concentration in reparative cartilage after autologous chondrocyte implantation: preliminary results. Radiology 2006;239(1):201–8.

76. Redfield AG. Nuclear spin thermodynamics in the rotating frame. Science 1969;164(3883):1015–23.

77. Duvvuri U, Goldberg AD, Kranz JK, et al. Water magnetic relaxation dispersion in biological systems: the contribution of proton exchange and

implications for the noninvasive detection of cartilage degradation. Proc Natl Acad Sci U S A 2001;98(22):12479–84.

78. Regatte RR, Akella SV, Wheaton AJ, et al. 1 rho-relaxation mapping of human femoral-tibial cartilage in vivo. J Magn Reson Imaging 2003;18(3):336–41.

79. Duvvuri U, Charagundla SR, Kudchodkar SB, et al. Human knee: in vivo T1(rho)-weighted MR imaging at 1.5 T–preliminary experience. Radiology 2001;220(3):822–6.

80. Wheaton AJ, Borthakur A, Kneeland JB, et al. In vivo quantification of T1rho using a multislice spin-lock pulse sequence. Magn Reson Med 2004;52(6):1453–8.

81. Li X, Han ET, Ma CB, et al. In vivo 3T spiral imaging based multi-slice T(1rho) mapping of knee cartilage in osteoarthritis. Magn Reson Med 2005;54(4):929–36.

82. Pakin SK, Xu J, Schweitzer ME, et al. Rapid 3D-T1rho mapping of the knee joint at 3.0T with parallel imaging. Magn Reson Med 2006;56(3):563–71.

83. Zuo J, Li X, Banerjee S, et al. Parallel imaging of knee cartilage at 3 Tesla. J Magn Reson Imaging 2007;26(4):1001–9.

84. Mosher TJ, Zhang Z, Reddy R, et al. Knee articular cartilage damage in osteoarthritis: analysis of MR image biomarker reproducibility in ACRIN-PA 4001 multicenter trial. Radiology 2011;258(3):832–42.

85. Li X, Wyatt C, Rivoire J, et al. Simultaneous acquisition of T and T quantification in knee cartilage: repeatability and diurnal variation. J Magn Reson Imaging 2013;39(5):1287–93.

86. Wheaton AJ, Casey FL, Gougoutas AJ, et al. Correlation of T1rho with fixed charge density in cartilage. J Magn Reson Imaging 2004;20(3):519–25.

87. Wheaton AJ, Dodge GR, Elliott DM, et al. Quantification of cartilage biomechanical and biochemical properties via T1rho magnetic resonance imaging. Magn Reson Med 2005;54(5):1087–93.

88. Regatte RR, Akella SV, Borthakur A, et al. Proteoglycan depletion-induced changes in transverse relaxation maps of cartilage: comparison of T2 and T1rho. Acad Radiol 2002;9(12):1388–94.

89. Wheaton AJ, Dodge GR, Borthakur A, et al. Detection of changes in articular cartilage proteoglycan by T(1rho) magnetic resonance imaging. J Orthop Res 2005;23(1):102–8.

90. Duvvuri U, Reddy R, Patel SD, et al. T1rho-relaxation in articular cartilage: effects of enzymatic degradation. Magn Reson Med 1997;38(6):863–7.

91. Menezes NM, Gray ML, Hartke JR, et al. T2 and T1rho MRI in articular cartilage systems. Magn Reson Med 2004;51(3):503–9.

92. Keenan KE, Besier TF, Pauly JM, et al. Prediction of glycosaminoglycan content in human cartilage by age, T1rho and T2 MRI. Osteoarthritis Cartilage 2011;19(2):171–9.

93. Li X, Cheng J, Lin K, et al. Quantitative MRI using T1rho and T2 in human osteoarthritic cartilage specimens: correlation with biochemical measurements and histology. Magn Reson Imaging 2011;29(3):324–34.

94. Souza RB, Baum T, Wu S, et al. Effects of unloading on knee articular cartilage T1rho and T2 magnetic resonance imaging relaxation times: a case series. J Orthop Sports Phys Ther 2012;42(6):511–20.

95. Goto H, Yuki I, Fujii M, et al. The natural degenerative course of T1rho values of normal knee cartilage. Kobe J Med Sci 2011;57(4):155–70.

96. Witschey WR, Borthakur A, Fenty M, et al. T1rho MRI quantification of arthroscopically confirmed cartilage degeneration. Magn Reson Med 2010;63(5):1376–82.

97. Regatte RR, Akella SV, Lonner JH, et al. T1rho relaxation mapping in human osteoarthritis (OA) cartilage: comparison of T1rho with T2. J Magn Reson Imaging 2006;23(4):547–53.

98. Li X, Benjamin Ma C, Link TM, et al. In vivo T(1rho) and T(2) mapping of articular cartilage in osteoarthritis of the knee using 3 T MRI. Osteoarthritis Cartilage 2007;15(7):789–97.

99. Stahl R, Luke A, Li X, et al. T1rho, T2 and focal knee cartilage abnormalities in physically active and sedentary healthy subjects versus early OA patients–a 3.0-Tesla MRI study. Eur Radiol 2009;19(1):132–43.

100. Carballido-Gamio J, Stahl R, Blumenkrantz G, et al. Spatial analysis of magnetic resonance T1rho and T2 relaxation times improves classification between subjects with and without osteoarthritis. Med Phys 2009;36(9):4059–67.

101. Schooler J, Kumar D, Nardo L, et al. Longitudinal evaluation of T and T spatial distribution in osteoarthritic and healthy medial knee cartilage. Osteoarthritis Cartilage 2013;22(1):51–62.

102. Theologis AA, Kuo D, Cheng J, et al. Evaluation of bone bruises and associated cartilage in anterior cruciate ligament-injured and -reconstructed knees using quantitative t(1rho) magnetic resonance imaging: 1-year cohort study. Arthroscopy 2011;27(1):65–76.

103. Bolbos RI, Ma CB, Link TM, et al. In vivo T1rho quantitative assessment of knee cartilage after anterior cruciate ligament injury using 3 Tesla magnetic resonance imaging. Invest Radiol 2008;43(11):782–8.

104. Li X, Ma BC, Bolbos RI, et al. Quantitative assessment of bone marrow edema-like lesion and overlying cartilage in knees with osteoarthritis and anterior cruciate ligament tear using MR imaging and spectroscopic imaging at 3 Tesla. J Magn Reson Imaging 2008;28(2):453–61.

105. Li X, Kuo D, Theologis A, et al. Cartilage in anterior cruciate ligament-reconstructed knees: MR imaging T1{rho} and T2–initial experience with 1-year follow-up. Radiology 2011;258(2):505–14.

106. Su F, Hilton JF, Nardo L, et al. Cartilage morphology and T1rho and T2 quantification in ACL-reconstructed knees: a 2-year follow-up. Osteoarthritis Cartilage 2013;21(8):1058–67.

107. Theologis AA, Schairer WW, Carballido-Gamio J, et al. Longitudinal analysis of T1rho and T2 quantitative MRI of knee cartilage laminar organization following microfracture surgery. Knee 2012;19(5):652–7.

108. Holtzman DJ, Theologis AA, Carballido-Gamio J, et al. T(1rho) and T(2) quantitative magnetic resonance imaging analysis of cartilage regeneration following microfracture and mosaicplasty cartilage resurfacing procedures. J Magn Reson Imaging 2010;32(4):914–23.

109. Boulby PA, Rugg FJ. T2: the transverse relaxation time. Hoboken, New Jersey: John Wiley & Sons Ltd; 2003. p. 143–201.

110. Liess C, Lusse S, Karger N, et al. Detection of changes in cartilage water content using MRI T2-mapping in vivo. Osteoarthritis Cartilage 2002;10(12):907–13.

111. Nishioka H, Hirose J, Nakamura E, et al. T1rho and T2 mapping reveal the in vivo extracellular matrix of articular cartilage. J Magn Reson Imaging 2012; 35(1):147–55.

112. Watrin-Pinzano A, Ruaud JP, Olivier P, et al. Effect of proteoglycan depletion on T2 mapping in rat patellar cartilage. Radiology 2005;234(1):162–70.

113. Wong CS, Yan CH, Gong NJ, et al. Imaging biomarker with T1rho and T2 mappings in osteoarthritis - in vivo human articular cartilage study. Eur J Radiol 2013;82(4):647–50.

114. Goodwin DW, Wadghiri YZ, Zhu H, et al. Macroscopic structure of articular cartilage of the tibial plateau: influence of a characteristic matrix architecture on MRI appearance. AJR Am J Roentgenol 2004;182(2):311–8.

115. Nieminen MT, Rieppo J, Toyras J, et al. T2 relaxation reveals spatial collagen architecture in articular cartilage: a comparative quantitative MRI and polarized light microscopic study. Magn Reson Med 2001;46(3):487–93.

116. Xia Y, Moody JB, Burton-Wurster N, et al. Quantitative in situ correlation between microscopic MRI and polarized light microscopy studies of articular cartilage. Osteoarthritis Cartilage 2001;9(5):393–406.

117. Apprich S, Mamisch TC, Welsch GH, et al. Quantitative T2 mapping of the patella at 3.0T is sensitive to early cartilage degeneration, but also to loading of the knee. Eur J Radiol 2012;81(4):e438–43.

118. Mosher TJ, Liu Y, Torok CM. Functional cartilage MRI T2 mapping: evaluating the effect of age and training on knee cartilage response to running. Osteoarthritis Cartilage 2010;18(3):358–64.

119. Mosher TJ, Smith HE, Collins C, et al. Change in knee cartilage T2 at MR imaging after running: a feasibility study. Radiology 2005;234(1):245–9.

120. Xia Y. Magic-angle effect in magnetic resonance imaging of articular cartilage: a review. Invest Radiol 2000;35(10):602–21.

121. Rubenstein JD, Kim JK, Morova-Protzner I, et al. Effects of collagen orientation on MR imaging characteristics of bovine articular cartilage. Radiology 1993;188(1):219–26.

122. Mlynarik V, Degrassi A, Toffanin R, et al. Investigation of laminar appearance of articular cartilage by means of magnetic resonance microscopy. Magn Reson Imaging 1996;14(4):435–42.

123. Xia Y, Farquhar T, Burton-Wurster N, et al. Origin of cartilage laminae in MRI. J Magn Reson Imaging 1997;7(5):887–94.

124. Goodwin DW, Wadghiri YZ, Dunn JF. Micro-imaging of articular cartilage: T2, proton density, and the magic angle effect. Acad Radiol 1998;5(11): 790–8.

125. Foster JE, Maciewicz RA, Taberner J, et al. Structural periodicity in human articular cartilage: comparison between magnetic resonance imaging and histological findings. Osteoarthritis Cartilage 1999;7(5):480–5.

126. Xia Y, Moody JB, Alhadlaq H. Orientational dependence of T2 relaxation in articular cartilage: a microscopic MRI (microMRI) study. Magn Reson Med 2002;48(3):460–9.

127. Alhadlaq HA, Xia Y, Moody JB, et al. Detecting structural changes in early experimental osteoarthritis of tibial cartilage by microscopic magnetic resonance imaging and polarised light microscopy. Ann Rheum Dis 2004;63(6):709–17.

128. Bi X, Yang X, Bostrom MP, et al. Fourier transform infrared imaging and MR microscopy studies detect compositional and structural changes in cartilage in a rabbit model of osteoarthritis. Anal Bioanal Chem 2007;387(5):1601–12.

129. Grunder W, Wagner M, Werner A. MR-microscopic visualization of anisotropic internal cartilage structures using the magic angle technique. Magn Reson Med 1998;39(3):376–82.

130. Reiter DA, Lin PC, Fishbein KW, et al. Multicomponent T2 relaxation analysis in cartilage. Magn Reson Med 2009;61(4):803–9.

131. Reiter DA, Roque RA, Lin PC, et al. Mapping proteoglycan-bound water in cartilage: improved specificity of matrix assessment using multiexponential transverse relaxation analysis. Magn Reson Med 2011;65(2):377–84.

132. Reiter DA, Roque RA, Lin PC, et al. Improved specificity of cartilage matrix evaluation using multiexponential transverse relaxation analysis applied to pathomimetically degraded cartilage. NMR Biomed 2011;24(10):1286–94.

133. Wang N, Xia Y. Dependencies of multi-component T2 and T1rho relaxation on the anisotropy of collagen fibrils in bovine nasal cartilage. J Magn Reson 2011;212(1):124–32.

134. Zheng S, Xia Y. On the measurement of multi-component T2 relaxation in cartilage by MR spectroscopy and imaging. Magn Reson Imaging 2010;28(4):537–45.

135. Mlynarik V. Magic angle effect in articular cartilage. AJR Am J Roentgenol 2002;178(5):1287 [author reply:1287–8].

136. Wayne JS, Kraft KA, Shields KJ, et al. MR imaging of normal and matrix-depleted cartilage: correlation with biomechanical function and biochemical composition. Radiology 2003;228(2):493–9.

137. Nieminen MT, Toyras J, Rieppo J, et al. Quantitative MR microscopy of enzymatically degraded articular cartilage. Magn Reson Med 2000;43(5):676–81.

138. Koff MF, Amrami KK, Felmlee JP, et al. Bias of cartilage T2 values related to method of calculation. Magn Reson Imaging 2008;26(9):1236–43.

139. Paul PK, Jasani MK, Sebok D, et al. Variation in MR signal intensity across normal human knee cartilage. J Magn Reson Imaging 1993;3(4):569–74.

140. Maier CF, Tan SG, Hariharan H, et al. T2 quantitation of articular cartilage at 1.5 T. J Magn Reson Imaging 2003;17(3):358–64.

141. Smith HE, Mosher TJ, Dardzinski BJ, et al. Spatial variation in cartilage T2 of the knee. J Magn Reson Imaging 2001;14(1):50–5.

142. Pai A, Li X, Majumdar S. A comparative study at 3 T of sequence dependence of T2 quantitation in the knee. Magn Reson Imaging 2008;26(9):1215–20.

143. Balamoody S, Williams TG, Wolstenholme C, et al. Magnetic resonance transverse relaxation time T2 of knee cartilage in osteoarthritis at 3-T: a cross-sectional multicentre, multivendor reproducibility study. Skeletal Radiol 2013;42(4):511–20.

144. Dardzinski BJ, Schneider E. Radiofrequency (RF) coil impacts the value and reproducibility of cartilage spin-spin (T2) relaxation time measurements. Osteoarthritis Cartilage 2013;21(5):710–20.

145. Mosher TJ, Collins CM, Smith HE, et al. Effect of gender on in vivo cartilage magnetic resonance imaging T2 mapping. J Magn Reson Imaging 2004; 19(3):323–8.

146. Mosher TJ, Dardzinski BJ, Smith MB. Human articular cartilage: influence of aging and early symptomatic degeneration on the spatial variation of T2–preliminary findings at 3 T. Radiology 2000; 214(1):259–66.

147. Dunn TC, Lu Y, Jin H, et al. T2 relaxation time of cartilage at MR imaging: comparison with severity of knee osteoarthritis. Radiology 2004;232(2):592–8.

148. Apprich S, Welsch GH, Mamisch TC, et al. Detection of degenerative cartilage disease: comparison of high-resolution morphological MR and quantitative T2 mapping at 3.0 Tesla. Osteoarthritis Cartilage 2010;18(9):1211–7.

149. Koff MF, Amrami KK, Kaufman KR. Clinical evaluation of T2 values of patellar cartilage in patients with osteoarthritis. Osteoarthritis Cartilage 2007; 15(2):198–204.

150. Stahl R, Blumenkrantz G, Carballido-Gamio J, et al. MRI-derived T2 relaxation times and cartilage morphometry of the tibio-femoral joint in subjects with and without osteoarthritis during a 1-year follow-up. Osteoarthritis Cartilage 2007;15(11): 1225–34.

151. Kijowski R, Blankenbaker DG, Munoz Del Rio A, et al. Evaluation of the articular cartilage of the knee joint: value of adding a T2 mapping sequence to a routine MR imaging protocol. Radiology 2013; 267(2):503–13.

152. Joseph GB, Baum T, Carballido-Gamio J, et al. Texture analysis of cartilage T2 maps: individuals with risk factors for OA have higher and more heterogeneous knee cartilage MR T2 compared to normal controls–data from the osteoarthritis initiative. Arthritis Res Ther 2011;13(5):R153.

153. Baum T, Stehling C, Joseph GB, et al. Changes in knee cartilage T2 values over 24 months in subjects with and without risk factors for knee osteoarthritis and their association with focal knee lesions at baseline: data from the osteoarthritis initiative. J Magn Reson Imaging 2012;35(2):370–8.

154. Friedrich KM, Shepard T, de Oliveira VS, et al. T2 measurements of cartilage in osteoarthritis patients with meniscal tears. AJR Am J Roentgenol 2009; 193(5):W411–5.

155. Bining HJ, Santos R, Andrews G, et al. Can T2 relaxation values and color maps be used to detect chondral damage utilizing subchondral bone marrow edema as a marker? Skeletal Radiol 2009;38(5): 459–65.

156. Baum T, Joseph GB, Arulanandan A, et al. Association of magnetic resonance imaging-based knee cartilage T2 measurements and focal knee lesions with knee pain: data from the Osteoarthritis Initiative. Arthritis Care Res (Hoboken) 2012;64(2): 248–55.

157. Joseph GB, Baum T, Alizai H, et al. Baseline mean and heterogeneity of MR cartilage T2 are associated with morphologic degeneration of cartilage, meniscus, and bone marrow over 3 years–data from the Osteoarthritis Initiative. Osteoarthritis Cartilage 2012;20(7):727–35.

158. Van Ginckel A, Verdonk P, Victor J, et al. Cartilage status in relation to return to sports after anterior cruciate ligament reconstruction. Am J Sports Med 2013;41(3):550–9.

159. Kai B, Mann SA, King C, et al. Integrity of articular cartilage on T2 mapping associated with meniscal signal change. Eur J Radiol 2011;79(3):421–7.

160. Welsch GH, Mamisch TC, Domayer SE, et al. Cartilage T2 assessment at 3-T MR imaging: in vivo differentiation of normal hyaline cartilage from reparative tissue after two cartilage repair procedures–initial experience. Radiology 2008;247(1):154–61.

161. Welsch GH, Mamisch TC, Marlovits S, et al. Quantitative T2 mapping during follow-up after matrix-associated autologous chondrocyte transplantation (MACT): full-thickness and zonal evaluation to visualize the maturation of cartilage repair tissue. J Orthop Res 2009;27(7):957–63.

162. Welsch GH, Mamisch TC, Zak L, et al. Evaluation of cartilage repair tissue after matrix-associated autologous chondrocyte transplantation using a hyaluronic-based or a collagen-based scaffold with morphological MOCART scoring and biochemical T2 mapping: preliminary results. Am J Sports Med 2010;38(5):934–42.

163. Welsch GH, Trattnig S, Hughes T, et al. T2 and T2* mapping in patients after matrix-associated autologous chondrocyte transplantation: initial results on clinical use with 3.0-Tesla MRI. Eur Radiol 2010; 20(6):1515–23.

164. Welsch GH, Trattnig S, Scheffler K, et al. Magnetization transfer contrast and T2 mapping in the evaluation of cartilage repair tissue with 3T MRI. J Magn Reson Imaging 2008;28(4):979–86.

165. Du J, Takahashi AM, Chung CB. Ultrashort TE spectroscopic imaging (UTESI): application to the imaging of short T2 relaxation tissues in the musculoskeletal system. J Magn Reson Imaging 2009; 29(2):412–21.

166. Gatehouse PD, Thomas RW, Robson MD, et al. Magnetic resonance imaging of the knee with ultrashort TE pulse sequences. Magn Reson Imaging 2004;22(8):1061–7.

167. Young IR, Bydder GM. Magnetic resonance: new approaches to imaging of the musculoskeletal system. Physiol Meas 2003;24(4):R1–23.

168. Du J, Bydder M, Takahashi AM, et al. Short T2 contrast with three-dimensional ultrashort echo time imaging. Magn Reson Imaging 2011;29(4):470–82.

169. Rahmer J, Bornert P, Groen J, et al. Three-dimensional radial ultrashort echo-time imaging with T2 adapted sampling. Magn Reson Med 2006;55(5): 1075–82.

170. Du J, Takahashi AM, Bydder M, et al. Ultrashort TE imaging with off-resonance saturation contrast (UTE-OSC). Magn Reson Med 2009;62(2):527–31.

171. Du J, Takahashi AM, Bae WC, et al. Dual inversion recovery, ultrashort echo time (DIR UTE) imaging: creating high contrast for short-T(2) species. Magn Reson Med 2010;63(2):447–55.

172. Williams A, Qian Y, Bear D, et al. Assessing degeneration of human articular cartilage with ultra-short echo time (UTE) T2* mapping. Osteoarthritis Cartilage 2010;18(4):539–46.

173. Du J, Diaz E, Carl M, et al. Ultrashort echo time imaging with bicomponent analysis. Magn Reson Med 2012;67(3):645–9.

174. Qian Y, Williams AA, Chu CR, et al. Multicomponent T2* mapping of knee cartilage: technical feasibility ex vivo. Magn Reson Med 2010;64(5):1426–31.

175. Bae WC, Dwek JR, Znamirowski R, et al. Ultrashort echo time MR imaging of osteochondral junction of the knee at 3 T: identification of anatomic structures contributing to signal intensity. Radiology 2010; 254(3):837–45.

176. Oegema TR Jr, Carpenter RJ, Hofmeister F, et al. The interaction of the zone of calcified cartilage and subchondral bone in osteoarthritis. Microsc Res Tech 1997;37(4):324–32.

177. Pauli C, Bae WC, Lee M, et al. Ultrashort-echo time MR imaging of the patella with bicomponent analysis: correlation with histopathologic and polarized light microscopic findings. Radiology 2012;264(2): 484–93.

178. Henkelman RM, Stanisz GJ, Graham SJ. Magnetization transfer in MRI: a review. NMR Biomed 2001; 14(2):57–64.

179. Gray ML, Burstein D, Lesperance LM, et al. Magnetization transfer in cartilage and its constituent macromolecules. Magn Reson Med 1995;34(3):319–25.

180. Kim DK, Ceckler TL, Hascall VC, et al. Analysis of water-macromolecule proton magnetization transfer in articular cartilage. Magn Reson Med 1993; 29(2):211–5.

181. Laurent D, Wasvary J, Yin J, et al. Quantitative and qualitative assessment of articular cartilage in the goat knee with magnetization transfer imaging. Magn Reson Imaging 2001;19(10):1279–86.

182. Henkelman RM, Stanisz GJ, Menezes N, et al. Can MTR be used to assess cartilage in the presence of Gd-DTPA2-? Magn Reson Med 2002;48(6):1081–4.

183. Yao W, Qu N, Lu Z, et al. The application of T1 and T2 relaxation time and magnetization transfer ratios to the early diagnosis of patellar cartilage osteoarthritis. Skeletal Radiol 2009;38(11):1055–62.

184. Lee JS, Parasoglou P, Xia D, et al. Uniform magnetization transfer in chemical exchange saturation transfer magnetic resonance imaging. Sci Rep 2013;3:1707.

185. Ling W, Regatte RR, Navon G, et al. Assessment of glycosaminoglycan concentration in vivo by chemical exchange-dependent saturation transfer (gagCEST). Proc Natl Acad Sci U S A 2008;105(7):2266–70.

186. Wei W, Jia G, Flanigan D, et al. Chemical exchange saturation transfer MR imaging of articular cartilage glycosaminoglycans at 3 T: accuracy of B0 Field Inhomogeneity corrections with gradient echo method. Magn Reson Imaging 2014;32(1):41–7.

187. Singh A, Haris M, Cai K, et al. Chemical exchange saturation transfer magnetic resonance imaging of human knee cartilage at 3 T and 7 T. Magn Reson Med 2012;68(2):588–94.

188. Schmitt B, Zbyn S, Stelzeneder D, et al. Cartilage quality assessment by using glycosaminoglycan chemical exchange saturation transfer and (23)Na MR imaging at 7 T. Radiology 2011;260(1):257–64.

189. Stejskal EO, Tanner JE. Spin diffusion measurements: spin echoes in the presence of a time-dependent field gradient. J Chem Phys 1965;42(1):288–92.

190. Miller KL, Hargreaves BA, Gold GE, et al. Steady-state diffusion-weighted imaging of in vivo knee cartilage. Magn Reson Med 2004;51(2):394–8.

191. Staroswiecki E, Granlund KL, Alley MT, et al. Simultaneous estimation of T(2) and apparent diffusion coefficient in human articular cartilage in vivo with a modified three-dimensional double echo steady state (DESS) sequence at 3 T. Magn Reson Med 2012;67(4):1086–96.

192. Le Bihan D, Mangin JF, Poupon C, et al. Diffusion tensor imaging: concepts and applications. J Magn Reson Imaging 2001;13(4):534–46.

193. Basser PJ, Pierpaoli C. A simplified method to measure the diffusion tensor from seven MR images. Magn Reson Med 1998;39(6):928–34.

194. Meder R, de Visser SK, Bowden JC, et al. Diffusion tensor imaging of articular cartilage as a measure of tissue microstructure. Osteoarthritis Cartilage 2006;14(9):875–81.

195. Deng X, Farley M, Nieminen MT, et al. Diffusion tensor imaging of native and degenerated human articular cartilage. Magn Reson Imaging 2007; 25(2):168–71.

196. Raya JG, Melkus G, Adam-Neumair S, et al. Change of diffusion tensor imaging parameters in articular cartilage with progressive proteoglycan extraction. Invest Radiol 2011;46(6):401–9.

197. de Visser SK, Bowden JC, Wentrup-Byrne E, et al. Anisotropy of collagen fibre alignment in bovine cartilage: comparison of polarised light microscopy and spatially resolved diffusion-tensor measurements. Osteoarthritis Cartilage 2008;16(6): 689–97.

198. Raya JG, Arnoldi AP, Weber DL, et al. Ultra-high field diffusion tensor imaging of articular cartilage correlated with histology and scanning electron microscopy. MAGMA 2011;24(4): 247–58.

199. Raya JG, Melkus G, Adam-Neumair S, et al. Diffusion-tensor imaging of human articular cartilage specimens with early signs of cartilage damage. Radiology 2013;266(3):831–41.

200. Raya JG, Horng A, Dietrich O, et al. Articular cartilage: in vivo diffusion-tensor imaging. Radiology 2012;262(2):550–9.

Magnetic Resonance Imaging of Cartilage Repair Procedures

Michael C. Forney, MD[a],*, Amit Gupta, MD[a],
Tom Minas, MD[b], Carl S. Winalski, MD[a,c]

KEYWORDS

- Magnetic resonance imaging • Cartilage repair • Knee

KEY POINTS

- Current cartilage repair strategies in the knee.
- Magnetic resonance (MR) imaging appearance of cartilage repair procedures in the knee.
- Reporting MR imaging findings of cartilage repair in the knee.

Videos of microfracture procedure and autologous chondrocyte implantation procedure accompany this article at http://www.mri.theclinics.com/

INTRODUCTION

Articular cartilage lesions occur frequently and can be a common source of pain, especially in the knee. Up to 36% of athletic injuries have an associated chondral injury,[1,2] more so in women. A study of 31,516 arthroscopies identified chondral injuries in 63% of patients.[3] When left untreated, chondral lesions can accelerate the development of osteoarthritis and result in permanent dysfunction.[4,5] Mature articular cartilage has limited capability for repair because of poor vascularity, inability to recruit undifferentiated cells, and limitations on cell replication and migration by the dense extracellular matrix.[6] Some investigators have suggested that a subset of cartilage defects in humans may heal spontaneously,[7] and spontaneous cartilage repair has been shown in some animal models.[8,9] However, even in animal models, the repair tissue is imperfect and dependent on the age of the animal.[9,10] For these reasons, there has been intense research in the development of techniques to repair or restore articular cartilage surfaces.

Imaging plays an increasingly important role in both the initial detection of chondral lesions and the postoperative evaluation of chondral repair procedures. Magnetic resonance (MR) imaging, with its ability to directly image cartilage and chondral repair tissue, is particularly valuable and with proper use may help patients avoid unnecessary arthroscopic or even open surgery. Because an increasing number of cartilage repair procedures

Disclosures: no relevant disclosures (M.C. Forney, A. Gupta); T. Minas is on Speakers Bureau and is a consultant for The Sanofi Group; has stock ownership in ConforMIS, Inc.; has royalties,patents with Elsevier BV and ConforMIS, Inc; C.S. Winalski has no relevant financial disclosures. He has interpreted clinical trial studies for BioClinica, Sanofi Biosurgery and CartiHeal in the course of his employment at Cleveland Clinic. He owns stock in Pfizer and General Electric.
[a] Section of Musculoskeletal Imaging, Imaging Institute, Cleveland Clinic, Mail Code: A21, 9500 Euclid Avenue, Cleveland, OH 44195, USA; [b] Department of Orthopedic Surgery, Cartilage Repair Center, Brigham and Women's Hospital, 850 Boylston Street, Suite 112, Chestnut Hill, MA 02467, USA; [c] Department of Biomedical Engineering, Lerner Research Institute, Cleveland Clinic, 9500 Euclid Avenue, Cleveland, OH 44195, USA
* Corresponding author.
E-mail address: forneym@ccf.org

are being performed, the radiologist must have an understanding of the surgical techniques involved, the expected postoperative appearances of these repairs, and the possible complications associated with repair strategies. The basic approaches to the treatment of cartilage damage include nonoperative conservative measures, lavage and debridement, marrow stimulation techniques, synthetic scaffolds, biological tissue grafting, and cell-based therapies. Many cartilage repair techniques are not approved by the US Food and Drug Administration and are available only outside the United States or through clinical trials.

The following sections provide an overview of current cartilage repair strategies and their normal and abnormal MR imaging appearances. Guidelines for reporting postoperative imaging findings are discussed also.

NONOPERATIVE CONSERVATIVE THERAPY, LAVAGE, AND DEBRIDEMENT

Nonperative conservative treatments include symptomatic relief options such as nonsteroidal antiinflammatory drugs, braces, oral nutriceuticals such as chondroitin sulfate, intra-articular visco-supplementation with hyaluronic acid (HA), and injection with platelet-rich plasma (PRP). No studies have shown a significant improvement in the MR imaging appearance of chondral surfaces after HA or PRP injection.[11–13] This finding could, in part, relate to the short follow-up interval of these studies (1–2 years). In 1 randomized controlled study, clinical outcome scores were better for patients who underwent PRP injection than for those who received HA injection.[14,15]

Lavage and debridement are usually performed arthroscopically and involve the removal of unstable cartilage, loose bodies, and osteophytes. After debridement, lesions may appear larger and may have sharper margins on MR imaging. Some lesions may appear to fill, either from attempted self-repair or because of differences in slice position and partial volume averaging artifacts. MR imaging is usually performed after these therapies to assess the joint for progression of the cartilage defect or development of new structural damage.

SURGICAL TECHNIQUES FOR CARTILAGE REPAIR

All of the surgical techniques begin with complete removal of the damaged cartilage. This procedure may involve debridement of the cartilage to the calcified cartilage or subchondral bone. Bone and cartilage may also be removed en bloc or as a plug (as in osteochondral grafting). As a result,

all tissue within a cartilage repair site represents either newly grown or implanted tissue. Tissue grafting techniques use autograft or allograft tissue to provide a more optimal hyaline or hyaline-like cartilage repair tissue. Cell-based therapies are 2-step procedures in which chondrocytes harvested from the patient are cultured and then reimplanted as cells or as cell-seeded scaffolds. Acellular scaffolds may also be implanted into prepared cartilage defects. Nonbiological therapies can provide partial or complete resurfacing of a single compartment of a joint with metal or polyethylene, but these treatments are beyond the scope of this article. Patient compliance with a proper rehabilitation regimen is necessary to ensure a good outcome. A basic algorithm for these various procedures is shown in **Fig. 1**.

Bone Marrow Stimulation

Marrow stimulation techniques are probably the most common surgeries for chondral defects, with microfracture being the most common of these. The goal of stimulation procedures is to promote bleeding that forms a clot, which then fills the chondral defect with pluripotent cells derived from bone marrow. Cytokines are released, stimulating the formation of fibrocartilage within the lesion.[16] However, fibrocartilage does not have the same biomechanical properties as native hyaline cartilage, so this repair may be less durable.

Early marrow stimulation procedures removed the subchondral bone plate altogether. These procedures were then replaced by abrasion arthroplasty, a less invasive subchondral bone plate debriding technique. As time progressed, less invasive procedures were favored, such as subchondral bone drilling and microfracture. Although drilling and microfracture are similar, historically, drilling was theoretically believed to have a higher risk of tissue necrosis. However, a recent study in a rabbit model showed more osteocyte necrosis with microfracture than with microdrilling.[17]

Microfracture is appealing because it can be performed arthroscopically, is therefore relatively noninvasive, and has low morbidity. In this procedure, the chondral lesion is first debrided to sharp, stable margins, and an awl is then used to create 1-mm to 2-mm holes in the subchondral bone plate approximately 3 to 5 mm apart across the entire lesion area (**Fig. 2**, Video 1).[16] The recovery and rehabilitation time for microfracture is the same as for cartilage repair surgeries for small lesions (<4 cm^2): 6 weeks on crutches with partial weight bearing and continuous passive motion for 6 to 8 hours daily. No inline running for 6 to 9 months and no pivoting sports for 1 year are advised.

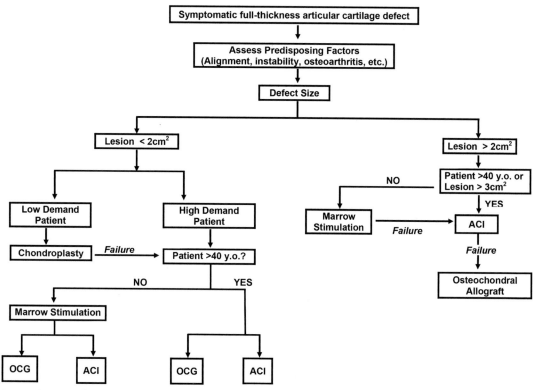

Fig. 1. Algorithm for surgical cartilage repair. ACI, autologous chondrocyte implantation; OCG, osteochondral graft.

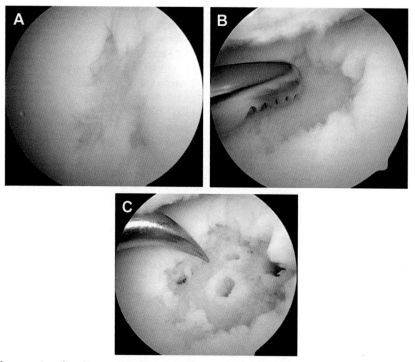

Fig. 2. Microfracture is a first-line option for small chondral defects less than 2 cm² and some larger lesions in patients younger than 40 years. This 1 cm² full-thickness cartilage defect (*A*) was first debrided (*B*) and then an awl used to make perforations in subchondral bone (*C*). After the tourniquet is released, bleeding from the marrow produces a clot that is rich in stem cells and matures into a fibrocartilaginous repair tissue. Video 1 shows a microfracture procedure.

Microfracture has the best outcomes when the patient age is younger than 40 years, the procedure is performed within 12 months of the initial injury, and the lesions are less than 2 cm^2.[18–20] Outcomes are not as good for microfracture performed in the patellofemoral compartment[20] and for lesions greater than 4 cm^2. The long-term durability of cartilage repair by microfracture seems to be limited; integrity has been shown to decline at approximately 18 to 36 months.[18] The formation of intralesional osteophytes has been described as a mode of failure.[21] Although failed microfracture repair sites can be revised with other cartilage repair techniques, there is evidence that postoperative changes in the subchondral bone plate may reduce the success rate of the second procedure.[22]

Recently, techniques have been proposed to improve the microfracture technique by adding a scaffold or polymer to the repair site. The purpose of the collagen matrix is to promote the formation of a higher-quality repair tissue. For an Autologous Matrix-Induced Chondrogenesis (AMIC) procedure, a collagen I/III porcine matrix is fixed within the defect with fibrin glue.[23,24] Alternatively, a chitosan-glycerol phosphate polymer (Piramal Healthcare, Laval, Quebec, Canada) (marketed as BST-CarGel in Europe) may be added to the microfracture site to help stabilize the blood clot and reduce contraction of the clot.[25] Additional methods of augmenting microfracture using biochemical modifiers such as growth factors and gene therapy have been proposed.[26–28]

TISSUE GRAFTS

Tissue grafting replaces the damaged articular surface with tissue from the same patient (ie, orthotopic autograft) or from a deceased donor (ie, allograft). With osteochondral grafts, bone and its overlying cartilage are transplanted, making the repair a true hyaline articular cartilage. More recently, particulated articular cartilage has been used for repair as an autograft (CAIS) or allograft juvenile cartilage (DeNovo NT).[29] Processed allograft tissue has also recently been used as an acellular biological scaffold to promote growth of bone and cartilage (eg, ChondroFix and ACS Articular Cartilage Scaffold).

Osteochondral Allograft

Osteochondral allograft uses cadaveric donor tissue to repair a bone-cartilage defect. This technique is most often used as a second-line salvage procedure for larger lesions, typically greater than 2.5 cm^2, which may have bone loss, but is also used for primary treatment of large defects in active

patients with high physiologic demands.[30] Chondrocyte viability in allograft material is dependent on tissue handling. The donor tissue must be harvested within 24 hours of death. Allografts may be fresh (stored at 4°C in culture) or frozen (stored at −40°C). Because freezing can kill chondrocytes, many surgeons prefer fresh over cryopreserved specimens.[31] The allograft bone is avascular and nonviable but provides a rigid structure to support the chondral allograft until it is incorporated by native bone.[31] Chondrocytes are believed to be immunoprivileged; however, there have been reports of immunoreactivity of chondrocytes after osteochondral allograft procedures.[32–34] Because the marrow elements are removed and the amount of transplanted bone is minimized, the risk of immunologic complications is decreased. In a review of the literature, Rihn and Harner[35] found no reports of clinically significant immune reactions after musculoskeletal allograft transplantation. For these reasons, donor tissue matching and immunosuppression therapy are not required for osteochondral allograft procedures. The risk of disease transmission is low, reported to be equivalent to that of a blood transfusion.[31] Buck and colleagues[36] reported that if the donors are properly screened for infection, the estimated risk of human immunodeficiency virus transmission is 1 in 1.6 million.

In the osteochondral allograft procedure (**Fig. 3**), the lesion is first debrided to healthy bone. Perforations are then created in the native bone to promote bleeding from the marrow space, which aids in native bone ingrowth. An allograft bone-cartilage segment is either tailored to the geometry of the lesion or consists of a large single round plug. If the allograft segment cannot be adequately press fit into the donor site, a screw or pin, often made of a bioabsorbable material, may be used. Overall, outcomes for this procedure are good, with high allograft survival rates: 85% at 4 years in 1 study and 72% at 7.7 years in another study for lesions averaging 8 cm^2.[37,38] For very large lesions greater than 10 cm^2, a unicompartmental prosthesis may be more appropriate.[39]

Osteochondral Autograft

Osteochondral autograft procedures make use of the patient's own bone-cartilage surfaces for donor material. Other commonly used terms for this procedure include generic names such as autogenous osteochondral transfer (AOT) and proprietary names such as osteochondral autograft transfer system (OATS) and mosaicplasty, which are frequently used as generic names. These procedures allow the defect to be resurfaced with native hyaline cartilage with no risk of disease

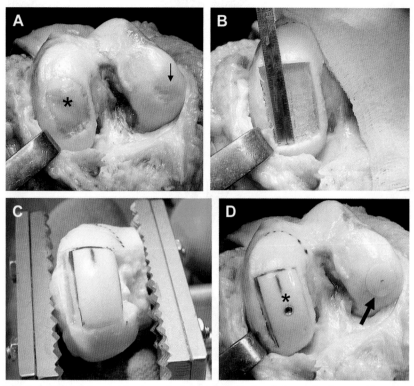

Fig. 3. Osteochondral allograft is used for large lesions (>3 cm²) after failure of other cartilage repair procedures such as ACI, or, by some surgeons, as a first-line treatment. This patient had a failed P-ACI on the medial femoral condyle (*asterisk*, *A*) and a full-thickness cartilage defect on the lateral femoral condyle (*arrow*, *A*). The lesions are first excised with minimal removal of bone (*B*). A matching osteochondral segment tailored to the defect is harvested from the donor knee (*C*) and fixed in the defect (*D*). Osteochondral allografts can be custom cut (*asterisk*, *D*) or cylindrical, similar to an osteochondral autograft transfer system plug (*arrow*, *D*). The allograft may be press fit or attached with a screw or pins, which may be metal or bioabsorbable.

transfer and no need to wait for donor tissue. Osteochondral autograft is typically used for lesions greater than 1 cm² but less than 4 to 5 cm² and up to 10 mm deep.[40]

The donor osteochondral material is typically harvested from the symptomatic joint from a relatively non–weight-bearing area, most often the lateral trochlea near the sulcus terminalis, but the margins of the intercondylar notch and medial trochlea are also options. Donor material may also be obtained from other joints (eg, treatment of a lesion of the talus or elbow with a donor site in the knee). When the lesion is small, it may be completely filled with 1 cylindrical osteochondral plug (**Fig. 4**). Larger lesions are typically filled with several plugs to better recreate the articular contour. Donor sites greater than 6 mm in diameter have higher rates of donor site morbidity.[40] Plugs of approximately 4.5 mm in diameter have a lower risk of breakage during implantation and a lower rate of donor site morbidity than larger plugs.[40] The term mosaicplasty has been coined for the use of multiple plugs because the repair

tissue resembles a mosaic, with a mixture of hyaline cartilage tiles and fibrocartilage grout filling the space between the transferred osteochondral plugs.[41] Typically, the donor sites are left as empty osteochondral defects, which fill over time with bone covered by fibrocartilage. Imaging evaluation of these osteochondral autografts should include both the donor and recipient sites.

Particulated Cartilage Tissue Graft

Chondrocytes within articular cartilage are embedded within a dense extracellular matrix and have a limited ability to migrate. However, when cartilage is cut into small particles, the cells are liberated from the matrix and proliferate.[42] A particulated or minced adult chondral autograft was first shown to effect a chondral repair in a rabbit model in Germany.[43] The combined change in local environment from the mincing process and fibrin glue and possibly the exposure to subchondral bleeding are believed to modify adult chondrocytes to behave more like juvenile

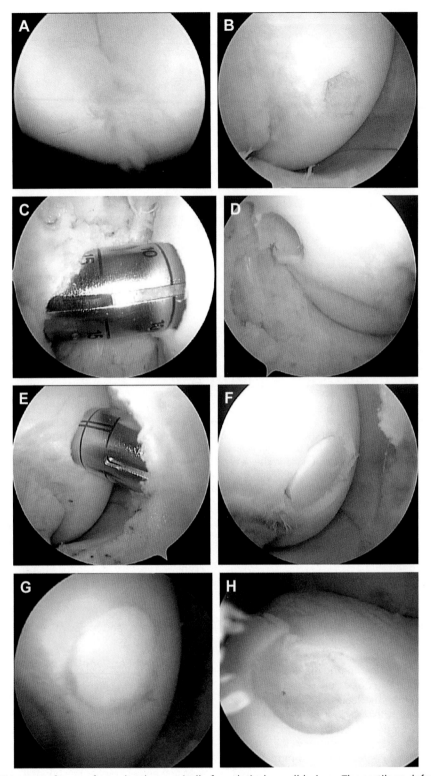

Fig. 4. OATS is most often performed arthroscopically for relatively small lesions. The cartilage defect (*A*) is debrided (*B*) and measured to determine the number of cylindrical grafts needed for repair. A tube harvester (*C*) is used to cut the donor plug from the trochlea. The donor site is usually left empty (*D*). A recipient hole is cut at the repair site (*E*) and the donor plug inserted and tamped to be level with the articular surface (*F*). At second-look arthroscopy 9 months after operation, the repair site shows good fill with fibrocartilage filling gaps around the plug (*G*) and fill of the donor site nearly to the level of the adjacent cartilage (*H*).

chondrocytes, thus producing extracellular matrix[42] and realizing a hyalinelike repair. Unlike the hyaline cartilage that is transferred with osteochondral grafts, the cartilage repair tissue that grows from particulated cartilage becomes incorporated into the surrounding articular cartilage.[29]

As an autograft procedure performed through a miniarthrotomy, CAIS is a 1-step procedure in which roughly 200 mg of the patient's own cartilage is harvested from the margin of the intercondylar notch as minced cartilage particles.[44] These particles are deposited uniformly onto a biodegradable scaffold and covered with fibrin glue. The coated scaffold is then trimmed to fit the debrided lesion and affixed to the defect with bioabsorbable staples, with the particulated cartilage facing the subchondral bone. CAIS is limited by the amount of donor cartilage that may be harvested and the potential of donor site morbidity.[29] This procedure is available in Europe but has not been approved in the United States.

An allograft approach to particulated cartilage transplantation, DeNovo NT, has been developed using juvenile donor cartilage. DeNovo NT is harvested from donors ranging in age from 29 days to 12 years (mean age, 4.2 years).[29] The method exploits the potential advantage of providing cartilage particles with a greater cell density, which may produce more extracellular matrix.[45,46] In addition, a greater amount of cartilage may be grafted, because there is no potential for donor site morbidity, as there is with autograft techniques. As mentioned earlier, cartilage is immunoprivileged; no immunologic reactions to chondral allograft have been reported.[47] This material is considered to be minimally manipulated tissue and is approved for use in the United States. During the single-stage procedure, the lesion is debrided, with removal of the calcified layer of cartilage and with efforts made to keep the subchondral bone plate intact.[48] Two methods for filling the debrided chondral defect have been suggested. One option is to create a mold of the debrided lesion with foil, fill the mold with evenly distributed tissue particles and fibrin glue, and allow the mixture to set for 3 to 10 minutes.[29] This cartilage–fibrin glue construct is then transferred and fixed within the chondral defect with fibrin glue. The alternative method is to fill the debrided chondral defect directly with evenly distributed particulated juvenile chondrocytes and fibrin glue. The DeNovo NT graft is intentionally underfilled by at least 1 mm, and usually 2 to 3 mm, to protect the new repair tissue in the immediate postoperative state.[29,48] DeNovo NT has been successfully used to fill bone defects less than 6 mm deep.[49]

Cell and Tissue Culture Therapies

Autologous chondrocyte implantation (ACI) was developed in the 1980s and spurred much of the interest in cell-based cartilage repair techniques.[16,50,51] Since the creation of the first generation of techniques, which used periosteum to cover the defect, several variations of ACI have been developed. ACI is a 2-step procedure. First, 250 to 300 mg of cartilage is harvested arthroscopically from a less weight-bearing portion of the joint; in the knee, this is typically the margin of the intercondylar notch or trochlea. The chondrocytes are extracted from the harvested cartilage and cultured ex vivo under special conditions for 3 to 4 weeks to expand the number of cells. During a second surgery (usually open), the lesion is debrided, a periosteal (first-generation, ACI-P) or synthetic collagen cover (eg, collagen-covered autologous chondrocyte implantation [second-generation CACI or ACI-C]) is sewn over the defect to the adjacent articular cartilage, and the cultured chondrocytes are implanted beneath the cover (**Fig. 5**, Video 2).[52] With this technique, large defects may be repaired, because the amount of harvested material does not significantly limit the number of cultured cells that may be provided. Although some have reserved ACI as a second-line therapy (ie, after failure of marrow stimulation procedures), increased failure rates have been seen with ACI when used as a second-line procedure. Larger cartilage defects may be best treated with primary ACI.[22] The best results have been seen in younger patients and in those with single medial femoral condyle lesions[18]; however, good results have also been seen in patients with multiple lesions, with greater than 92% of patients with osteoarthritis functioning well for greater than 5 years, delaying joint replacements.[53] The hyalinelike repair tissue seems to be durable, as shown by 2 case series of greater than 200 patients each; in these studies, 74% to 75% of patients had improved function greater than 10 years after surgery.[54]

More recently, scaffolds have been incorporated into ACI techniques to support the implanted chondrocytes and optimize repair. The chondrocytes extracted from the harvested cartilage are grown within a collagen matrix ex vivo and then inserted as a cultured tissue (**Fig. 6**). This third-generation technique is often referred to as matrix-assisted autologous chondrocyte implantation, although matrix-assisted chondrocyte implantation (MACI) is also a proprietary name for a specific technique. The scaffold may be made of one of several materials including collagen (MACI, NeoCart) or HA (Hyalograft C); each

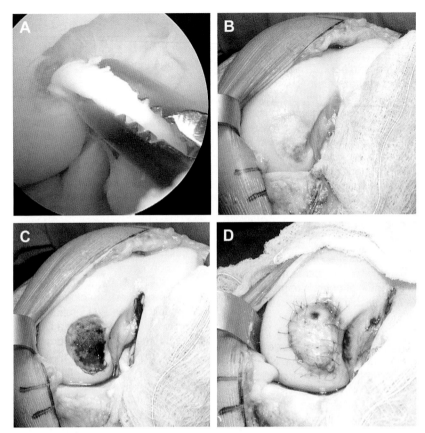

Fig. 5. ACI is a 2-step procedure used for larger cartilage defects. Cartilage harvest is performed at an initial arthroscopy (cartilage biopsy held by forceps, *A*). In vitro culture requires 3 to 4 weeks. At the second, open procedure, the lesion (*B*) is debrided to subchondral bone and stable cartilage margins (*C*), and the cultured chondrocytes are injected under a sewn periosteal (*D*) or collagen-based synthetic cover. Video 2 shows an ACI procedure.

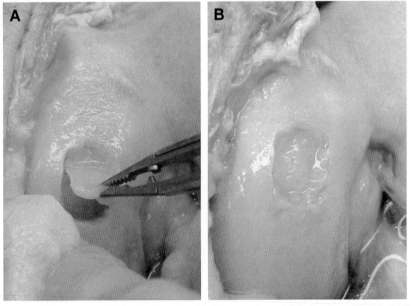

Fig. 6. Matrix-assisted chondrocyte implantation, the third generation of ACI, is also a 2-stage procedure. A matrix is seeded with the harvested cells and cultured in vitro. The chondral construct is implanted into the debrided defect without the need for a sewn cover, as shown in this cadaver knee (*A, B*).

product has proprietary culture techniques. The scaffold is stabilized in the repair site with fibrin glue or collagen-based glue and usually does not completely fill the depth of the defect.[16,55,56] Therefore, no suturing is required and no periosteal or collagen patch is needed. Furthermore, these procedures may be performed with smaller arthrotomies or arthroscopically.

With all of the chondrocyte implantation techniques, every effort is made to preserve the underlying subchondral bone to minimize cell contamination by subchondral marrow, which may induce a fibrocartilage repair tissue. Posttreatment evaluation of cell-based tissue implantation therapies shows the repair tissue to be hyalinelike with a mix of fibrocartilage compared with the more homogeneously fibrocartilage repair of marrow stimulation techniques.[57–59] Graft hypertrophy (overgrowth of the repair tissue above the level of the adjacent articular surface) was a common but treatable complication with first-generation ACI techniques, which was believed to be caused by the periosteal cover. The incidence of this complication has been greatly reduced with the use of a collagen membrane cover and with cultured scaffold techniques.

An allograft-seeded scaffold, RevaFlex (formerly DeNovo ET), currently in phase 3 clinical trials, combines strategies by culturing particulated allograft juvenile cartilage on a scaffold ex vivo for implantation in a 1-step procedure.[60] This engineered tissue is available in 22-mm to 24-mm disks, which can be tailored to fit the lesion at the time of implantation and are affixed to the lesion with fibrin glue.

Implanted Scaffold Therapies

In another strategy for cartilage repair, synthetic scaffolds engineered to promote cartilage or bone growth are implanted within the cartilage defect. Several different materials have been proposed for this use. These scaffolds may be cell seeded, loaded with growth factors or blood products, or acellular. The acellular scaffolds promise a 1-step off-the-shelf solution to cartilage repair. Most of these technologies are in development or in early trials. An acellular scaffold that is commercially available in Europe (TruFit CB or BGS) has shown conflicting short-term to intermediate-term results.[61,62] These cylindrical scaffolds are composed of 2 polymers: one designed to promote chondrocyte growth at the surface and the other designed to promote bone growth at the base. One study reported improved clinical scores, development of a cartilagelike surface based on delayed gadopentetate-enhanced MR imaging of cartilage (dGEMRIC) MR imaging features, and no damage to opposing articular surfaces.[62] However, another study comparing TruFit BGS scaffolds with mosaicplasty showed better clinical results at a mean of 22 to 30 months follow-up for mosaicplasty.[63] By MR criteria, good incorporation of the bone and cartilage repair to the surrounding tissues has been reported in patients but was shown to be ongoing at 16 months (**Fig. 7**).[64] Although patients may return to weight-bearing activities relatively quickly after these procedures are performed, the imaging appearance of these repair sites may appear concerning for years while the tissue ingrowth matures.[65] A study by Barber and Dockery[66] indicates that bony incorporation or ingrowth into this scaffold is either extremely slow or incomplete, with persistent areas of the scaffold without bone, as shown by computed tomography (CT) scans, even after 5 years. A trilayer nanostructured biomimetic scaffold (MaioRegen, FinCeramica Faenza SpA, Faenza, Italy) has shown promising results in the experimental stages. The 2-year and 5-year follow-up studies have shown good clinical outcomes with statistically significant clinical improvements when compared with preoperative and 2-year time points, respectively.[67,68] The magnetic resonance observation of cartilage repair tissue (MOCART) scores, although shown to significantly improve with time, were not as favorable as clinical findings, and no correlation was noted between clinical outcomes and MR imaging findings even after 5 years.[67] As mentioned in the section on allografts, treated acellular allogeneic cartilage-bone cylinders that serve as scaffolds are also available for implantation.

MR IMAGING ASSESSMENT OF SURGICAL CARTILAGE REPAIR

Arthroscopy is considered the gold standard for postoperative assessment of surgical cartilage repair; however, this procedure is invasive and relatively expensive. Arthroscopic evaluation may include the degree of filling of the defect, the integration of the edge (border zone) of the repair tissue to the surrounding articular cartilage, the macroscopic appearance of the repair tissue (smooth, fraying/fissuring), the color of the tissue, and the stiffness of the tissue on probing. The International Cartilage Repair Society macroscopic evaluation of cartilage repair and Oswestry Arthroscopy Score are semiquantitative scoring systems that provide an overall grade of the success of the cartilage repair and are useful for research and clinical trials.[69]

Although MR imaging cannot provide an accurate assessment of some of the arthroscopic

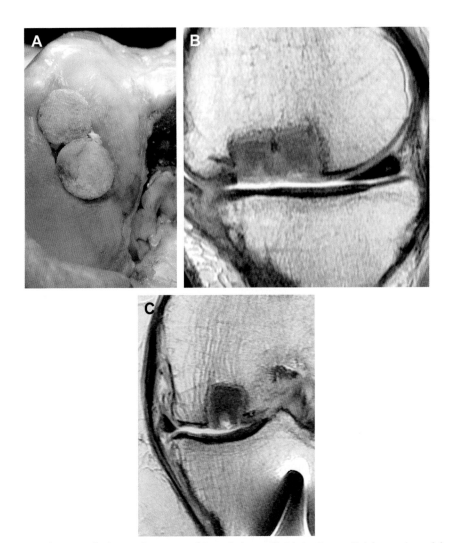

Fig. 7. Operative photograph shows placement of 2 acellular scaffolds in the medial femoral condyle for treatment of an osteochondral lesion (*A*). Sagittal (*B*) and coronal (*C*) images 7 months postoperatively show the typical appearance with early signal changes at the periphery of the scaffolds as bone in growth occurs. The superficial repair cartilage layer is high signal and irregular. It may take years before the scaffold incorporates, and although the imaging appearance is concerning for failure, the patient may be doing well clinically.

features of cartilage repair tissue such as color, stiffness, and fine fibrillations, it can provide information about the defect fill and integration along with additional information about the subchondral bone. Because this technique is noninvasive and easily repeated, imaging is generally a more practical way to assess surgical success than arthroscopy. MR imaging is now used frequently in clinical trials of new cartilage repair techniques. Although follow-up MR imaging at regular intervals is commonly performed in clinical trials, in clinical practice, MR imaging is reserved for symptomatic patients and is often the one of the first steps, because it provides valuable information about the repair site structure. The information provided can help clinicians to plan surgical or nonsurgical

interventions. Blackman and colleagues[70] reviewed 26 studies assessing the correlation between MR imaging and clinical outcomes, concluding that imaging findings at 6 and 36 months postoperatively correlated best with clinical outcomes. In the very early postoperative phase, many repairs are immature, and imaging before 6 months after surgery may confuse the clinical picture, unless warranted by acute symptoms or to assess for non–repair site complications. Often, repair site findings found on MR do not correlate with symptoms, but the structural abnormalities identified by imaging may have prognostic implications. Some surgeons may request MR imaging for asymptomatic patients when the patient is considering a change in activity level. MR findings of an immature repair may factor into a decision to delay their return to high-demand activities.

Several MR scoring systems have been developed to help standardize postoperative cartilage assessment. Most of these systems judge many parameters, and although these systems are useful in gathering objective data for clinical trials, they may not be practical for daily radiology reports. However, a review of these systems can help provide the basis for an effective clinical radiology report.

In 2003, Henderson and colleagues[37] reported on the use of an MR scoring system to assess cartilage repair tissue after ACI. The Henderson scoring system assigns a score of 1 to 4 points in 4 categories, with lower scores indicating a better result, the opposite of arthroscopic scoring systems. The Henderson MR imaging parameters are defect filling (complete fill = 1 point; >50% = 2; <50% = 3; full-thickness defect = 4), repair tissue signal intensity (normal = 1; near normal = 2; abnormal = 3; absent signal = 4), bone marrow edema (absent = 1; mild edema = 2; moderate edema = 3; severe edema = 4), and joint effusion (absent = 1; mild = 2; moderate = 3; severe = 4). In this study, significant improvements in appearance were seen postoperatively at 12 months compared with 3 months. For 15 patients who also had a postoperative arthroscopy, moderate correlation between the Henderson score and the arthroscopic visual data was reported. No single parameter or total score correlated well with the clinical outcomes. Another MR imaging scoring system reported by Roberts and colleagues[71] in the same year also used 4 categories, assigning either 0 (abnormal) or 1 (normal or nearly normal) point for each category, with a score of 4 points indicating the best possible result.[51] The 4 MR parameters in this system are surface integrity and contour, signal intensity of the repair tissue, repair cartilage thickness, and changes in the underlying bone. The study reported a correlation between MR scoring and histologic scoring of postoperative biopsy specimens. Although this system is simpler, it does not provide many gradations for abnormalities.

In 2004, Marlovits and colleagues[72] defined the MR parameters of the MOCART scoring system, which showed sensitivity to changes between 6 and 12 months after surgery for 45 patients who had undergone surgical cartilage repair with microfracture, MACI, or autologous osteochondral transplantation. Nine parameters were defined to assess the quality of the repair: defect filling, repair tissue integration, repair tissue surface, repair tissue structure, repair tissue signal intensity, subchondral lamina status, subchondral bone status,

presence or absence of adhesions, and presence or absence of synovitis. In 2009, Welsch and colleagues[73] proposed 3D-MOCART as a modified version of the MOCART system adapted for higher-resolution imaging, including isotropic three-dimensional acquisitions. This version refined gradations for some parameters, included localization and degree of involvement relative to the repair site, divided repair tissue integration into cartilage and bone interfaces, added parameters for chondral osteophytes and bone marrow edema, eliminated adhesions, and replaced synovitis with effusion. The MOCART systems are the most commonly used MR scoring systems for clinical trials of cartilage repair.

A recent publication[74] suggests that 1 scoring system may not be optimal for all cartilage repair procedures. The investigators indicate that the MOCART system, although comprehensive for marrow stimulation and cell-based therapies, may not include adequate assessment of the bony changes to fully evaluate osteochondral allografts. The Osteochondral Allograft MRI Scoring System (OCAMRISS), on the other hand, grades 5 cartilage parameters, 4 bone parameters, and 4 additional joint findings and was compared with micro-CT and histopathologic evaluations in a goat model with substantial agreement for almost all parameters.

The number of MR scoring systems for cartilage repair and the detailed parameters discussed earlier can present a challenge for a high-volume clinical radiologist. Distilling the necessary features to generate a radiology report that is useful to the cartilage repair surgeon is important for optimal patient care. **Table 1** summarizes the important features that we recommend be mentioned in the report, and the following sections describe the details of these features.

DEFECT FILL

Because all of the cartilage is removed from the cartilage repair site before treatment, anything visualized postoperatively within the operative site should represent newly grown or transplanted/implanted repair tissue. The degree of filling is considered complete if the repair tissue fills the entire defect and is level with the adjacent native cartilage (**Fig. 8**). At times, the repair tissue surface may extend above the expected level of the articular surface (ie, be proud), indicating repair tissue hypertrophy (**Fig. 9**). If filling is incomplete, the report should include an estimate of the volume and thickness of the repair site that is filled as well as the degree of restoration of the articular contour. Both descriptors are important, because

Table 1
Practical considerations for MR reports on chondral repair

Chondral Repair Findings	Considerations for the MR Report
Defect fill	Volume and thickness Surface contour and character
Integration	With underlying bone With native cartilage
Subchondral bone status	Edemalike marrow signal Cyst formation Osteophyte formation within the repair site
Repair tissue character	Signal intensity of repair tissue
Non–repair site complications	New cartilage defects Joint adhesions, arthrofibrosis Meniscus, ligaments, and so forth Donor site appearance (if applicable)

a repair with 50% fill by volume could have either a uniform level at 50% the thickness of adjacent cartilage or be filled to normal articular surface over half of the repair site and completely empty over the other half. As with native articular cartilage, the underfilled surface contour may be easily characterized as greater than 50% of adjacent cartilage, less than 50%, or exposed subchondral bone. The description of any full-thickness defects or deep fissures is important, because these may indicate failure of the repair tissue.

The time evolution of defect fill varies with the type of surgery performed. With osteochondral grafts and periosteal or collagen-assisted ACI, there is usually complete defect fill immediately after surgery. For techniques that rely on repair tissue growth, including marrow stimulation, matrix-assisted ACI, and particulated cartilage, MR images most often show initial underfilling, with progressive filling of the defect as the tissue grows. The final level of tissue growth may not be achieved for as long as 24 months with some techniques.[75]

INTEGRATION

A successful cartilage repair should integrate with the surrounding native articular cartilage and with the underlying bone. On MR images, if there is no discernible interface with adjacent native cartilage, integration is usually considered complete.

However, because transplanted intact mature, adult articular cartilage does not integrate with mature articular cartilage, integration of the repair-cartilage interface at the border zone of autologous or allogeneic osteochondral grafts usually does not occur, despite appearances.[74] MR imaging can miss regions of incomplete edge integration, because the repair-cartilage interface in osteochondral grafts may be indiscernible or appear as a dark line. The presence of a slitlike or wide fluidlike interface may indicate failure of repair-cartilage integration. However, care must be taken in the early postoperative period, because the border zone of the repair tissue may have an initially bright interface that normalizes in signal intensity over time (**Fig. 10**). In such cases, the bright line most likely represents loosely arranged tissue or fluid that matures and integrates over time. When a fluidlike repair-cartilage interface is encountered, the presence of focal edemalike marrow signal or a subchondral cyst immediately beneath the border zone usually indicates failure of integration.

Cartilage repair tissue must also successfully integrate with the subchondral bone if the surgery is to be successful. In the case of osteochondral grafts, the transplanted bone must integrate to the surrounding cancellous bone; the transplanted cartilage is already naturally integrated to the subchondral bone. Bony integration of osteochondral grafts is discussed in detail later. Failure of repair-bone integration may result in detachment or delamination of a portion or all of the repair tissue (**Fig. 11**). When the separated repair tissue is dislodged from the repair site (displaced delamination), there is a full-thickness defect at the repair site and, potentially, a loose body elsewhere in the joint (**Fig. 12**). However, when the nonintegrated repair tissue remains in place (delamination in situ), a bright linear signal at the deep interface between the subchondral bone and the overlying repair is often seen. Frequently, a delamination in situ shows accompanying edemalike marrow signal. Delamination in situ has the same appearance as an articular cartilage nondisplaced delamination or cartilage flap.

SUBCHONDRAL BONE STATUS

Reactive edemalike marrow changes beneath cartilage repair sites may be seen in the early postoperative period. The abnormal signal may be intense and deep and may extend beyond the repair site. Over time, the edemalike marrow signal normalizes by fading in intensity and, to a variable extent, decreasing in volume. The rate of regression of the reactive postoperative marrow signal

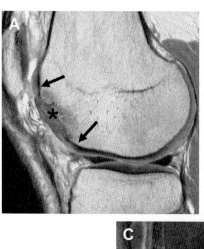
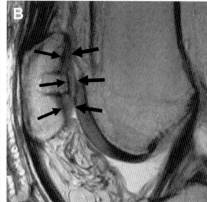
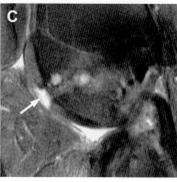

Fig. 8. Fill of the repair site should be judged by restoration of the articular contour. Sagittal (*A*) proton density–weighted image 15 months after P-ACI of a trochlear osteochondral defect shows complete defect fill with a congruent articular surface, even though the repair tissue is thicker (*asterisk*) than adjacent native cartilage (*arrows*). Images from another patient (*B*) 4 months after OATS of the patella show an incongruent subchondral bone plate (*thin arrows*) of the allograft and native bone, but congruent articular surface (*thick arrows*), indicating appropriate fill of the repair site. Because donor and recipient cartilage are often of different thicknesses, this is a relatively common finding, although particularly prominent in this patient. A third patient (*C*) shows lack of repair site fill 6 months after marrow stimulation (*arrow*). There is persistent, intense marrow edema and cyst formation.

is variable with the type of repair, but in general, the abnormal marrow signal returns to normal or near normal 12 to 18 months after surgery. Persistence beyond 18 months, worsening, or reappearance of abnormal marrow signal beneath the repair site should raise concern that there is a problem. The abnormal edemalike marrow signal may be seen with poor integration to the cartilage or bone, poor-quality (soft) repair tissue, or, in the case of osteochondral grafts, failure of the bony portion of the graft to integrate or revascularize (eg, necrosis of the plug). When focal, the abnormal marrow signal usually localizes the problem within the repair site. A brief description of the amount and intensity of edemalike marrow signal beneath a repair site should be included in the radiology report. If comparison studies are available, the change in the degree of any marrow abnormality is the most important factor.

Subchondral cysts may form beneath the repair sites. These cysts often appear beneath the border zone of the repair and may reflect poor repair-cartilage integration. Although these cysts may be asymptomatic, if a revision of the repair is performed, they may require bone grafting. Because these cysts are most often not visible from the surface, a description of the location within the repair site (eg, the anterior edge of the repair) and the size/depth of the cysts can provide useful information to the surgeon.

Thickening of the subchondral bone plate may develop after cartilage repair either as sclerosis (ie, new bone deep to the subchondral bone plate) or as a subchondral or central osteophyte (ie, new bone above the level of the subchondral bone plate). Thickening of the subchondral bone plate has been implicated in the greater number of ACIs that fail when performed as second-line therapy after marrow stimulation versus ACIs performed as first-line treatment.[22] The osteophytes are most likely caused by advancement of the subchondral bone plate or ossification of nonhyaline repair tissue at the base of the repair. They extend from the subchondral bone plate to a variable height, sometimes

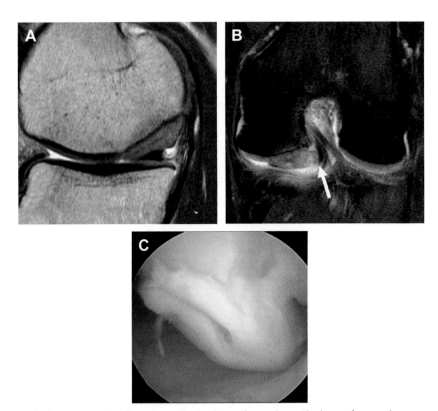

Fig. 9. Hypertrophy is overgrowth of repair cartilage above the native articular surface and may occur after any type of repair except osteochondral grafting but is most commonly seen after P-ACI. Sagittal (A) and oblique coronal (B) images 1 year after revision P-ACI show hypertrophy of the medial femoral condyle repair tissue with arthroscopic correlation (C). Hypertrophy greater than 150% of normal cartilage thickness is often symptomatic. In this case, the hypertrophic tissue may be snapping on the posterior cruciate ligament with flexion (arrow, B).

reaching the level of the articular surface, and can result in a repair site that is biomechanically harder than normal cartilage, which may adversely affect the opposing articular surface.

REPAIR TISSUE CHARACTER

The signal intensity of the repair cartilage reflects the structure of the extracellular matrix of the repair tissue. Except for the true articular cartilage transplanted with osteochondral grafts, the repair tissue differs in signal intensity when compared with the adjacent nonoperated cartilage. Most newly grown repair tissue has an inhomogeneous microstructure and thus inhomogeneous signal intensity on MR images. Repair tissue usually appears brighter than articular cartilage shortly after surgery, with diminishing signal intensity over time, eventually appearing similar to articular cartilage. The cartilage layer of osteochondral grafts usually has the same appearance as adjacent cartilage, with no change in signal intensity over time. However, the cartilage signal intensity of osteochondral grafts may be different from that of adjacent cartilage, because the collagen of the

grafted cartilage may be oriented differently from that of the adjacent cartilage.

To the best of our knowledge, there is no definitive method for predicting the histology or biomechanical character of repair tissue based on the MR appearance on images obtained with typical clinical acquisitions. Several specialized, quantitative techniques have been studied to determine the histologic cartilage components of repair tissue, including T2 maps, dGEMRIC, T1rho, magnetization transfer contrast, diffusion imaging, sodium imaging, and glycosaminoglycan chemical exchange saturation transfer imaging.[76–78] However, these techniques are infrequently used in clinical practice and are not reviewed in this article.

NON–REPAIR SITE EVALUATION

Along with careful assessment of the cartilage repair site, it is important to evaluate the entire joint. Symptoms in the postoperative knee are often related to new abnormalities that may or may not be directly related to the surgery. Postoperative injuries may result in injury to the ligaments and menisci or cause cartilage defects at remote sites.

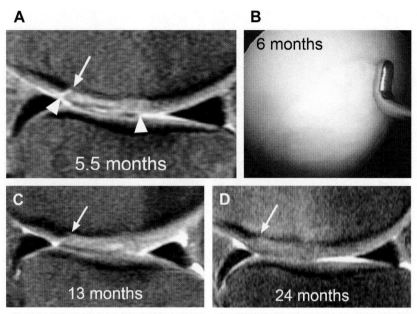

Fig. 10. Maturation of the cartilage repair tissue border zone. (*A*) 5.5 months after P-ACI the cartilage–repair tissue interface is bright (*arrowheads* bracket repair tissue) with the appearance of a fissure (*A, arrow*); however, on arthroscopy at 6 months (*B*), no defect can be found (note mild hypertrophy); 13 months postoperatively (*C*), the interface (*arrow*) has lower signal, indicating progression of the tissue incorporation. At 24 months postoperatively (*D*), the interface (*arrow*) has fully matured and is no longer visible. ([*A, B*] *From* Alparslan L, Minas T, Winalski CS. Magnetic resonance imaging of autologous chondrocyte implantation. Semin Ultrasound CT MR 2001;22(4):341–51.)

New cartilage abnormalities immediately adjacent to a repair site may develop even without failure of the initial operative site. It is unclear whether these abnormalities represent progression of the initial injury to osteoarthritis or incomplete debridement of damaged tissue during surgery. With further study, preoperative quantitative imaging measures may prove useful in determining the amount of tissue that should be debrided.

As with other surgeries, intra-articular adhesions and arthrofibrosis may develop after cartilage repair, resulting in a clinically stiff joint. When this situation occurs, MR imaging commonly shows thickening of the joint capsule or the articular surface of the infrapatellar (Hoffa) fat pad. The bands of fibrous tissue commonly extend from the inferior patella to the tibia, potentially interfering with patellar motion (**Fig. 13**). Adhesions may be

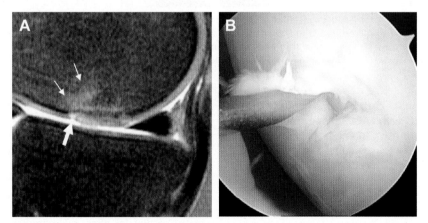

Fig. 11. Edge delamination. Fat-suppressed proton density–weighted sagittal image (*A*) shows a near fluid signal intensity cleft at the anterior margin of the P-ACI site (*large arrow, A*) with subjacent subchondral bone marrow edema (*small arrows, A*). An arthroscopic image of this patient (*B*) shows a probe lifting the delaminated anterior edge ACI tissue. Focal subchondral bone marrow edema may point to a site of abnormal repair tissue or integration.

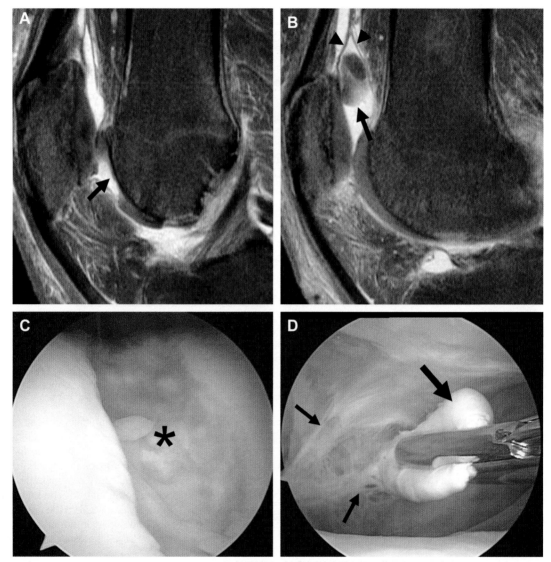

Fig. 12. Eight weeks after P-ACI, sagittal fat-suppressed proton density–weighted image shows an empty repair site (*arrow*, *A*). The displaced cartilage repair tissue is seen in the suprapatellar recess as a similar sized intra-articular body (*arrow*, *B*) adjacent to thin adhesions (*arrowheads*, *B*). Arthroscopy confirmed the presence of an empty repair site (*asterisk*, *C*) and the intra-articular body (*arrow*, *D*) seen attached to adhesions (*small arrows*, *D*) was removed.

directly attached to cartilage repair tissue (**Fig. 14**), as described with ACI; these require open debridement to avoid damage to the repair site as the patient increases activity or as the joint is manipulated.[79]

MR IMAGING APPEARANCES AFTER SPECIFIC PROCEDURES

Within the general reporting categories summarized in **Table 1**, there are some specific MR findings that are more commonly observed after each of the various repair techniques. These expected outcomes or commonly encountered complications are discussed in the following sections.

MARROW STIMULATION PROCEDURES

Little has been reported on MR appearance after abrasion arthroplasty or drilling.[80] Microfracture is more frequently performed, and the MR appearance of tissue after microfracture has been reported in many articles. Initially, after microfracture, the repair tissue is usually thin and commonly intermediate to fluidlike in signal intensity. The defect fill usually improves over time (≤2 years),

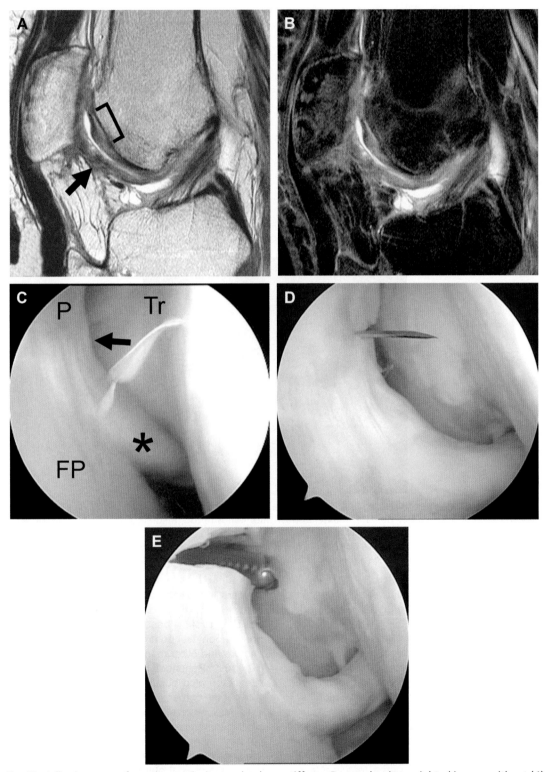

Fig. 13. Adhesions away from the repair site causing knee stiffness. Proton density–weighted images without (*A*) and with fat suppression (*B*) from an intravenous MR arthrogram 3 months after P-ACI of the trochlea (*brackets indicate repair site*) show a thick adhesion (*arrow*) on the surface of the infrapatellar fat pad extending from the intercondylar notch to the inferior pole of the patella. Arthroscopic image 4 months postoperatively (*C*) shows the adhesion (*asterisk*) exiting the notch anterior to the trochlea (Tr) joining the fat pad (FP) and its attachment (*arrow*) to the patella (P). The adhesion was cut with a scalpel (*D*) and shaver (*E*).

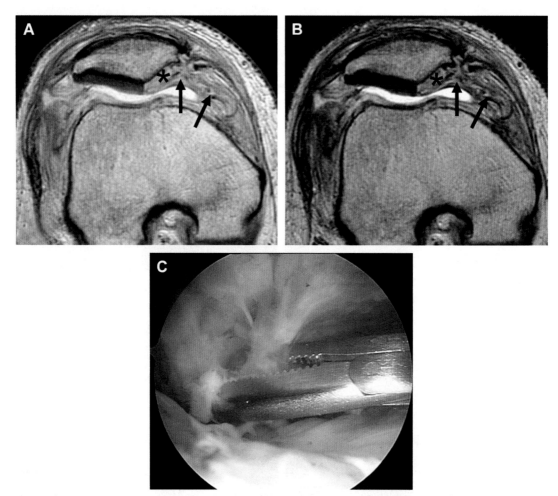

Fig. 14. Adhesion attached to the repair site/tissue. Axial proton density–weighted (*A*) and T2-weighted (*B*) images at 3 weeks after P-ACI of the lateral patella show thick bands of intermediate signal tissue (*arrows, A, B*) extending from the capsule attaching to the surface of the repair tissue (*asterisk, A, B*). Arthroscopic lysis of the adhesions was performed 5 weeks postoperatively (*C*). It is important to identify these adhesions with imaging, because they require surgical lysis to avoid damage of the repair tissue with joint movement.

and the repair tissue shows a lower signal intensity, appearing heterogeneous and often showing a higher signal intensity than native cartilage (**Fig. 15**).[81] Should the patient be imaged shortly after surgery, subchondral marrow edema beneath the entire repair site is expected. This subchondral marrow edema has been shown to progressively decrease over the first few postoperative months.[82] Persistent marrow edema after microfracture is of unclear significance, because this finding can be seen in asymptomatic patients and may be present for years.[17] However, in our experience, persistent marrow edema after 18 months that is intense, localized to a portion of the repair site, or worse than on earlier postoperative images is unexpected and may indicate a complication or future treatment failure. Because the subchondral bone plate is violated as part of the procedure, this structure appears irregular and remains less distinct than normal in the region of the repair on MR imaging. Ossification of the base of the repair tissue (ie, central osteophytes) commonly develops after microfracture and other marrow stimulation procedures (**Fig. 16**).[81] Peripheral fissures from failure of edge integration also occur frequently[81]; however, fissures at the border zone on early postoperative images may resolve with time as the repair–native cartilage interface matures and presumably incorporates. Incomplete filling of the defect on MR imaging may indicate clinical failure. Studies comparing clinical outcome and MR scores after microfracture have shown good to excellent correlation with respect to defect fill.[70,81,83]

For the matrix-assisted microfracture technique AMIC, 1 study reported that most lesions showed greater than 50% lesion fill at a mean follow-up

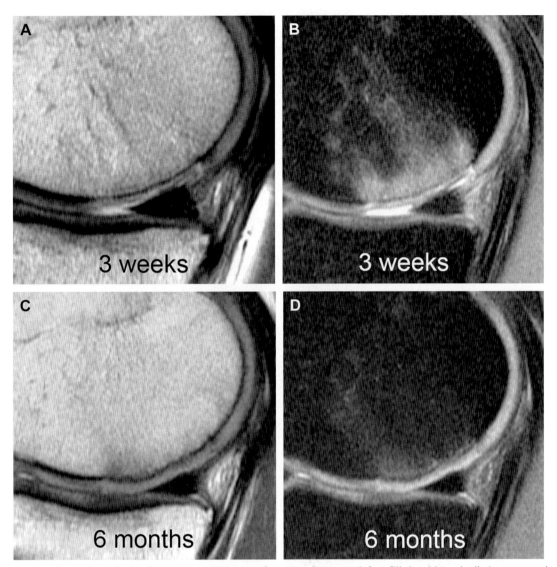

Fig. 15. Maturation of microfracture repair tissue. After microfracture, defect fill should gradually increase and subchondral marrow edema decrease, as seen from 3 weeks to 26 months (*A–H*). Between 36 and 48 months, the marrow edema has returned, which may indicate that the repair tissue has begun to fail (*arrows, J*). The subchondral bone plate (best evaluated on non–fat-suppressed images) has an irregular appearance after marrow stimulation because the subchondral bone plate is disrupted. By 36 months, a central osteophyte (*asterisk, G–J*) has formed.

time of 37 months, with 47% of these cases showing bone marrow edema and 60% showing central osteophytes at the repair site at follow-up.[24] In another study of augmented microfracture, BST-CarGel was shown by MR imaging to produce greater lesion fill than standard microfracture.[84] Although the clinical improvement at 12 months was equivalent for the 2 groups, the repair tissue in the BST-CarGel group had a lower T2 value than the tissue in the standard microfracture group, which was interpreted as indicating a more hyalinelike character.[84]

OSTEOCHONDRAL GRAFTS

The postoperative MR appearances of allografts and autografts have many common features. The chondral surface of the graft material should be congruent with the adjacent native cartilage. Incongruity of the native subchondral bone plate and graft subchondral bone may be present, because the donor cartilage thickness is often different from the thickness of the cartilage at the recipient site (see **Fig. 8B; Fig. 17**). Abnormal grafts may protrude above (ie, proud) or below

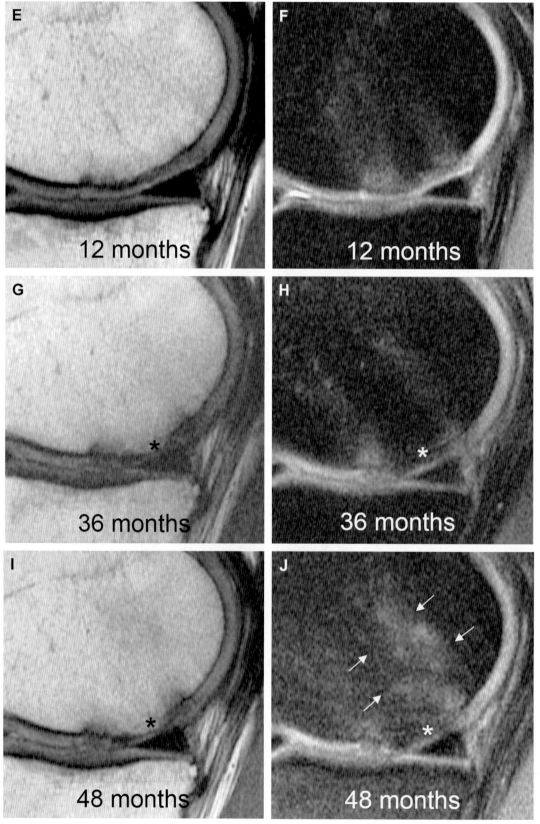

Fig. 15. (*continued*)

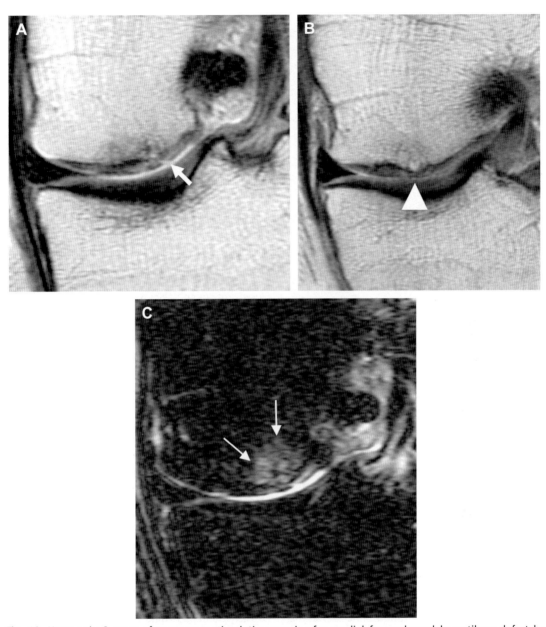

Fig. 16. Knee pain 3 years after marrow stimulation repair of a medial femoral condyle cartilage defect by abrasion arthroplasty. The repair site shows signs of tissue failure with fissures (*arrow, A*), central osteophyte (*arrowhead, B*), and marrow edema (*thin arrows, C*).

(ie, sunken) the level of adjacent cartilage. This surface incongruity may occur during initial placement, result from early weight bearing, or, when delayed, indicate poor bony incorporation of the graft. The appearance of the osteochondral graft cartilage should be normal; any signal abnormality or defect should be reported. When multiple autograft cylinders are placed, there may also be incongruities among the grafts. These incongruities

may improve with time.[82] In an animal model, resolution of the incongruities occurred because of deformation of surrounding tissue or overgrowth by fibrous tissue, depending on the degree of incongruity.[85]

Transplanted adult articular cartilage does not usually incorporate into adjacent cartilage.[57,67] Despite this fact, it is unusual to identify fluid signal at the interfaces. After placement of multiple

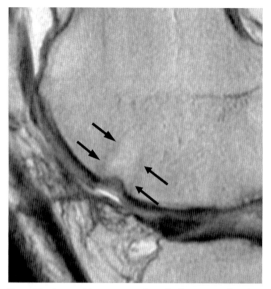

Fig. 17. A trochlear osteochondral autograft plug 11 months after surgery with normal appearance on sagittal proton density–weighted imaging (*arrows*). The articular surface of the autograft may be left countersunk with respect to the adjacent native cartilage or may be congruent.

cylindrical grafts, the gaps between the grafts are usually filled with fibrocartilage grout, which has variable, but most commonly intermediate, signal intensity.[76] Rarely, the cartilage cap of a cylindrical graft may become displaced, leaving a round, full-thickness defect in the articular cartilage of the graft. Subchondral cyst formation beneath the border zone is likely caused by fluid entering the bone through the unincorporated interface; these cysts may be asymptomatic and may not require immediate attention.

MR evaluation of osteochondral grafts must also include the appearance of the bony portion of the graft and its interface with native bone. In the initial postoperative state, it is normal to see edemalike marrow signal within the grafted bone and in the surrounding native bone. Over time, the marrow signal normalizes, and ideally, the interface between the grafted and native bone becomes indistinct or indiscernible, showing normal marrow fat and trabeculations within the grafted bone (**Fig. 18**). Grafted bone that becomes low in signal on all pulse sequences (ie, sclerotic appearing) is abnormal and suggests poor viability or failure.[86]

With autologous grafts, marrow edema within the repair usually resolves over the first year[76]; mild persistent edema has been reported up to 2 years after implantation.[87,88] A good rule of thumb for autografts is that the marrow signals of the donor and repair sites often normalize with a similar time course. When cylindrical autografts

are used, there may be regions without trabeculae deep to the graft, because the surgeon may cut the recipient site deeper than the length of the graft to avoid an inadvertently proud graft at the articular surface.

With allografts, the junction between the grafted bone and native bone may have an appearance reminiscent of the reactive interface of avascular necrosis of the femoral head.[89] The entire interface initially appears bright on T2-weighted images and may widen over time[89]; however, the interface becomes indistinguishable from adjacent marrow. This appearance is more striking with allografts that have thick regions of bone. It has been hypothesized that this appearance may represent the process of creeping substitution of the host osteocytes into the allograft bone.[78] Unique among the cartilage repair procedures, osteochondral allografts have the potential to incite an immunologic response. Clinically significant responses are unusual; however, patients with antibody positivity toward a bone allograft have shown a greater degree of bone marrow edema in the graft, a thicker interface at the graft site, and a greater proportion of chondral surface collapse compared with patients without antibodies.[32] Formation of cysts at the allograft-host interface is abnormal and suggests instability.

The donor sites for osteochondral autografts are usually harvested from the ipsilateral knee joint and should also be evaluated on postoperative imaging. The peripheral trochlea, usually immediately superior to the junction of the patellofemoral and femorotibial articulations (sulcus terminalis) and the superior intercondylar notch are typical harvest sites. Because the knee is a common place for graft harvest when other joints are repaired, a donor site may be rarely encountered without the repair site being found. Edemalike signal is expected in the harvest site and surrounding bone marrow on early postoperative images; this signal usually decreases after 6 to 9 months.[76] The harvest site fills, initially appearing high to intermediate in signal intensity and returning to normal fatty marrow signal with or without visible trabeculations over time as bone forms.[76,81,82] Most often, there is a cap of fibrous or fibrocartilaginous tissue, which fills below the adjacent articular surface overlying bone. Donor sites may become symptomatic, although this is unusual. In patients with osteochondral harvest from asymptomatic knees for transfer to a different joint, studies have shown reduced knee scores after surgery.[82] Persistent pain at the donor site has been reported as a complication of osteochondral autografting, often without imaging correlation. Exuberant fibrocartilage filling above the articular contour can also

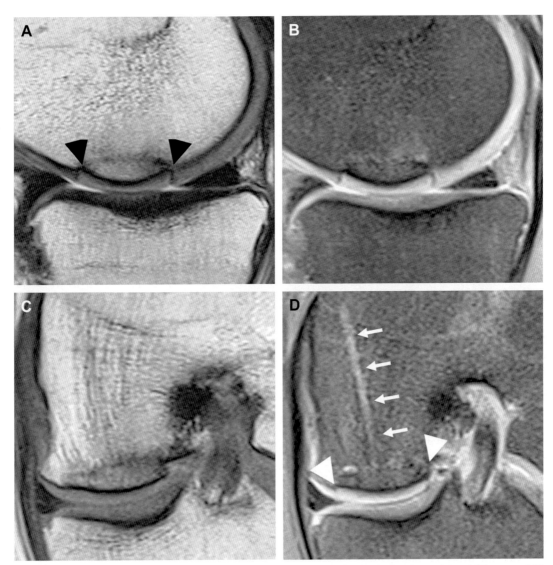

Fig. 18. Sagittal proton density–weighted (*A*), sagittal fat-suppressed proton density–weighted (*B*), coronal T1-weighted (*C*), and fat-suppressed coronal proton density–weighted (*D*) images of an osteochondral allograft of the medial femoral condyle (*arrowheads, A, D*) 1 year after surgery. The grafted cartilage has normal signal intensity, with restoration of the articular surface. The marrow signal of the graft has returned to near normal and the deep bone interface is becoming indistinct. The thin bright line seen on the coronal fat-suppressed proton density–weighted (*arrows, D*) image is from the bioabsorbable pin that was used to fix the graft in place.

occur and be symptomatic.[70] In our experience, persistent, intense edemalike marrow signal within the donor site indicates a complication (**Fig. 19**).

PARTICULATED CARTILAGE GRAFTS

Because particulated chondral grafting has been introduced only recently, there are few reports on the postoperative MR appearance of these grafts. One study evaluating the outcomes of CAIS reported variable lesion fill at 3 weeks, with progressively increased fill over 2 years (**Fig. 20**).[44] At a 2-year follow-up, approximately 80% of the repair sites showed 75% to 100% fill.[44] Central osteophyte and subchondral cyst formation at the CAIS repair sites were seen.[44] One study of 4 patients who received DeNovo NT grafts[29] reported good filling of the lesions on MR images obtained up to 2 years after surgery. Another study[60] evaluating 9 cases of DeNovo ET (now RevaFlex) found that MR findings correlated well with repair tissue fill and quality on a 1-

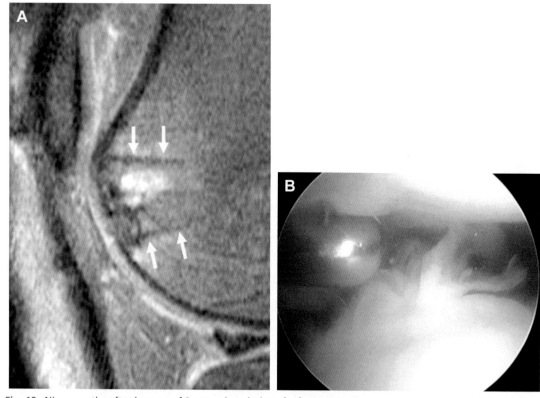

Fig. 19. Nine months after harvest of 2 osteochondral grafts for repair of a talar osteochondral defect, the knee was painful. MR images show bright marrow edema at the donor sites in the superior aspect of the lateral trochlea (*arrows, A*). At arthroscopy (*B*), hypertrophic fibrous tissue was found at the donor site.

year follow-up arthroscopy. In a case report, a patient who underwent DeNovo NT repair of a patellar apex lesion showed near complete defect filling at 21 months and resolution of preoperative subchondral marrow edema.[87] As more of these procedures are performed, more information regarding the expected MR imaging appearance will be available.

CELL-BASED CHONDRAL REPAIR

The appearance of the repair site after the use of cell-based therapies is dependent on the particular procedure and changes as the repair tissue matures.[90] After first-generation and second-generation ACI-P or ACI-C procedures, the defect usually appears filled or even overfilled when imaged soon after surgery (**Fig. 21**). With third-generation MACI, there may be initial underfilling, because the implanted scaffold may not be as thick as the adjacent cartilage. Over the next 2 years, the MACI tissue usually grows to fill the defect.[68] Mild underfilling of the defect may be asymptomatic; symptoms are more often seen in patients with defect filling of less than 50%.[91] In the early postoperative period, the repair tissue

with all techniques frequently appears brighter than normal cartilage, sometimes similar to joint fluid. As the cells form extracellular matrix, the signal intensity of the repair becomes similar to that of native cartilage. However, the tissue often has a persistent heterogeneous appearance,[76] most likely because of the mixed histology and relatively disorganized collagen structure.

Overfill (hypertrophy) has been reported in cases of ACI performed with a sewn periosteal cover and with seeded matrix techniques.[92] When the patient is symptomatic, the hypertrophic tissue may be trimmed arthroscopically without revision of the entire repair site. Kreuz and colleagues[92] studied 102 patients who underwent ACI-P and found that hypertrophy greater than double the thickness of native cartilage caused symptoms and required a surgical intervention, whereas only 50% of patients with hypertrophic tissue 150% to 200% the thickness of native cartilage needed surgery, and none of the patients with hypertrophy less than 150% required treatment. Although measurable hypertrophy can be seen in about one-quarter of all patients who undergo ACI,[92,93] it is more likely to be severe and require intervention with ACI-P than with the cell-seeded

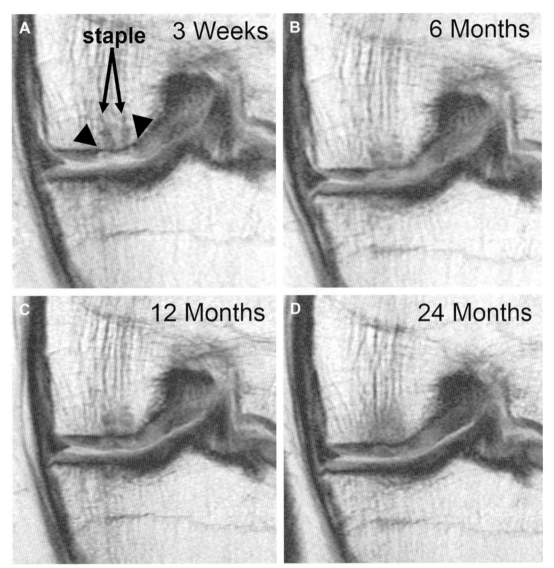

Fig. 20. Postoperative appearance after minced cartilage autograft (CAIS) on coronal proton density–weighted images. The repair construct containing minced autograft cartilage fragments (*arrowheads* mark graft margins, *A*) is secured with a bioabsorbable staple (*arrows*, *A*). With time, there is improved filling of the defect, and repair tissue gradually appears more homogeneous and intermediate in signal intensity (*A–D*). Associated bone marrow signal changes also improve, and the staple appears resorbed by 24 months (*D*). (*From* Cole BJ, Farr J, Winalski CS, et al. Outcomes after a single-stage procedure for cell-based cartilage repair: a prospective clinical safety trial with 2-year follow-up. Am J Sports Med 2011;39(6):1170–9.)

matrix techniques.[75,93] Mild degrees of hypertrophy can regress spontaneously.[92,93]

In the immediate postoperative state, fluidlike signal intensity may be seen at the interfaces of the repair tissue with the subchondral bone and the border zone with the native cartilage, but this should resolve over time.[75] Persistent or new bright or fluid signal intensity at either the bone-repair tissue or repair-cartilage interface is abnormal and may represent failure of the repair

tissue to integrate. Delamination of the repair tissue from the subchondral bone may be partial or complete and the tissue that has separated from the bone may remain in place (ie, delamination in situ) or may become displaced into the joint (**Fig. 22**). Delamination of the periosteal or biologic patch can also occur.

Although the subchondral bone plate is preserved during ACI procedures, edemalike signal in the bone marrow edema beneath the

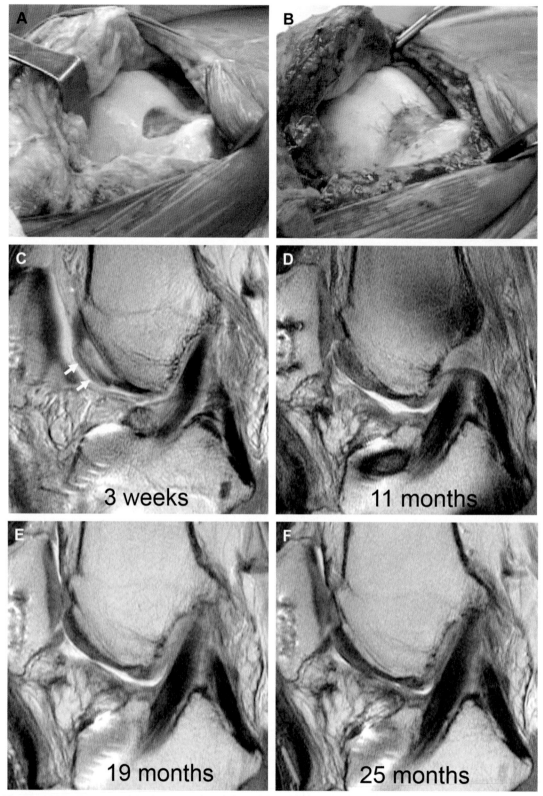

Fig. 21. MR appearance of P-ACI maturation. (*A*) Trochlear cartilage defect after debridement; (*B*) final P-ACI; C. 3 weeks postoperatively, the repair tissue is high signal, and the periosteal cover is visible as a lower signal (*arrows, C*); (*D*) 11 months postoperatively, the repair tissue appears similar to native cartilage with minimal hypertrophy; (*E*) 19 months postoperatively, there has been some ossification of the base of the repair tissue; (*F*) 25 months postoperatively no further change in the repair is shown.

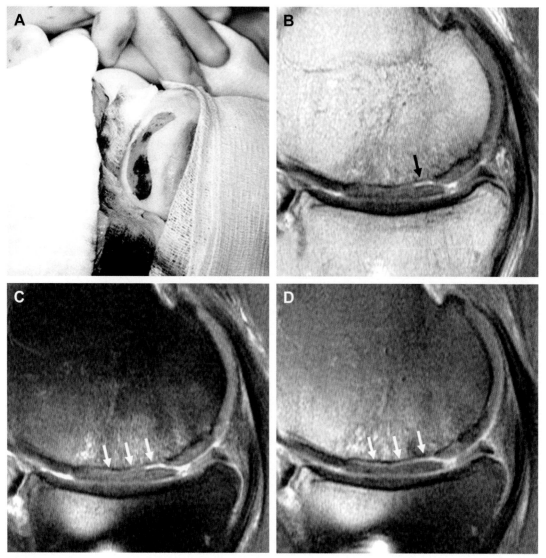

Fig. 22. Partial delamination in situ. Large defect of the medial femoral condyle was treated with P-ACI; (*A*) shows the debrided lesion before periosteal patch. Seven years after surgery, indirect (intravenous) MR arthrogram shows a bright line at the repair-bone interface beneath much of the repair site (*arrows, B–D*). The delamination is best seen on the fat-suppressed T1-weighted image (*D*) for this patient.

postoperative site is universally seen in the early postoperative period. This bone marrow edema should resolve with time. Although the exact time course for resolution is unclear, persistent edema beyond 1 to 1.5 years after the procedure should be of concern, and increasing edema or reappearance of edema may be seen with complications or treatment failure. Subchondral cysts and sclerosis around the repair site are abnormal and often occur beneath the cartilage border zone, likely an indicator of poor repair tissue–cartilage integration or delamination at the edge of the repair site.

Because subchondral cysts cannot be seen during surgery, it is important to describe their size and location relative to the repair site in MR reports so they can be easily treated when necessary.

The harvest site for the chondrocytes used in cell-based therapies often remains occult on follow-up MR imaging. This situation is likely because only a small amount of cartilage is removed and the subchondral bone is not violated during the harvest. Signal changes may be seen at the periosteal harvest site in the case of first-generation ACI procedures. These findings should resolve with time; however, cases of periosteal harvest site morbidity have been reported.[94]

SUMMARY

The variety of chondral repair procedures has increased rapidly over the past 2 decades, and the radiologist's role in the management of patients undergoing these procedures has increased. Imaging physicians need to understand these surgical procedures and the normal and abnormal postoperative imaging appearances of these chondral repairs. When radiologists are presented with unusual cases, it is helpful to fall back on the principles outlined in arthroscopic and MR imaging reporting systems. The clinical significance of many MR imaging findings after chondral repair remains to be determined, but a report including the basic postoperative findings not only helps in standardizing report information but also assists the clinician and patient in follow-up.

ACKNOWLEDGMENTS

We would like to sincerely thank Megan Griffiths, MA, for her help in the preparation and submission of this article.

SUPPLEMENTARY DATA

Supplementary data related to this article can be found online at http://dx.doi.org/10.1016/j.mric.2014.07.008.

REFERENCES

1. Flanigan DC, Harris JD, Trinh TQ, et al. Prevalence of chondral defects in athletes' knees: a systematic review. Med Sci Sports Exerc 2010;42(10):1795–801.
2. Levy AS, Lohnes J, Sculley S, et al. Chondral delamination of the knee in soccer players. Am J Sports Med 1996;24(5):634–9.
3. Curl WW, Krome J, Gordon ES, et al. Cartilage injuries: a review of 31,516 knee arthroscopies. Arthroscopy 1997;13(4):456–60.
4. Drawer S, Fuller CW. Propensity for osteoarthritis and lower limb joint pain in retired professional soccer players. Br J Sports Med 2001;35(6):402–8.
5. Roos EM. Joint injury causes knee osteoarthritis in young adults. Curr Opin Rheumatol 2005;17(2):195–200.
6. Buckwalter JA, Mankin HJ. Articular cartilage: degeneration and osteoarthritis, repair, regeneration, and transplantation. Instr Course Lect 1998;47:487–504.
7. Heywood HK, Nalesso G, Lee DA, et al. Culture expansion in low-glucose conditions preserves chondrocyte differentiation and enhances their subsequent capacity to form cartilage tissue in three-dimensional culture. Biores Open Access 2014;3(1):9–18.
8. DePalma AF, McKeever CD, Subin DK. Process of repair of articular cartilage demonstrated by histology and autoradiography with tritiated thymidine. Clin Orthop Relat Res 1966;48:229–42.
9. Convery FR, Akeson WH, Keown GH. The repair of large osteochondral defects. An experimental study in horses. Clin Orthop Relat Res 1972;82:253–62.
10. Tsuruoka H, Sasho T, Yamaguchi S, et al. Maturation-dependent spontaneous healing of partial thickness cartilage defects in infantile rats. Cell Tissue Res 2011;346(2):263–71.
11. Halpern BC, Chaudhury S, Rodeo SA. The role of platelet-rich plasma in inducing musculoskeletal tissue healing. Hss J 2012;8(2):137–45.
12. Halpern B, Chaudhury S, Rodeo SA, et al. Clinical and MRI outcomes after platelet-rich plasma treatment for knee osteoarthritis. Clin J Sport Med 2013;23(3):238–9.
13. Hart R, Safi A, Komzak M, et al. Platelet-rich plasma in patients with tibiofemoral cartilage degeneration. Arch Orthop Trauma Surg 2013;133(9):1295–301.
14. Sampson S, Reed M, Silvers H, et al. Injection of platelet-rich plasma in patients with primary and secondary knee osteoarthritis: a pilot study. Am J Phys Med Rehabil 2010;89(12):961–9.
15. Sanchez M, Anitua E, Orive G, et al. Platelet-rich therapies in the treatment of orthopaedic sport injuries. Sports Med 2009;39(5):345–54.
16. Farr J, Cole B, Dhawan A, et al. Clinical cartilage restoration: evolution and overview. Clin Orthop Relat Res 2011;469(10):2696–705.
17. Chen H, Sun J, Hoemann CD, et al. Drilling and microfracture lead to different bone structure and necrosis during bone-marrow stimulation for cartilage repair. J Orthop Res 2009;27(11):1432–8.
18. Mithoefer K. Complex articular cartilage restoration. Sports Med Arthrosc 2013;21(1):31–7.
19. Knutsen G, Engebretsen L, Ludvigsen TC, et al. Autologous chondrocyte implantation compared with microfracture in the knee. A randomized trial. J Bone Joint Surg Am 2004;86-A(3):455–64.
20. Kreuz PC, Erggelet C, Steinwachs MR, et al. Is microfracture of chondral defects in the knee associated with different results in patients aged 40 years or younger? Arthroscopy 2006;22(11):1180–6.
21. Gomoll AH, Madry H, Knutsen G, et al. The subchondral bone in articular cartilage repair: current problems in the surgical management. Knee Surg Sports Traumatol Arthrosc 2010;18(4):434–47.
22. Minas T, Gomoll AH, Rosenberger R, et al. Increased failure rate of autologous chondrocyte implantation after previous treatment with marrow

stimulation techniques. Am J Sports Med 2009; 37(5):902–8.

23. Gille J, Behrens P, Volpi P, et al. Outcome of autologous matrix induced chondrogenesis (AMIC) in cartilage knee surgery: data of the AMIC Registry. Arch Orthop Trauma Surg 2013;133(1):87–93.

24. Gille J, Schuseil E, Wimmer J, et al. Mid-term results of autologous matrix-induced chondrogenesis for treatment of focal cartilage defects in the knee. Knee Surg Sports Traumatol Arthrosc 2010; 18(11):1456–64.

25. Hoemann CD, Sun J, McKee MD, et al. Chitosan-glycerol phosphate/blood implants elicit hyaline cartilage repair integrated with porous subchondral bone in microdrilled rabbit defects. Osteoarthritis Cartilage 2007;15(1):78–89.

26. Neumann K, Dehne T, Endres M, et al. Chondrogenic differentiation capacity of human mesenchymal progenitor cells derived from subchondral cortico-spongious bone. J Orthop Res 2008; 26(11):1449–56.

27. Morisset S, Frisbie DD, Robbins PD, et al. IL-1ra/IGF-1 gene therapy modulates repair of microfractured chondral defects. Clin Orthop Relat Res 2007;462:221–8.

28. Kuo AC, Rodrigo JJ, Reddi AH, et al. Microfracture and bone morphogenetic protein 7 (BMP-7) synergistically stimulate articular cartilage repair. Osteoarthritis Cartilage 2006;14(11):1126–35.

29. Farr J, Cole BJ, Sherman S, et al. Particulated articular cartilage: CAIS and DeNovo NT. J Knee Surg 2012;25(1):23–9.

30. Cole BJ, Pascual-Garrido C, Grumet RC. Surgical management of articular cartilage defects in the knee. J Bone Joint Surg Am 2009;91(7):1778–90.

31. Shasha N, Aubin PP, Cheah HK, et al. Long-term clinical experience with fresh osteochondral allografts for articular knee defects in high demand patients. Cell Tissue Bank 2002;3(3):175–82.

32. Sirlin CB, Brossmann J, Boutin RD, et al. Shell osteochondral allografts of the knee: comparison of MR imaging findings and immunologic responses. Radiology 2001;219(1):35–43.

33. Revell CM, Athanasiou KA. Success rates and immunologic responses of autogenic, allogenic, and xenogenic treatments to repair articular cartilage defects. Tissue Eng Part B Rev 2009;15(1):1–15.

34. Phipatanakul WP, VandeVord PJ, Teitge RA, et al. Immune response in patients receiving fresh osteochondral allografts. Am J Orthop (Belle Mead NJ) 2004;33(7):345–8.

35. Rihn JA, Harner CD. The use of musculoskeletal allograft tissue in knee surgery. Arthroscopy 2003;19(Suppl 1):51–66.

36. Buck BE, Malinin TI, Brown MD. Bone transplantation and human immunodeficiency virus. An estimate of risk of acquired immunodeficiency

syndrome (AIDS). Clin Orthop Relat Res 1989;(240):129–36.

37. Henderson IJ, Tuy B, Connell D, et al. Prospective clinical study of autologous chondrocyte implantation and correlation with MRI at three and 12 months. J Bone Joint Surg Br 2003;85(7):1060–6.

38. Hayter C, Potter H. Magnetic resonance imaging of cartilage repair techniques. J Knee Surg 2011; 24(4):225–40.

39. Giorgini A, Donati D, Cevolani L, et al. Fresh osteochondral allograft is a suitable alternative for wide cartilage defect in the knee. Injury 2013; 44(Suppl 1):S16–20.

40. McCoy B, Miniaci A. Osteochondral autograft transplantation/mosaicplasty. J Knee Surg 2012; 25(2):99–108.

41. Hangody L, Kish G, Karpati Z, et al. Arthroscopic autogenous osteochondral mosaicplasty for the treatment of femoral condylar articular defects. A preliminary report. Knee Surg Sports Traumatol Arthrosc 1997;5(4):262–7.

42. Lu Y, Dhanaraj S, Wang Z, et al. Minced cartilage without cell culture serves as an effective intraoperative cell source for cartilage repair. J Orthop Res 2006;24(6):1261–70.

43. Albrecht F, Roessner A, Zimmermann E. Closure of osteochondral lesions using chondral fragments and fibrin adhesive. Arch Orthop Trauma Surg 1983;101(3):213–7.

44. Cole BJ, Farr J, Winalski CS, et al. Outcomes after a single-stage procedure for cell-based cartilage repair: a prospective clinical safety trial with 2-year follow-up. Am J Sports Med 2011;39(6): 1170–9.

45. Adkisson HD 4th, Martin JA, Amendola RL, et al. The potential of human allogeneic juvenile chondrocytes for restoration of articular cartilage. Am J Sports Med 2010;38(7):1324–33.

46. Namba RS, Meuli M, Sullivan KM, et al. Spontaneous repair of superficial defects in articular cartilage in a fetal lamb model. J Bone Joint Surg Am 1998;80(1):4–10.

47. Tompkins M, Hamann JC, Diduch DR, et al. Preliminary results of a novel single-stage cartilage restoration technique: particulated juvenile articular cartilage allograft for chondral defects of the patella. Arthroscopy 2013;29(10):1661–70.

48. Farr J, Yao J. Chondral defect repair with particulated juvenile cartilage allograft. Cartilage 2011;2: 346–53. Available at: http://car.sagepub.com/content/2/4/346.abstract.

49. Tompkins M, Adkisson DH, Bonner KF. DeNovo NT allograft. Oper Tech Sports Med 2013;21:82–9. Available at: http://www.optechsportsmed.com/article/S1060-1872(13)00028-2/abstract.

50. Brittberg M, Lindahl A, Nilsson A, et al. Treatment of deep cartilage defects in the knee with

autologous chondrocyte transplantation. N Engl J Med 1994;331(14):889–95.

51. Grande DA, Pitman MI, Peterson L, et al. The repair of experimentally produced defects in rabbit articular cartilage by autologous chondrocyte transplantation. J Orthop Res 1989;7(2):208–18.

52. Minas T. A primer in cartilage repair. J Bone Joint Surg Br 2012;94(11 Suppl A):141–6.

53. Minas T, Gomoll AH, Solhpour S, et al. Autologous chondrocyte implantation for joint preservation in patients with early osteoarthritis. Clin Orthop Relat Res 2010;468(1):147–57.

54. Minas T, Von Keudell A, Bryant T, et al. The John Insall Award: a minimum 10-year outcome study of autologous chondrocyte implantation. Clin Orthop Relat Res 2014;472(1):41–51.

55. McNickle AG, Provencher MT, Cole BJ. Overview of existing cartilage repair technology. Sports Med Arthrosc 2008;16(4):196–201.

56. Takazawa K, Adachi N, Deie M, et al. Evaluation of magnetic resonance imaging and clinical outcome after tissue-engineered cartilage implantation: prospective 6-year follow-up study. J Orthop Sci 2012;17(4):413–24.

57. Horas U, Pelinkovic D, Herr G, et al. Autologous chondrocyte implantation and osteochondral cylinder transplantation in cartilage repair of the knee joint. A prospective, comparative trial. J Bone Joint Surg Am 2003;85-A(2):185–92.

58. Krishnan SP, Skinner JA, Carrington RW, et al. Collagen-covered autologous chondrocyte implantation for osteochondritis dissecans of the knee: two- to seven-year results. J Bone Joint Surg Br 2006;88(2):203–5.

59. Peterson L, Minas T, Brittberg M, et al. Treatment of osteochondritis dissecans of the knee with autologous chondrocyte transplantation: results at two to ten years. J Bone Joint Surg Am 2003;85-A-(Suppl 2):17–24.

60. McCormick F, Cole B, Nwachukwu B, et al. Treatment of focal cartilage defects with a juvenile allogenic 3-dimensional articular cartilage graft. Oper Tech Sports Med 2013;21:95–9. Available at: http://www.optechsportsmed.com/article/S1060-1872(13)00030-0/abstract.

61. Melton JT, Wilson AJ, Chapman-Sheath P, et al. TruFit CB bone plug: chondral repair, scaffold design, surgical technique and early experiences. Expert Rev Med Devices 2010;7(3):333–41.

62. Bekkers JE, Bartels LW, Vincken KL, et al. Articular cartilage evaluation after TruFit plug implantation analyzed by delayed gadolinium-enhanced MRI of cartilage (dGEMRIC). Am J Sports Med 2013;41(6):1290–5.

63. Hindle P, Hendry JL, Keating JF, et al. Autologous osteochondral mosaicplasty or TruFit plugs for

cartilage repair. Knee Surg Sports Traumatol Arthrosc 2014;22(6):1235–40.

64. Bedi A, Foo LF, Williams RJ, et al. The maturation of synthetic scaffolds for osteochondral donor sites of the knee: an MRI and T2-mapping analysis. Cartilage 2010;1(1):20–8.

65. Carmont MR, Carey-Smith R, Saithna A, et al. Delayed incorporation of a TruFit plug: perseverance is recommended. Arthroscopy 2009;25(7):810–4.

66. Barber FA, Dockery WD. A computed tomography scan assessment of synthetic multiphase polymer scaffolds used for osteochondral defect repair. Arthroscopy 2011;27(1):60–4.

67. Kon E, Filardo G, Di Martino A, et al. Clinical results and MRI evolution of a nano-composite multilayered biomaterial for osteochondral regeneration at 5 years. Am J Sports Med 2014;42(1):158–65.

68. Kon E, Filardo G, Perdisa F, et al. A one-step treatment for chondral and osteochondral knee defects: clinical results of a biomimetic scaffold implantation at 2 years of follow-up. J Mater Sci Mater Med 2014. [Epub ahead of print].

69. van den Borne MP, Raijmakers NJ, Vanlauwe J, et al. International Cartilage Repair Society (ICRS) and Oswestry macroscopic cartilage evaluation scores validated for use in autologous chondrocyte implantation (ACI) and microfracture. Osteoarthritis Cartilage 2007;15(12):1397–402.

70. Blackman AJ, Smith MV, Flanigan DC, et al. Correlation between magnetic resonance imaging and clinical outcomes after cartilage repair surgery in the knee: a systematic review and meta-analysis. Am J Sports Med 2013;41(6):1426–34.

71. Roberts S, McCall IW, Darby AJ, et al. Autologous chondrocyte implantation for cartilage repair: monitoring its success by magnetic resonance imaging and histology. Arthritis Res Ther 2003;5(1):R60–73.

72. Marlovits S, Striessnig G, Resinger CT, et al. Definition of pertinent parameters for the evaluation of articular cartilage repair tissue with high-resolution magnetic resonance imaging. Eur J Radiol 2004;52(3):310–9.

73. Welsch GH, Zak L, Mamisch TC, et al. Three-dimensional magnetic resonance observation of cartilage repair tissue (MOCART) score assessed with an isotropic three-dimensional true fast imaging with steady-state precession sequence at 3.0 Tesla. Invest Radiol 2009;44(9):603–12.

74. Chang EY, Pallante-Kichura AL, Bae WC, et al. Development of a comprehensive osteochondral allograft MRI scoring system (OCAMRISS) with histopathologic, micro-computed tomography, and biomechanical validation. Cartilage 2014;5(1):16–27.

75. Ebert JR, Robertson WB, Woodhouse J, et al. Clinical and magnetic resonance imaging-based outcomes to 5 years after matrix-induced autologous chondrocyte implantation to address articular

cartilage defects in the knee. Am J Sports Med 2011;39(4):753–63.

76. Trattnig S, Domayer S, Welsch GW, et al. MR imaging of cartilage and its repair in the knee–a review. Eur Radiol 2009;19(7):1582–94.

77. Trattnig S, Zbyn S, Schmitt B, et al. Advanced MR methods at ultra-high field (7 Tesla) for clinical musculoskeletal applications. Eur Radiol 2012; 22(11):2338–46.

78. Trattnig S, Welsch GH, Juras V, et al. 23Na MR imaging at 7 T after knee matrix-associated autologous chondrocyte transplantation preliminary results. Radiology 2010;257(1):175–84.

79. Alparslan L, Winalski CS, Boutin RD, et al. Postoperative magnetic resonance imaging of articular cartilage repair. Semin Musculoskelet Radiol 2001;5(4):345–63.

80. Polster J, Recht M. Postoperative MR evaluation of chondral repair in the knee. Eur J Radiol 2005; 54(2):206–13.

81. Mithoefer K, Williams RJ 3rd, Warren RF, et al. The microfracture technique for the treatment of articular cartilage lesions in the knee. A prospective cohort study. J Bone Joint Surg Am 2005;87(9): 1911–20.

82. Recht M, White LM, Winalski CS, et al. MR imaging of cartilage repair procedures. Skeletal Radiol 2003;32(4):185–200.

83. Riyami M, Rolf C. Evaluation of microfracture of traumatic chondral injuries to the knee in professional football and rugby players. J Orthop Surg Res 2009;4:13.

84. Stanish WD, McCormack R, Forriol F, et al. Novel scaffold-based BST-CarGel treatment results in superior cartilage repair compared with microfracture in a randomized controlled trial. J Bone Joint Surg Am 2013;95(18):1640–50.

85. Huang FS, Simonian PT, Norman AG, et al. Effects of small incongruities in a sheep model of osteochondral autografting. Am J Sports Med 2004; 32(8):1842–8.

86. Williams RJ 3rd, Ranawat AS, Potter HG, et al. Fresh stored allografts for the treatment of osteochondral defects of the knee. J Bone Joint Surg Am 2007;89(4):718–26.

87. Sanders TG, Mentzer KD, Miller MD, et al. Autogenous osteochondral "plug" transfer for the treatment of focal chondral defects: postoperative MR appearance with clinical correlation. Skeletal Radiol 2001;30(10):570–8.

88. Akens MK, Weishaupt D, Nadler D, et al. Integration of osteochondral grafts: comparison of MR imaging and histological results in osteochondral photooxidized grafts and allografts in sheep. International Cartilage Repair Society Symposium. Toronto, June 15–18, 2002.

89. Collins M, Stuart MJ. Magnetic resonance imaging osteonecrosis pattern within an osteochondral dowel allograft. J Knee Surg 2010;23(1):45–50.

90. Alparslan L, Minas T, Winalski CS. Magnetic resonance imaging of autologous chondrocyte implantation. Semin Ultrasound CT MR 2001;22(4): 341–51.

91. Moradi B, Schonit E, Nierhoff C, et al. First-generation autologous chondrocyte implantation in patients with cartilage defects of the knee: 7 to 14 years' clinical and magnetic resonance imaging follow-up evaluation. Arthroscopy 2012;28(12):1851–61.

92. Kreuz PC, Steinwachs M, Erggelet C, et al. Classification of graft hypertrophy after autologous chondrocyte implantation of full-thickness chondral defects in the knee. Osteoarthritis Cartilage 2007; 15(12):1339–47.

93. Pietschmann MF, Niethammer TR, Horng A, et al. The incidence and clinical relevance of graft hypertrophy after matrix-based autologous chondrocyte implantation. Am J Sports Med 2012;40(1): 68–74.

94. Matricali GA, Dereymaeker GP, Luyten FP. Donor site morbidity after articular cartilage repair procedures: a review. Acta Orthop Belg 2010;76(5): 669–74.

MR Imaging Assessment of Arthritis of the Knee

 CrossMark

Donald J. Flemming, MD[a],*, Thomas W. Hash II, MD[b], Stephanie A. Bernard, MD[a], Pamela S. Brian, MD[a]

KEYWORDS

- Synovitis • Rheumatoid arthritis • Psoriatic arthritis • Septic arthritis • Lyme arthritis
- Pigmented villonodular synovitis • Synovial chondromatosis • Osteoarthritis

KEY POINTS

- Synovitis is a nonspecific finding that may be confused with effusion.
- Erosions in the knee occur in tight recesses. Multiple ill-defined erosions are an indication of an aggressive arthropathy.
- Enthesitis may be an indication of a seronegative spondyloarthropathy.
- Correlation with radiography is important for evaluation of low T2-signal intra-articular or periarticular processes.
- Accurate diagnosis of an arthropathy on magnetic resonance imaging is possible when imaging findings are correlated with distribution of disease and clinical presentation.

INTRODUCTION

Radiologists must be able to recognize and characterize the magnetic resonance (MR) imaging manifestations of arthropathies of the knee regardless of whether the diagnosis is known, suspected, or unsuspected, because arthropathies are an important source of knee pain. In some instances, the referring clinician may presume internal derangement as the cause of joint symptoms and not be aware of an underlying arthritis, in which case the radiologist can provide a helpful differential diagnosis. In other situations, the diagnosis of arthritis is suspected or known and the radiologist's role changes from suggesting a diagnosis to defining the extent of disease. The purpose of this article is to discuss the general MR imaging manifestations of arthritis in the knee and to review their presentation in specific diseases.

BASIC PRINCIPLES

The key presentation of arthritis, both clinically and radiologically, is that the disease is centered on the joint and typically involves both sides of it. Arthritis can solely involve the synovium, ligaments, tendons, cartilage, or bone of an involved joint, but more commonly the disease affects multiple components of the joint. The character of the involvement of these structures not only permits the gross characterization of an arthropathy but also may lead to a specific diagnosis.

Synovium/Synovitis

The synovium is the lining of the joint and is normally only a few cell layers thick. Therefore, the synovium should not be visible in the normal patient. Inflammation leads to thickening of the synovium at histology and on imaging. The diseased

Disclosures: None.
[a] Department of Radiology, Penn State Milton S. Hershey Medical Center, 500 University Drive, Hershey, PA 17033, USA; [b] Department of Radiology, Duke University Hospital, DUMC Box 3808, Durham, NC 27710, USA
* Corresponding author.
E-mail address: dflemming@hmc.psu.edu

Magn Reson Imaging Clin N Am 22 (2014) 703–724
http://dx.doi.org/10.1016/j.mric.2014.07.012
1064-9689/14/$ – see front matter © 2014 Elsevier Inc. All rights reserved.

synovium is leaky, and effusion commonly accompanies synovitis. Synovitis is a nonspecific finding that can be seen in many arthropathies including inflammatory, crystal-induced, septic, and degenerative etiology. The radiologist needs to recognize the MR imaging manifestations of synovitis and characterize both its imaging features and extent, because the presence of synovitis commonly correlates with pain.

Synovitis may manifest diffusely, focally, or in a mass-like pattern in any location in the knee joint. Diffuse inflammatory synovitis is most commonly recognized in the posterior aspect of the knee (posterior cruciate ligament recess), The Hoffa fat pad, and the suprapatellar bursa.[1,2] On T1-weighted images, inflammatory synovitis may be visualized as thickening of the joint capsule that can be differentiated from the lower signal of adjacent joint fluid (**Fig. 1**).[3] Inflammatory synovitis is typically high in signal on fluid-sensitive sequences. Sometimes in more advanced stages, one can manipulate window and level on a PACS (Picture Archiving and Communication System) workstation to recognize synovitis as fronds that have lower signal than adjacent high-signal effusion on fat-suppressed proton-density or T2-weighted sequences (**Fig. 2**).[3] Noncontrast depiction of the extent of synovitis in a joint can be improved with diffusion-weighted imaging.[4] However, the true extent of synovitis is characterized best with intravenous gadolinium.[5] Normal synovium enhances,[6] but this enhancement should not be visible to the naked eye. Active synovitis enhances rapidly, and the extent of inflammation can be characterized on dynamic contrast-enhanced sequences.[7] The true extent

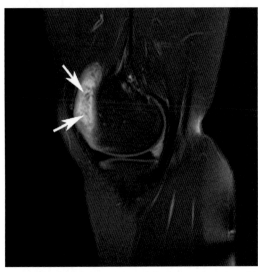

Fig. 2. Sagittal fat-suppressed fast spin-echo T2-weighted image through the medial knee shows intermediate signal of frond-like projections of synovitis in the suprapatellar bursa (*arrows*).

of synovitis should be assessed within 10 minutes following the administration of intravenous contrast, because rapid diffusion of gadolinium into the adjacent effusion may preclude distinction of synovitis adjacent to the effusion later.[8]

The signal characteristics of the thickened synovium also should be assessed for patterns that deviate from the typical intermediate T1 and high T2 signal of acute synovitis. Synovitis that is low in signal on T2-weighted images is usually an indication of either increased collagen in chronic synovitis or hemosiderin in the synovium in entities such as pigmented villonodular synovitis (PVNS)

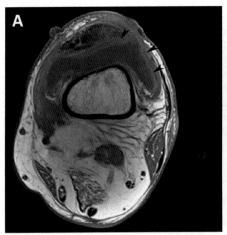
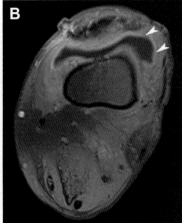

Fig. 1. Septic arthritis of the right knee in a 74-year-old man. Axial T1-weighted image (*A*) through suprapatellar bursa shows thickened synovium (*arrowheads*) that has slightly higher signal than knee effusion. Axial fat-suppressed T1-weighted image through suprapatellar bursa (*B*) following intravenous contrast administration shows enhancement of the thickened synovium (*arrowheads*).

or chronic hemorrhage in the joint from a coagulopathy (eg, hemophilia) (**Fig. 3**).[9] Hemosiderin is the most likely cause of low T2-signal synovitis if blooming artifact is appreciated on a gradient-echo sequence. Amyloid should also be considered in the differential diagnosis of low T2-signal synovitis.[10] It is very important to review a radiograph to ensure that calcification is not the source of low T2 signal.

Chronic synovitis also may demonstrate fat signal pattern (high T1 and low on fat-suppressed sequence).[11] Fatty replacement of the synovitis is reported as lipoma arborescens (**Fig. 4**). This nonspecific pattern of chronic synovitis is most commonly seen in the setting of osteoarthritis (OA), but can also be seen in patients with burned-out inflammatory arthritis.[12]

Bone Manifestations

Arthropathies may affect the osseous components of an involved articulation. Osseous manifestations of arthritis may include erosions, bone marrow edema–like lesions, subchondral cysts, and osteonecrosis.

Erosion is a relatively uncommon manifestation of an arthropathy in the knee because of the capacious nature of this joint. Acute erosions are usually a manifestation of an aggressive inflammatory arthritis such as septic arthritis, rheumatoid arthritis (RA), or reactive arthritis. Acute erosions have ill-defined margins and are seen adjacent to tight spaces in the joint such as the meniscal recesses, on the articular surfaces, or superior to the posterior condyles (**Fig. 5**). The cortical disruption and replacement of adjacent normal fat marrow is best recognized on T1-weighted images. Increased T2 signal on fat-suppressed images in the marrow adjacent to an erosion is an indication of an aggressive process.[13]

Chronic erosions that are well corticated suggest a slowly progressive process such as gout, PVNS, synovial chondromatosis, or amyloidosis. Chronic erosions also usually are appreciated in the tight recesses of the joint rather than adjacent to the suprapatellar bursa.

Bone marrow edema–like lesions may be seen in the inflammatory arthropathies or OA. In the setting of OA, bone marrow edema–like lesions correlate with pain in most patients,[14–16] and may be an indication of remodeling of subchondral bone in response to abnormal mechanics. Subchondral cysts are also a nonspecific finding that can be appreciated in many arthropathies. Their development can be due to direct erosion or be a reparative response to subchondral microfracture.

Bone infarction or osteonecrosis can be a secondary manifestation resulting from steroid therapy. Systemic lupus erythematosus should be considered in the setting of suspected rheumatologic disease, particularly when the infarcts are multiple and there is no history of steroid administration.

Tendons and Ligaments

Careful evaluation of the tendons and ligaments is important in the setting of atraumatic knee pain. Diffuse or mass-like infiltration of a tendon or ligament of the knee may be an indication of crystal deposition disease such as gout, hydroxyapatite deposition disease (HADD), or, less commonly, calcium pyrophosphate deposition disease. The signal characteristics of crystal deposition disease are variable (see later more detailed discussion).

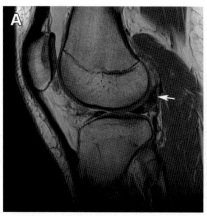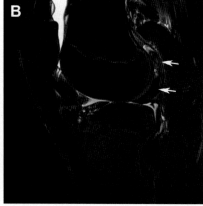

Fig. 3. A 17-year-old man with hemophilia. Sagittal fast spin-echo proton-density (*A*) and fat-suppressed fast spin-echo T2-weighted (*B*) images through the lateral knee show low-signal hemosiderin-stained synovitis posterior to the lateral femoral condyle (*arrows*), evidence of repeated hemarthrosis.

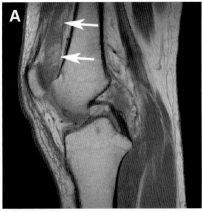
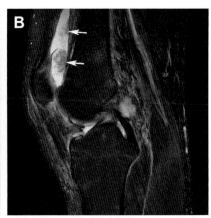

Fig. 4. A 58-year-old man with osteoarthritis and lipoma arborescens. Sagittal fast spin-echo proton-density (*A*) and fat-suppressed fast spin-echo T2-weighted (*B*) images through the intercondylar notch show fat signal in chronic synovitis in the suprapatellar bursa (*arrows*). Typical fronds of high T1 and low signal on fat-suppressed T2-weighted images are diagnostic of lipoma arborescens.

Enthesopathic changes at the attachment of ligaments and tendons to bone are classically associated with a seronegative spondyloarthropathy such as reactive arthritis or psoriatic arthritis (PsA). Increased T2 signal in the bone at the site of attachment of the tendon or ligament is an indication of enthesitis.[17]

Cartilage

Loss of articular cartilage is a nonspecific indicator of an arthropathy. The articular cartilage of

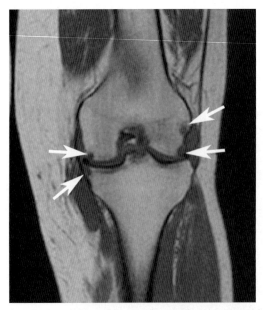

Fig. 5. A 39-year-old woman with rheumatoid arthritis. Coronal T1-weighted image through the knee shows erosions at the margin of the joint adjacent to the meniscal recesses (*arrows*).

the knee is adequately evaluated in most cases on a fat-suppressed fast spin-echo proton-density sequence or steady-state gradient-echo sequence. Diffuse loss of articular cartilage is usually an indication of an inflammatory arthritis. Focal loss of articular cartilage is most commonly an indication of OA.

MR IMAGING MANIFESTATIONS IN SPECIFIC ARTHROPATHIES

Arthritis can be subdivided into major categories: inflammatory, deposition disease, OA, neuropathic, collagen vascular disease, and mass-like arthropathies. The MR imaging findings associated with specific arthropathies are discussed, but MR imaging features of neuropathic and collagen vascular disease involving the knee are not covered in this article.

Inflammatory Arthropathies

Inflammatory arthropathy includes septic arthritis, RA, PsA, and reactive arthritis. Much research has been directed at identification of MR imaging features that can differentiate septic from other inflammatory arthritides.[13,18–23] Many of the findings have demonstrated too much overlap to allow a specific diagnosis by imaging alone. Both infectious and noninfectious joint inflammation results in the development of varying degrees of joint effusion, pericapsular edema, synovial hypertrophy, and enhancement, all of which can lead to the development of marginal erosions and cartilage loss. The features that may help to narrow the differential diagnosis and direct further diagnostic evaluation are covered in this section. The number of joints involved, distribution of disease, and clinical features of the disease presentation are all crucial factors in arriving at a correct diagnosis.

Septic arthritis

Septic arthritis of the knee presents with one of two primary clinical pictures. With pyogenic organisms a swollen, red, painful joint develops within days of inoculation. In nonpyogenic infections, the presentation may be more indolent with swelling and pain occurring over the course of weeks to months. Though septic arthritis must be excluded in any monoarticular arthropathy, 2 or more joints are involved simultaneously in up to 19% of cases. This oligoarticular involvement, especially in nonpyogenic infections, can result in confusion of the diagnosis with inflammatory arthritis.[18] The classic clinical and laboratory features of septic arthritis, which include fever, rigors, increased systemic white blood cell count, and elevated sedimentation rate, are each only present in about one-half to two-thirds of patients.[20,24] The appropriate initial imaging study is conventional radiography. However, radiographs are often normal or show only nonspecific joint effusion and symmetric soft tissue swelling in the early phase of disease. Even joint effusion may be absent in as many as one-third of infected joints.[13] As such, a lack of joint effusion should not be used to exclude septic arthritis. Joint aspiration remains the primary means of diagnosis of septic arthritis. The most important predictor of morbidity is the time from symptom development to initiation of treatment, with improved outcomes when treatment is initiated in the first 7 days.[25]

MR imaging is a sensitive means of additional evaluation of the joint and surrounding soft tissues when the diagnosis is unable to be established through aspiration or when complicating features are of concern. The most helpful imaging sequences include T1-weighted and fat-suppressed T2-weighted imaging, or short-tau inversion recovery (STIR) imaging followed by fat-suppressed T1-weighted imaging after intravenous gadolinium administration.

Pyogenic septic arthritides

Fifty percent of cases of septic arthritis of the knee are bacterial.[20] Most bacterial cases of septic arthritis are the result of a single organism, with Staphylococcus aureus the causative organism in 50% to 80% of cases across all age groups. Intravenous drug use, the presence of indwelling catheters, and underlying immunocompromised states in addition to preexisting joint arthropathy, such as RA, serve as predisposing factors for the development of a septic arthritis.[26,27] Beyond S aureus, a variety of organisms should be considered, based on patient age and clinical scenario (**Table 1**), some of which have special culture requirements or lower diagnostic yields on synovial fluid evaluation.

On MR imaging, bone erosions, cartilage loss, bone marrow edema, and erosion enhancement are more often seen in the setting of bacterial infection (**Fig. 6**). Development of adjacent osteomyelitis may be difficult to exclude on MR imaging. Most cases progressing to osteomyelitis demonstrate diffuse marrow edema on T2-weighted imaging adjacent to the septic joint, but this finding can also present in one-third of cases of septic arthritis without osteomyelitis. Although abnormal intermediate T1 signal increases specificity, normal T1 marrow signal does not exclude osteomyelitis.[13]

Nonpyogenic arthritides

Lyme arthritis Lyme disease is the result of the tick-transmitted infection with the spirochete Borrelia burgdorferi.[28,29] The disease has been reported throughout the United States but with the highest incidence in the mid-Atlantic and northeast states during the spring and summer months. Up to half of individuals will manifest the pathognomonic erythema chronicum migrans rash within days to a month from the time of the tick bite. Left untreated, carditis, neurologic symptoms, and an oligoarthritis may develop within weeks to years.[28,29] The knee is involved in Lyme arthritis in 80% of patients. Massive recurrent joint effusions are a classic presentation, with few

Table 1
Septic arthritis: organisms other than *S aureus* to consider, based on the patient population

Patient Population	Organisms
Children <2 y old	*Kingella kingae, Haemophilus influenzae*, group A *Streptococcus*
Young adult	*Neisseria gonorrhoeae, Streptococcus*
Infectious diarrhea	*Shigella, Salmonella, Campylobacter, Yersinia*
Human immunodeficiency virus	*Streptococcus pneumoniae, Mycobacterium*, fungal
Joint prosthesis in place >3 mo	*Streptococcus*, gram-negative aerobes, anaerobic infections

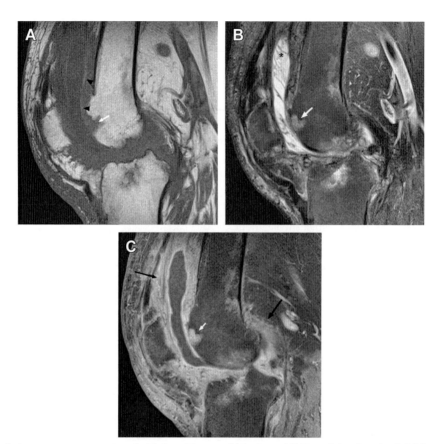

Fig. 6. *Staphylococcus aureus* septic arthritis in a 64-year-old woman. (*A*) T1-weighted sagittal, (*B*) fat-suppressed T2-weighted sagittal, and (*C*) fat-suppressed T1-weighted sagittal images following intravenous gadolinium administration. A heterogeneous joint effusion containing debris (*B, asterisk*) with mild increased T1 signal of the synovial lining (*black arrowheads*) and thick enhancement on postgadolinium images is apparent. There is intermediate signal replacement of the perisynovial soft tissues with patchy T2 signal but marked perisynovial enhancement (*C, black arrows*). An irregular erosion with intermediate T1 signal, intermediate to increased T2 signal, and enhancement is seen in the trochlea (*white arrows*). Additional tibial plateau and lateral femoral condylar erosions are present, associated with cartilage loss.

patients progressing to chronic synovitis. The massive joint effusions may be associated with large popliteal cysts.[30] Progression from marginal erosions to uniform cartilage loss from all compartments can occur. Enthesitis at the patella attachments of the quadriceps and patella tendons also has been described occasionally, and is conjectured to be related to traction as a result of recurrent massive joint effusions.[30]

MR imaging features that have been reported more frequently in Lyme arthritis than in other arthritides are the presence of popliteal fossa lymphadenopathy and popliteus muscle myositis (**Fig. 7**).[19] Pericapsular soft-tissue edema is reported as occurring less commonly in Lyme arthritis than in other infections.[19] Serologic tests or polymerase chain reaction of synovial fluid can be confirmatory, and treatment with oral or intravenous antibiotics is curative in most cases.

Tuberculous arthritis The musculoskeletal system is involved in 1% to 3% of patients with extrapulmonary *Mycobacterium tuberculosis* (TB), most cases involving the spine. The hip and knee joints are the 2 most common sites for extraspinal musculoskeletal infection with TB.[31] The clinical presentation is often indolent and nonspecific, and may mimic an inflammatory arthritis such as rheumatoid or juvenile inflammatory arthritis.[18] A history of travel to endemic areas should be sought. Although the diagnosis of tuberculous arthritis is not possible based solely on the clinical or imaging findings, there are features that may suggest the diagnosis. The classic radiographic findings (Phemister's triad) of juxta-articular osteoporosis, marginal erosions, and gradual joint space loss may be seen radiographically. At MR imaging, in addition to the nonspecific findings of synovial thickening, perisynovial edema, joint

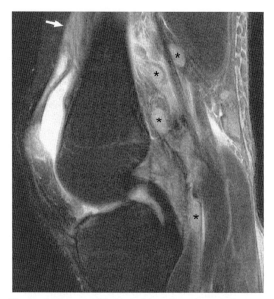

Fig. 7. A 27-year-old man with polymerase chain reaction test positive for Lyme disease. Intermediate signal thickening of the synovium can be seen about the suprapatellar bursa and at the anterior joint line. Myositis is seen in the distal quadriceps musculature (*white arrow*), and lymphadenopathy (*asterisks*) is present along the popliteal vasculature.

effusion, and marginal erosions, fibrinoid "rice bodies," similar to what may be seen in RA, may be encountered. The synovitis present may also demonstrate a relatively low T2 signal, which may help suggest TB arthritis.[32] Periarticular "cold abscesses" presenting as soft-tissue fluid collections or fluid extensions from the joint may be seen, with an appearance similar to that of synovial cysts encountered in RA. Over time, these collections may form marginally enhancing draining sinus tracts to the skin surface,[33] which is not a common development in synovial cysts in other inflammatory arthropathies.

Rheumatoid arthritis

RA is a chronic systemic inflammatory disorder producing synovitis and cartilage destruction. Since the advent of disease-modifying antirheumatic drugs (DMARDs), early diagnosis and initiation of treatment, before radiographically evident erosive changes, has demonstrated a significant impact on slowing disease progression and the long-term disability associated with RA. Though classically a bilateral symmetric polyarthropathy with wrist or metacarpal phalangeal joint involvement, RA also frequently involves the knees and may serve as an initial site of involvement in 13% of patients.[34] Involvement of a single joint may occur for weeks to months before presentation of classic polyarticular involvement.[35] As in septic arthritides, during flares of acute inflammation elevation of nonspecific inflammatory serum markers (C-reactive protein, erythrocyte sedimentation rate) can occur. Seropositivity for rheumatoid factor (RF) is seen in 70% to 80% of cases.

MR imaging not only permits early identification of synovitis but also allows for reproducible quantification of the synovitis that is a strong predictor for the development of future erosions.[36] MR imaging has also demonstrated usefulness in assessing the response to therapy or reactivation of disease.[37] Postcontrast imaging most accurately demonstrates the extent of synovitis (**Fig. 8**). Dynamic gadolinium enhancement in an

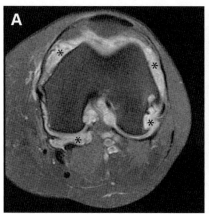
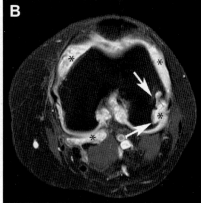

Fig. 8. A 39-year-old woman with rheumatoid arthritis and knee pain. Axial fat-suppressed fast spin-echo proton-density image (*A*) through the knee shows hyperintense signal in the synovial recesses of the joint. It is difficult to appreciate whether it is due to synovitis or effusion. Axial fat-suppressed T1-weighted image (*B*) obtained at the same level soon after administration of intravenous gadolinium shows extensive enhancement of synovitis (*asterisks*). Note the erosion of the lateral femoral condyle (*white arrows*).

early phase (30–60 seconds) has been shown to accurately correlate with active synovial inflammation.[38] When not performing dynamic gadolinium imaging, images should be acquired within 10 minutes of gadolinium injection because contrast will diffuse into the joint fluid, thus limiting the reliable distinction of synovium from effusion.[8]

Besides the common features of infectious or inflammatory arthropathies already described, additional features that may suggest RA include the following. (1) Rice bodies consist of sloughed fibrinous material and necrotic debris. These rod-shaped (1–3 mm) intermediate T1 and T2 signal bodies may be seen in the joints or involved bursae. Though also seen in tuberculous arthritis, rice bodies are most frequently encountered in RA and are less common in other inflammatory arthritides (**Fig. 9**).[39,40] (2) Synovial cysts are synovial lined fluid collections that may have long extensions from the joint into the adjacent soft tissues. About the knee, these most commonly originate from popliteal Baker cyst. Synovial cysts may also gain access to the medullary cavity of the bones through erosions and create lytic, endosteal eroding lesions that will image as low T1,

high T2 central fluid signal with peripheral rim enhancement, as would be expected of a cyst. The cysts are not specific and may develop with any long-standing large joint effusion, but in the setting of a polyarthropathy are most common in RA. (3) Low T2-signal synovitis. Most inflammatory synovitis demonstrates low to intermediate T1 and intermediate to increased T2 signal. Chronic RA may result in fibrosis within the pannus that shows low signal on both T1 and T2 imaging.[10]

Seronegative arthropathies

Psoriatic and reactive arthritis PsA is an HLA B27–associated arthropathy that has several diverse clinical presentations. The most common (70%) is that of an asymmetric oligoarthritis that frequently includes involvement of the knee.[41] Approximately 5% to 8% of patients with psoriatic skin changes will develop PsA, at a mean age of diagnosis of 40 years.[41,42] Conversely, at the time of PsA development, most patients will have dermatologic findings of psoriasis, although in 15% arthritis will precede visible skin changes.[43] Similar to other inflammatory arthropathies, PsA

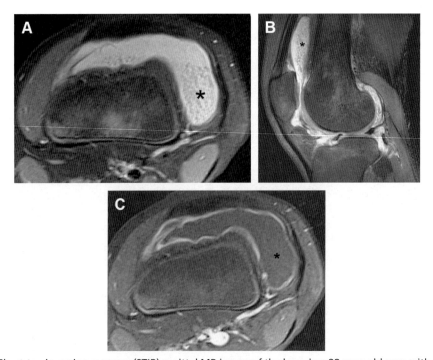

Fig. 9. (*A*) Short-tau inversion recovery (STIR) sagittal MR image of the knee in a 28-year-old man with a diagnosis of rheumatoid arthritis. (*B*) Axial proton-density fat-suppressed (PDFS) image and (*C*) Fat-suppressed T1-weighted axial image following intravenous gadolinium administration in an 18-year-old woman with rheumatoid arthritis. In both patients there are small irregular to rod-shaped intra-articular "rice bodies" (*asterisks*) that show intermediate signal on STIR and PDFS images. Although the postgadolinium imaging demonstrates a rim of abnormal synovial thickening about the suprapatellar recess, the nonvascularized fibrinous debris making up the rice bodies lacks enhancement.

produces synovitis, marginal erosions, and often pericapsular inflammatory changes.

Reactive arthritis (formerly Reiter syndrome) is an HLA B27–associated autoimmune inflammatory arthropathy that is triggered by a genitourinary or gastrointestinal infection. The result is a triad of clinical symptoms that includes (1) arthropathy, in association with (2) urethritis and (3) conjunctivitis or uveitis. Joint involvement is typically an oligoarthropathy that is more common in the lower extremities.

On MR imaging, the seronegative arthropathies may demonstrate synovitis and erosions, beginning marginally, with progression to diffuse cartilage destruction. As is seen with other infectious or inflammatory arthropathies, varying degrees of perisynovial edema signal on T2 images and enhancement in addition to adjacent soft-tissue and marrow edema may be seen. Relatively unique to the seronegative arthropathies, the inflammation at the joint may begin first in the entheses, resulting in increased T2-signal inflammatory changes and postgadolinium enhancement at or in these tendinoligamentous insertions, and within the underlying marrow and adjacent soft tissues (**Fig. 10**).[44] When present, this enthesitis may help to differentiate the seronegative arthropathies from RA.[45–47] Manifestation of enthesitis may be limited to peritendinous or periligamentous edema.[48]

Deposition Disease

Deposition of material such as crystal, amyloid, or hemosiderin into a joint or periarticular structure can lead to the development of an arthropathy. The deposition of urate crystal (gout) and hydroxyapatite crystal (HADD) are the most common rheumatologic disorders of this type that have characteristic MR imaging findings.

Gout

Gout classically presents in the great toe in patients as intense pain, redness, and swelling. If the patient also has hyperuricemia, the clinical diagnosis is relatively straightforward. The prevalence of gout in the United States is increasing, likely attributable to growing numbers of patients with obesity and metabolic syndrome.[49] Gout should be in the differential for the acute onset of any monoarticular arthropathy, even in young adult males.

Previously unrecognized gout may first be diagnosed on MR imaging of the knee. Moreover, false-negative results on joint aspiration are known to occur secondarily to suboptimal laboratory quality control, so the diagnosis of gout cannot be entirely excluded based on lack of crystals on joint aspiration.[50] It is therefore important for the interpreting radiologist to suggest this diagnosis when typical MR imaging findings are present. A painless tophus may infiltrate the patellar or quadriceps tendon, leading to evaluation for possible neoplasm. Intra-articular tophus may also cause clicking and pain that can be clinically confused with meniscal tear.[51]

The MR imaging manifestations of gout are variable.[52] Tophaceous gout can be appreciated as a

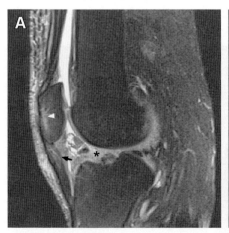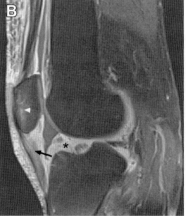

Fig. 10. (*A*) STIR sagittal and (*B*) fat-suppressed T1-weighted sagittal image following intravenous gadolinium administration in a 42-year-old man with known psoriatic arthritis of the knee and ankle. There is thickening and abnormal increased T2 signal and postcontrast enhancement in the patellar tendon (*black arrows*), with increased T2 signal in the marrow and enhancement at the anterior superficial attachment of the quadriceps and patella tendons (*white arrowheads*). T2 edema and enhancement is seen in the soft tissues anterior to the patella tendon and in infrapatellar fat. Synovitis, showing intermediate signal on STIR imaging and enhancement, is seen in the joint (*asterisks*). The patient progressed to tendon rupture.

rounded mass in the foot or hand, but in the knee it more commonly infiltrates tendons and ligaments, resulting in enlargement of these structures. These findings may be confused with tendon degeneration or ligament injury (**Fig. 11**).[53,54] The tophus will demonstrate intermediate to low signal on T1-weighted images and may range from high to very low in signal on T2-weighted sequences.[52,55] Low signal on T2-weighted sequences can lead to an erroneous diagnosis of PVNS. A tophus has a more amorphous appearance on T2-weighted images than the well-defined mass-like pattern of PVNS. Synovial deposition is nonspecific, but is visualized as small masses with irregular margins and intermediate T1 and T2 signal. Contrast enhancement is variable, ranging from little to marked increased signal following the administration of intravenous gadolinium.[52]

Gout has a predilection to involve the patellar and quadriceps tendons.[54] It has been suggested that this tendency may be related to the relatively low temperature of these structures, encouraging crystal deposition there. The tophus may erode the underlying bone and lead to fracture of the patella.[56] Gout also has a curious predilection for the popliteus tendon near its insertion on the lateral aspect of the femoral condyle. The possibility of gout should be considered in the setting of atraumatic knee pain in a middle-aged or older patient with an enlarged and irregular popliteus tendon.

Hydroxyapatite deposition disease
HADD is a common malady that most commonly affects the shoulder. Knee involvement is relatively uncommon. In practice, the disorder can be seen in asymptomatic patients as an incidental finding or in symptomatic persons who complain of acute onset of pain about the involved joint. Uncommonly HADD may be clinically confused with fracture, infection,[57] or neoplasm.[58] Rarely deposition may lead to locking symptoms.[59]

HADD has variable appearance on MR imaging.[58] The focal deposit will usually be low in signal on T1-weighted and T2-weighted images. Small deposits may be difficult to appreciate because their signal is similar to that of tendon and ligament. Edema surrounding a HADD deposit increases the likelihood of detection but may lead to the erroneous diagnosis of muscle strain, ligamentous injury, or fracture (**Fig. 12**). Detection may be facilitated with postcontrast or gradient-echo sequences. The deposit shows no enhancement following administration of intravenous contrast, and will demonstrate very low signal on gradient-echo images. It is imperative to review conventional radiographs if HADD is suspected, because even small calcifications are readily appreciated on conventional radiographs despite the sometimes confusing MR imaging presentation.

Mass-Like Arthropathies

The mass-like arthropathies are neoplastic disorders of the knee that lead to focal or diffuse intra-articular masses, pain, and variable joint-space narrowing. The 2 most common mass-like arthropathies are PVNS and synovial chondromatosis.

Pigmented villonodular synovitis
PVNS is a hyperplastic synovial process that can be intra-articular or extra-articular; in the latter case it presents in tendon sheaths or bursae.

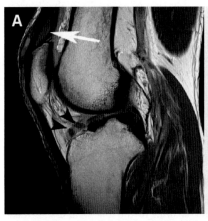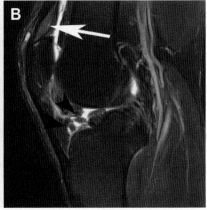

Fig. 11. A 45-year-old man with clinically undiagnosed gout and knee pain. Sagittal fast spin-echo proton-density (*A*) and sagittal fat-suppressed T2-weighted (*B*) images of the knee show intermediate signal of tophaceous gout in the distal quadriceps tendon (*white arrow*). Tophus is also seen at the posterior aspect of the Hoffa fat pad (*arrowheads*). The significance of these findings was not recognized at initial image interpretation. Tophaceous gout was diagnosed at arthroscopy.

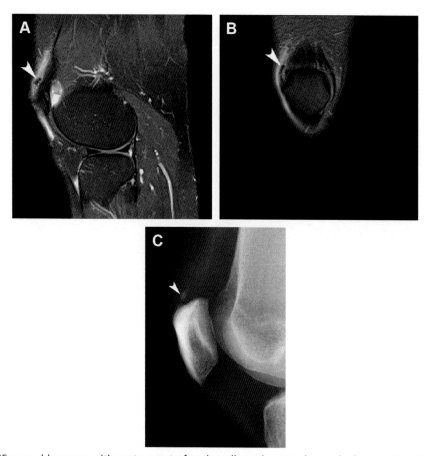

Fig. 12. A 45-year-old woman with acute onset of peripatellar pain secondary to hydroxyapatite deposition disease (HADD) involving the distal quadriceps tendon. Sagittal (*A*) and coronal (*B*) fat-suppressed T2-weighted images of the knee show comma-shaped focus of low signal (*arrowhead*) in the distal lateral quadriceps tendon that is surrounded by high-signal edema. Lateral view of the knee (*C*) confirms the presence of amorphous calcification in a comet shape that is typical of HADD involving a tendon (*arrowhead*).

The etiology of PVNS is uncertain, although most investigators believe it is a neoplastic process given the frequent cytogenetic tissue abnormalities, overexpression of colony-stimulating factor 1, and rare malignant transformation.[60–63]

PVNS is nearly always monoarticular, and affects the knee in approximately 66% to 80% of patients.[63–65] Affected patients are most frequently in their third to fifth decade of life at the time of diagnosis.[63] Males and females are affected equally.[66] PVNS presents in 2 forms in the knee: diffuse and localized. Diffuse PVNS in the knee is widespread, and frequently involves extra-articular ganglion cysts and/or extra-articular soft tissues. A joint effusion or hemarthrosis is frequently present. Diffuse PVNS often presents with chronic knee pain, swelling, and restricted motion.

Localized PVNS in the knee presents as a focal lobular or pedunculated mass, located anywhere in the knee but most commonly in the anterior compartment.[63] A palpable mass may be present on physical examination. The synovium about the anterior horn of the medial meniscus is reported to be the most common site for localized PVNS.[66] Localized PVNS in the knee is often clinically misdiagnosed as a meniscus tear or loose intra-articular body, given the frequent symptoms of locking, catching, and instability. This form of PVNS is usually not associated with a joint effusion.

On MR imaging, PVNS manifests as an irregularly lobular, heterogeneous mass (the localized form) or masses (the diffuse form).[63] It is predominantly intermediate in signal on T1-weighted and fluid-sensitive sequences, with varying low signal (reflecting hemosiderin), which is the sine qua non of PVNS. It is not uncommon for slightly high signal to be present in the lesions on all pulse sequences (**Fig. 13**). Areas of high signal may be seen on T1-weighted images, possibly owing to

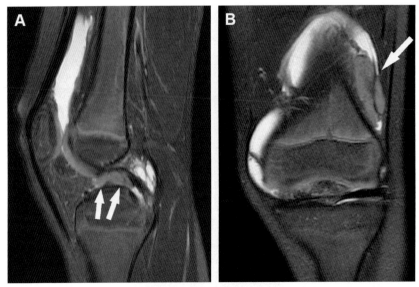

Fig. 13. Pigmented villonodular synovitis (PVNS). Sagittal (*A*) and coronal (*B*) fat-suppressed T2-weighted images of a 7-year-old girl show well-circumscribed masses (*arrows*) that have signal predominantly isointense to cartilage. Low signal within and at the margins of the masses reflect hemosiderin; nonmineralized synovial chondromatosis, though isointense to cartilage, would not contain such a low signal.

lipid-laden macrophages. Hemosiderin presence in the lesions is often more extensive in the diffuse form. However, low signal can predominate in localized PVNS as well (**Fig. 14**). Gradient-echo sequences exaggerate the paramagnetic effect of hemosiderin, causing the low signal to be more prominent (ie, "blooming") (**Fig. 15**). The hemosiderin in PVNS is accentuated when using higher-strength magnets and on pulse sequences with longer repetition times. PVNS typically enhances to a moderate or significant degree, although enhancement is nonspecific. The diffuse form often extends into extensive pericapsular ganglia. Any recess or ganglion can be involved (**Fig. 16**).

Subchondral and subcortical erosions and cystic areas can be seen, occasionally with an adjacent marrow edema pattern; these areas are filled with signal similar to that of the remainder of the PVNS elsewhere in the joint. Joint effusion is much more prevalent in frequency and size in the diffuse form than in the localized form. It is uncommon for substantial periarticular soft-tissue edema to be present.

MR imaging in the detection of recurrent or residual disease is often more difficult, particularly after resection of diffuse PVNS, owing to postsurgical changes and, at times, magnetic susceptibility artifacts. In the setting of prior diffuse PVNS, close scrutiny of the entire joint, bursae, and extracapsular ganglia, particularly all sites of prior disease, should be made. Though uncommon, surgical sites, whether open or arthroscopic portal sites, can be seeded and act as sites of recurrence.[66]

There are several uncommon but important points about PVNS worth keeping in mind. PVNS can be found in persons of all ages, including the very young (reportedly as young as 2 years old); in young patients, PVNS is often misdiagnosed as juvenile idiopathic arthritis.[60] PVNS can occur both de novo and as a recurrent form after total knee arthroplasty,[67–69] either early (eg, 1 year) or late, presenting with pain and/or recurrent effusion or hemarthrosis. Rarely, PVNS can be bilateral or multifocal. Extra-articular PVNS can be seen about the knee,[63] and can be isolated to the tibiofibular joint.[70]

Malignant PVNS is rare but occurs over a wide range of ages. Extensive marrow involvement, though nonspecific, can be seen, and suspicion for malignant transformation should be raised.[63,71,72] A rapidly deteriorating clinical course and disease progression, though nonspecific, also suggest malignancy.[71]

Synovial chondromatosis

Primary synovial chondromatosis is a benign proliferative neoplastic synovial process that can involve joints, bursae, and tendon sheaths. It affects males 2 to 4 times more frequently than females, most commonly in their third to fifth decades of life. Patients frequently present with pain, swelling, and/or stiffness.

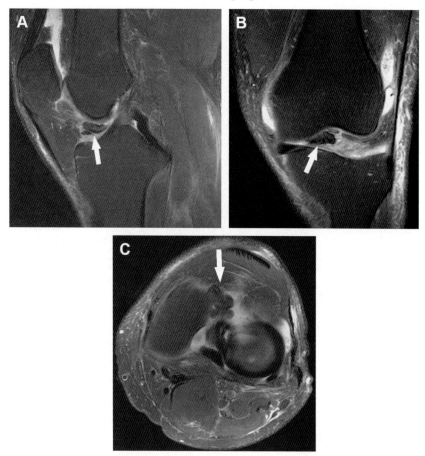

Fig. 14. Sagittal (*A*), coronal (*B*), and axial (*C*) fat-suppressed T2-weighted images show a well-circumscribed, lobular mass in the anterior intercondylar notch (*arrow*), which contains diffuse hemosiderin, consistent with localized PVNS.

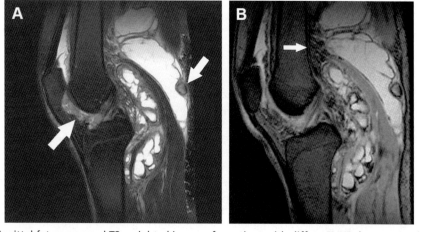

Fig. 15. (*A*) Sagittal fat-suppressed T2-weighted image of a patient with diffuse PVNS shows extensive conglomerate heterogeneous intermediate signal in the intercondylar notch extending into the adjacent anterior compartment (*anterior arrow*) with extensive posterior extracapsular ganglia containing similar signal material. A nodular focus of intermediate signal is present within a large popliteal cyst (*posterior arrow*). Thin low signal at the margins of the popliteal cyst and multiple extracapsular ganglia represent hemosiderin. Note the florid synovitis in the suprapatellar pouch. The visualized cartilage is normal. (*B*) Sagittal gradient-echo image accentuates the extensive, diffuse low-signal hemosiderin deposition. Note how the PVNS adjacent to the posterior femur (*arrow*) is better appreciated on this sequence.

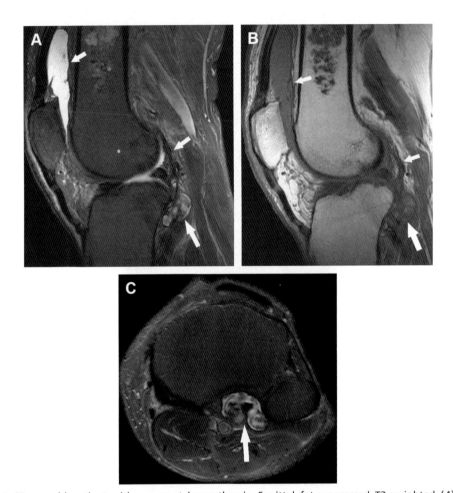

Fig. 16. A 67-year-old patient with recurrent hemarthrosis. Sagittal fat-suppressed T2-weighted (*A*) and T1-weighted (*B*) images show low signal of the capsular synovium (*small arrows*), reflecting hemosiderin deposition. Focal PVNS in the subpopliteal recess (*large arrow*) is a heterogeneously intermediate signal in *A* and heterogeneously high signal in *B*. The focal PVNS is better appreciated to have intermediate signal in addition to low-signal hemosiderin contents in the axial fat-suppressed T2-weighted image (*C*). Note the chondroid lesion in the distal femoral shaft.

As in PVNS, the knee is the most common site of synovial chondromatosis, involvement is rarely polyarticular, and it may not only be intra-articular but also extend into a popliteal cyst, ganglia, and other extra-articular soft tissues. Chronic erosions may be seen, although they are less frequent than in joints with less capacious capsules such as the hip. The cartilage masses calcify and ossify in the vast majority (70%–95%) of cases,[10,73,74] and thus are visible on radiographs in most patients. Whether calcified/ossified or nonmineralized synovial chondromatosis is present, the joint spaces are usually normal and periarticular osteopenia is usually absent.

On MR imaging the nonmineralized, radiographically occult form of the disease is seen as lobular, mass-like areas of cartilage signal. These masses manifest as low or, more frequently, intermediate signal on T1-weighted sequences (depending on the degree of cartilage hydration) and high signal on fluid-sensitive sequences (**Fig. 17**).[74] On fluid-sensitive sequences, the masses are slightly lower in signal than joint fluid. The foci may be slightly heterogeneous in signal and may contain punctate areas of low signal on all pulse sequences, reflecting early mineralization (**Figs. 18** and **19**). Larger low-signal areas are present on all pulse sequences when frank calcification of the masses is present on radiographs (**Fig. 20**). The low signal is often more well-defined and rounded in comparison with the more amorphous and elongated areas of low signal seen in PVNS. When the masses are ossified, the bodies will be often numerous and similar in size, displaying cortical

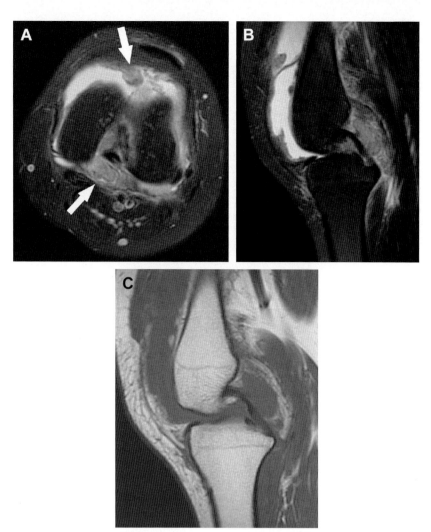

Fig. 17. Axial fat-suppressed T2-weighted image (*A*) shows well-defined slightly heterogeneous and high-signal mass-like foci in and about the intercondylar notch (*arrows*). Sagittal fat-suppressed T2-weighted image (*B*) shows diffuse synovial thickening with heterogeneous, intermediate signal masses in the posterior intercondylar notch and one in the anterior aspect of the suprapatellar pouch. On the sagittal T1-weighted image (*C*), masses are isointense to and indistinguishable from joint fluid in this patient with nonmineralized synovial chondromatosis.

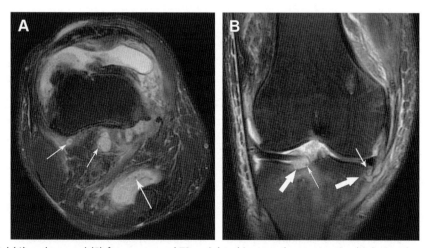

Fig. 18. Axial (*A*) and coronal (*B*) fat-suppressed T2-weighted images show extensive high signal mass-like thickening of the synovium, isointense to cartilage. Note the numerous punctate foci within the synovial thickening, some of which are low in signal, reflecting early mineralization (*thin arrows* in *A* and *B*). Note the associated erosions with adjacent marrow edema pattern in *B* (*thick arrows*).

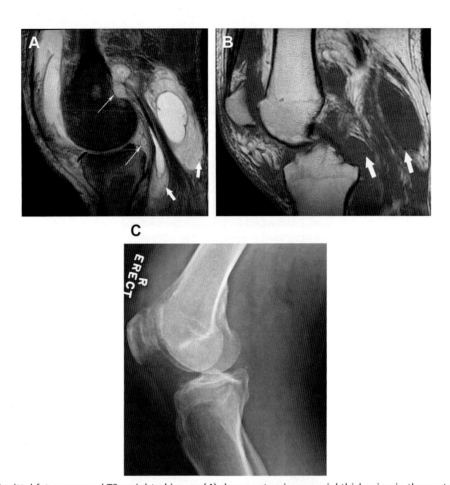

Fig. 19. Sagittal fat-suppressed T2-weighted image (*A*) shows extensive synovial thickening in the posterior knee containing foci of punctate low signal (*thick arrows*) and foci with a target-like appearance (*thin arrows*). Sagittal T1-weighted image (*B*) shows several punctate low-signal foci (*arrows*), reflecting early mineralization, to better advantage. Corresponding lateral radiograph (*C*) shows a large joint effusion with posterior soft-tissue opacities, corresponding to the bursal involvement on the MR scan. There are numerous scattered punctate calcified foci. Note the periarticular osteopenia, unusual for synovial chondromatosis.

low signal and internal fatty marrow. The calcifications will be more prominent (ie, blooming) on gradient-echo sequences.

Malignant transformation of synovial chondromatosis to synovial chondrosarcoma is very rare. Unfortunately, there are usually no distinguishing features between the two on MR imaging. As in PVNS, rapid growth and/or rapidly deteriorating clinical symptoms can be suggestive of malignant transformation.[74,75] Frank marrow invasion is atypical for benign disease, and thus should raise suspicion for malignant transformation.[74]

Osteoarthritis

OA, the most common form of arthritis,[76,77] is a chronic, progressive disorder of synovial joints characterized by degeneration of hyaline cartilage and its underlying bone, leading to pain, disability,

and possible clinically significant depression.[78] The knee is the joint with the highest prevalence of symptomatic OA.[79,80]

Development of OA is multifactorial. Risk of knee OA is higher in obese than in nonobese patients, higher in women than in men, and highest in non-Hispanic blacks.[79–83] Trauma, occupation, structural malalignment, and muscle weakness can contribute to the development of OA. Because MR imaging can detect the earliest stage of cartilage abnormality and other changes in the joint that may be causative or secondary to cartilage damage, it has become increasingly more popular in the clinical evaluation of OA and an important modality in research applications.

The MR imaging manifestations of knee OA are visible in the synovium, bone, cartilage, and ligaments of this articulation. The presence and extent of abnormalities in the synovium and bone have as

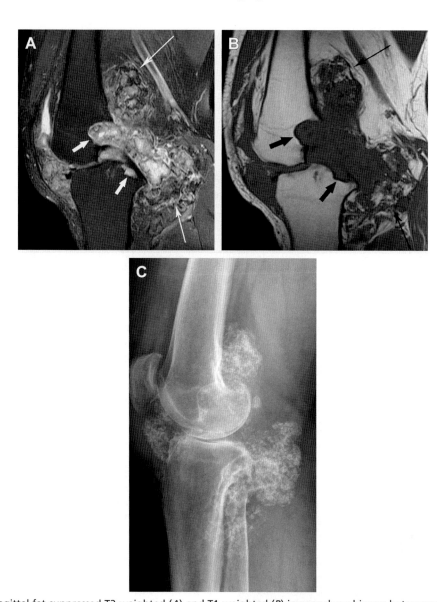

Fig. 20. Sagittal fat-suppressed T2-weighted (*A*) and T1-weighted (*B*) images show bizarre heterogeneous signal in large posterior capsular outpouchings, some of which (particularly superiorly and inferiorly, denoted by *thin arrows*) contains frank marrow signal. Extensive heterogeneous mass-like involvement anteriorly has signal predominantly isointense to cartilage. Note the associated well-defined erosions of the roof of the intercondylar notch and the posterior tibial plateau (*thick arrows*). The adjacent marrow is normal; marrow invasion, if present, would be highly concerning for sarcomatous transformation. Corresponding lateral radiograph (*C*) shows extensive conglomerate chondroid mineralization with numerous well-defined erosions of the adjacent posterior femur and tibia, the anterior proximal tibia, and the roof of the intercondylar notch.

much clinical relevance as the extent of cartilage defects in the typical clinical setting. Pain is the most common reason for patients with OA to undergo imaging evaluation. Although OA is primarily considered to be a mechanical arthritis, the inflammatory nature of this disorder and its clinical impact on both disease progression and pain is increasingly being recognized.[84–87]

Synovitis, a hallmark of joint inflammation, is commonly appreciated on MR imaging in OA and is a primary source of pain in these patients.[14,87] In fact, high signal in the recesses of the posterior knee joint seen on fat-suppressed proton-density sequences is often assumed to be effusion, but may be synovitis in patients with osteoarthritis (**Fig. 21**).[1] The true extent of synovitis is best appreciated on postcontrast images of the joint.[5] Joint effusion can extend into large periarticular cysts such as a popliteal cyst. These cysts may contain significant synovial and chondral debris,

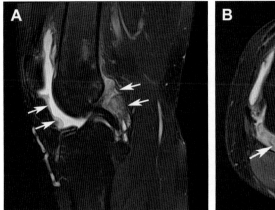
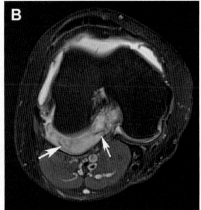

Fig. 21. Sagittal fat-suppressed fast spin-echo T2-weighted (*A*) and axial fat-suppressed fast spin-echo proton-density (*B*) images through the knee of a 42-year-old woman with patellar chondrosis (not shown) and reactive synovitis in the posterior cruciate ligament recess and posterior to the lateral femoral condyle (*arrows*).

leading to signal heterogeneity and confusion with soft-tissue neoplasm. Chronic synovitis may present with fatty infiltration typical of lipoma arborescens.[11] Chronic synovitis may also be mass-like and intermediate to low in signal, leading to concern for villonodular synovitis.

The bone manifestations of OA include osteophyte formation and subchondral bone remodeling. Early subchondral bone remodeling may be recognized on MR imaging as bone marrow edema (**Fig. 22**). Although the term bone marrow

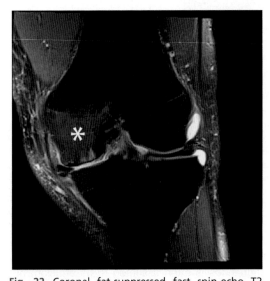

Fig. 22. Coronal fat-suppressed fast spin-echo T2-weighted image through the knee of a 58-year-old man with osteoarthritis and medial knee pain. Diffuse loss of articular cartilage in the medial compartment and medial extrusion of the body of the medial meniscus are associated with bone marrow edema–like lesion in the medial femoral condyle (*asterisk*).

edema is commonly used to describe high signal in the subchondral bone on fluid-sensitive sequences, histologic examination of these areas reveals edema to be a small component. A more accurate description of the area has been termed subchondral bone marrow edema–like lesion, which consists of, in descending order, normal bone, marrow necrosis, abnormal trabeculae, fibrosis, edema, and hemorrhage.[88] Although controversial, the presence of a bone marrow edema–like lesion correlates clinically with pain[14] in many studies.

Extensive subchondral remodeling can lead to the development of subarticular cysts.[89] These cysts can be fairly large, leading to concern for possible osseous neoplasm.[90] A sclerotic osseous rim and thin-walled enhancement on intravenous contrast administration of the cyst cavity are important clues to the nonneoplastic nature of these degenerative cysts.

Cartilage defects are important to recognize and characterize. These defects are best appreciated on fat-suppressed fast spin-echo proton-density or gradient-echo sequences such as 3-dimensional (3D) double-echo steady-state or 3D spoiled gradient-echo sequences. The defects can be graded using the International Cartilage Repair Society grading system (**Table 2**) or one of many other available grading systems.[91] Shedding of chondral fragments into the joint can lead to the development of secondary osteochondromatosis. In this setting, chondral fragments of degenerated cartilage in osteoarthritis are nourished by the synovial fluid and enlarge, eventually undergoing calcification and ossification. The bodies in the secondary form are usually of different shapes and sizes, and most often are much fewer in

Table 2
International Cartilage Repair Society grading system

Grade	Description
1	Superficial lesions and softening
2	Lesions involving <50% of the thickness of cartilage
3	Lesions involving >50% of the thickness of cartilage
4	Lesions extending to bone

number than in primary synovial chondromatosis.[74] When ossified, they may have concentric rings of compact bone, reflecting their continued growth, unlike those of the primary form of synovial chondromatosis.

SUMMARY

The radiologist has the opportunity to provide significant added value in the clinical diagnosis and management of patients with arthropathies. Therefore it is critically important to recognize the MR imaging manifestations of rheumatologic disorders and their effect on the synovium, bones, ligaments, tendons, and cartilage. Specific diagnoses should be provided when the imaging presentation is characteristic. Combining clinical information with MR imaging findings can often lead to the correct diagnosis when the MR imaging presentation is nonspecific.

REFERENCES

1. Roemer FW, Kassim Javaid M, Guermazi A, et al. Anatomical distribution of synovitis in knee osteoarthritis and its association with joint effusion assessed on non-enhanced and contrast-enhanced MRI. Osteoarthritis Cartilage 2010; 18(10):1269–74. Elsevier.

2. Roemer FW, Guermazi A, Zhang Y, et al. Hoffa's fat pad: evaluation on unenhanced MR images as a measure of patellofemoral synovitis in osteoarthritis. AJR Am J Roentgenol 2009;192(6):1696–700.

3. Bredella MA, Tirman PF, Wischer TK, et al. Reactive synovitis of the knee joint: MR imaging appearance with arthroscopic correlation. Skeletal Radiol 2000; 29(10):577–82.

4. Li X, Liu X, Du X, et al. Diffusion-weighted MR imaging for assessing synovitis of wrist and hand in patients with rheumatoid arthritis: a feasibility study. Magn Reson Imaging 2014;32(4):350–3. Elsevier.

5. Loeuille D, Sauliere N, Champigneulle J, et al. Comparing non-enhanced and enhanced sequences in the assessment of effusion and synovitis in knee OA: associations with clinical, macroscopic and microscopic features. Osteoarthr Cartil 2011;19(12):1433–9. Elsevier.

6. Winalski CS, Aliabadi P, Wright RJ, et al. Enhancement of joint fluid with intravenously administered gadopentetate dimeglumine: technique, rationale, and implications. Radiology 1993;187(1):179–85.

7. van de Sande MG, van der Leij C, Lavini C, et al. Characteristics of synovial inflammation in early arthritis analysed by pixel-by-pixel time-intensity curve shape analysis. Rheumatology (Oxford) 2012;51(7):1240–5.

8. Østergaard M, Klarlund M. Importance of timing of post-contrast MRI in rheumatoid arthritis: what happens during the first 60 minutes after IV gadolinium-DTPA? Ann Rheum Dis 2001;60(11):1050–4.

9. Goldman AB, DiCarlo EF. Pigmented villonodular synovitis. Diagnosis and differential diagnosis. Radiol Clin North Am 1988;26(6):1327–47.

10. Narváez JA, Narváez J, Ortega R, et al. Hypointense synovial lesions on T2-weighted images: differential diagnosis with pathologic correlation. AJR Am J Roentgenol 2003;181(3):761–9.

11. Ryu KN, Jaovisidha S, Schweitzer M, et al. MR imaging of lipoma arborescens of the knee joint. AJR Am J Roentgenol 1996;167(5):1229–32.

12. Howe BM, Wenger DE. Lipoma arborescens: comparison of typical and atypical disease presentations. Clin Radiol 2013;68(12):1220–6.

13. Karchevsky M, Schweitzer ME, Morrison WB, et al. MRI findings of septic arthritis and associated osteomyelitis in adults. AJR Am J Roentgenol 2004; 182(1):119–22.

14. Yusuf E, Kortekaas MC, Watt I, et al. Do knee abnormalities visualised on MRI explain knee pain in knee osteoarthritis? A systematic review. Ann Rheum Dis 2011;70(1):60–7.

15. Zhang Y, Nevitt M, Niu J, et al. Fluctuation of knee pain and changes in bone marrow lesions, effusions, and synovitis on magnetic resonance imaging. Arthritis Rheum 2011;63(3):691–9. Wiley Subscription Services, Inc., A Wiley Company.

16. Lo GH, McAlindon TE, Niu J, et al. Bone marrow lesions and joint effusion are strongly and independently associated with weight-bearing pain in knee osteoarthritis: data from the osteoarthritis initiative. Osteoarthr Cartil 2009;17(12):1562–9. Elsevier.

17. Emad Y, Ragab Y, Bassyouni I, et al. Enthesitis and related changes in the knees in seronegative spondyloarthropathies and skin psoriasis: magnetic resonance imaging case-control study. J Rheumatol 2010;37(8):1709–17.

18. Choi JA, Koh SH, Hong SH, et al. Rheumatoid arthritis and tuberculous arthritis: differentiating MRI features. AJR Am J Roentgenol 2009;193(5): 1347–53.

19. Ecklund K, Vargas S, Zurakowski D, et al. MRI features of Lyme arthritis in children. AJR Am J Roentgenol 2005;184(6):1904–9.

20. Goldenberg DL. Septic arthritis. Lancet 1998; 351(9097):197–202.

21. Graif M, Schweitzer ME, Deely D, et al. The septic versus nonseptic inflamed joint: MRI characteristics. Skeletal Radiol 1999;28(11):616–20.

22. Hong SH, Kim SM, Ahn JM, et al. Tuberculous versus pyogenic arthritis: MR imaging evaluation. Radiology 2001;218(3):848–53.

23. Hurd ER, Johns J, Chubick A. Comparative study of gonococcal arthritis and Reiter's syndrome. Ann Rheum Dis 1979;38(Suppl 1):suppl 55–8.

24. Pioro MH, Mandell BF. Septic arthritis. Rheum Dis Clin North Am 1997;23(2):239–58.

25. Javors JM, WM. Principles of diagnosis and treatment of joint infections. Arthritis and allied conditions a textbook of rheumatology. 15th edition. Baltimore (MD): Williams & Wilkins; 2005. p. 2253–66.

26. Kaandorp CJ, Van Schaardenburg D, Krijnen P, et al. Risk factors for septic arthritis in patients with joint disease. A prospective study. Arthritis Rheum 1995;38(12):1819–25.

27. Ryan MJ, Kavanagh R, Wall PG, et al. Bacterial joint infections in England and Wales: analysis of bacterial isolates over a four year period. Br J Rheumatol 1997;36(3):370–3.

28. Marques A. Chronic Lyme disease: a review. Infect Dis Clin North Am 2008;22(2):341–60, vii–viii.

29. Steere AC, Schoen RT, Taylor E. The clinical evolution of Lyme arthritis. Ann Intern Med 1987;107(5): 725–31.

30. Lawson JP, Rahn DW. Lyme disease and radiologic findings in Lyme arthritis. AJR Am J Roentgenol 1992;158(5):1065–9.

31. De Backer AI, Vanhoenacker FM, Sanghvi DA. Imaging features of extraaxial musculoskeletal tuberculosis. Indian J Radiol Imaging 2009;19(3): 176–86.

32. Sanghvi DA, Iyer VR, Deshmukh T, et al. MRI features of tuberculosis of the knee. Skeletal Radiol 2009;38(3):267–73.

33. Shah J, Patkar D, Parikh B, et al. Tuberculosis of the sternum and clavicle: imaging findings in 15 patients. Skeletal Radiol 2000;29(8):447–53.

34. Jacoby RK, Jayson MI, Cosh JA. Onset, early stages, and prognosis of rheumatoid arthritis: a clinical study of 100 patients with 11-year follow-up. Br Med J 1973;2(5858):96–100.

35. Mohana-Borges AV, Chung CB, Resnick D. Monoarticular arthritis. Radiol Clin North Am 2004; 42(1):135–49.

36. Østergaard M, Hansen M, Stoltenberg M, et al. Magnetic resonance imaging-determined synovial membrane volume as a marker of disease activity and a predictor of progressive joint destruction in the wrists of patients with rheumatoid arthritis. Arthritis Rheum 1999;42(5):918–29.

37. Creamer P, Keen M, Zananiri F, et al. Quantitative magnetic resonance imaging of the knee: a method of measuring response to intra-articular treatments. Ann Rheum Dis 1997;56(6):378–81.

38. Østergaard M, Stoltenberg M, Løvgreen-Nielsen P, et al. Quantification of synovitis by MRI: correlation between dynamic and static gadolinium-enhanced magnetic resonance imaging and microscopic and macroscopic signs of synovial inflammation. Magn Reson Imaging 1998;16(7):743–54.

39. Albrecht M, Marinetti GV, Jacox RF, et al. A biochemical and electron microscopy study of rice bodies from rheumatoid patients. Arthritis Rheum 1965;8(6):1053–63.

40. Popert AJ, Scott DL, Wainwright AC, et al. Frequency of occurrence, mode of development, and significance or rice bodies in rheumatoid joints. Ann Rheum Dis 1982;41(2):109–17.

41. Shbeeb M, Uramoto KM, Gibson LE, et al. The epidemiology of psoriatic arthritis in Olmsted County, Minnesota, USA, 1982-1991. J Rheumatol 2000;27(5):1247–50.

42. Thumboo J, Uramoto K, Shbeeb MI, et al. Risk factors for the development of psoriatic arthritis: a population based nested case control study. J Rheumatol 2002;29(4):757–62.

43. Klippel JH, Weyand CM, Wortmann R. Primer on the rheumatic diseases. Atlanta (GA): Arthritis Foundation; 1997.

44. McGonagle D, Conaghan PG, Emery P. Psoriatic arthritis: a unified concept twenty years on. Arthritis Rheum 1999;42(6):1080–6.

45. McGonagle D, Gibbon W, O'Connor P, et al. Characteristic magnetic resonance imaging entheseal changes of knee synovitis in spondylarthropathy. Arthritis Rheum 1998;41(4):694–700.

46. Taylor PW, Stoecker W. Enthesitis of the elbow in psoriatic arthritis. J Rheumatol 1997;24(11): 2268–9.

47. Jevtic V, Rozman B, Kos-Golja M, et al. MR imaging in seronegative spondyloarthritis. Radiologe 1996; 36(8):624–31 [in German].

48. Aydin SZ, Tan AL, Hodsgon R, et al. Comparison of ultrasonography and magnetic resonance imaging for the assessment of clinically defined knee enthesitis in spondyloarthritis. Clin Exp Rheumatol 2013; 31(6):933–6.

49. Pascual E, Pedraz T. Gout. Curr Opin Rheumatol 2004;16(3):282–6.

50. Essen von R, Hölttä AM, Pikkarainen R. Quality control of synovial fluid crystal identification. Ann Rheum Dis 1998;57(2):107–9.

51. Espejo-Baena A, Coretti SM, Fernandez JM, et al. Knee locking due to a single gouty tophus. J Rheumatol 2006;33(1):193–5.

52. Yu JS, Chung C, Recht M, et al. MR imaging of to-phaceous gout. AJR Am J Roentgenol 1997; 168(2):523–7.

53. Melloni P, Valls R, Yuguero M, et al. An unusual case of tophaceous gout involving the anterior cruciate ligament. Arthroscopy 2004;20(9): e117–21.

54. Recht MP, Seragini F, Kramer J, et al. Isolated or dominant lesions of the patella in gout: a report of seven patients. Skeletal Radiol 1994;23(2): 113–6.

55. Chen CK, Yeh LR, Pan HB, et al. Intra-articular gouty tophi of the knee: CT and MR imaging in 12 patients. Skeletal Radiol 1999;28(2):75–80.

56. Price MD, Padera RF, Harris MB, et al. Case reports: pathologic fracture of the patella from a gouty tophus. Clin Orthop Relat Res 2006;445: 250–3.

57. Doumas C, Vazirani RM, Clifford PD, et al. Acute calcific periarthritis of the hand and wrist: a series and review of the literature. Emerg Radiol 2007; 14(4):199–203.

58. Flemming DJ, Murphey MD, Shekitka KM, et al. Osseous involvement in calcific tendinitis: a retrospective review of 50 cases. AJR Am J Roentgenol 2003;181(4):965–72.

59. Tibrewal SB. Acute calcific tendinitis of the popliteus tendon–an unusual site and clinical syndrome. Ann R Coll Surg Engl 2002;84(5):338–41.

60. Baroni E, Russo BD, Masquijo JJ, et al. Pigmented villonodular synovitis of the knee in skeletally immature patients. J Child Orthop 2010; 4(2):123–7.

61. Kim HS, Kwon JW, Ahn JH, et al. Localized tenosynovial giant cell tumor in both knee joints. Skeletal Radiol 2010;39(9):923–6.

62. West RB, Rubin BP, Miller MA, et al. A landscape effect in tenosynovial giant-cell tumor from activation of CSF1 expression by a translocation in a minority of tumor cells. Proc Natl Acad Sci U S A 2006;103(3):690–5.

63. Murphey MD, Rhee JH, Lewis RB, et al. Pigmented villonodular synovitis: radiologic-pathologic correlation. Radiographics 2008;28(5):1493–518.

64. Stubbs AJ, Higgins LD. Pigmented villonodular synovitis of the knee: disease of the popliteus tendon and posterolateral compartment. Arthroscopy 2005;21(7):893–5.

65. Dorwart RH, Genant HK, Johnston WH, et al. Pigmented villonodular synovitis of synovial joints: clinical, pathologic, and radiologic features. AJR Am J Roentgenol 1984;143(4):877–85.

66. Tyler WK, Vidal AF, Williams RJ, et al. Pigmented villonodular synovitis. J Am Acad Orthop Surg 2006;14(6):376–85.

67. Ma X, Shi G, Xia C, et al. Pigmented villonodular synovitis: a retrospective study of seventy five cases (eighty one joints). Int Orthop 2013;37(6): 1165–70.

68. Chung BJ, Park YB. Pigmented villonodular synovitis after TKA associated with tibial component loosening. Orthopedics 2011;34(8):e418–20.

69. Oni JK, Cavallo RJ. A rare case of diffuse pigmented villonodular synovitis after total knee arthroplasty. J Arthroplasty 2011;26(6):978.e9–11.

70. Ryan RS, Louis L, O'Connell JX, et al. Pigmented villonodular synovitis of the proximal tibiofibular joint. Australas Radiol 2004;48(4):520–2.

71. Imakiire N, Fujino T, Morii T, et al. Malignant pigmented villonodular synovitis in the knee - report of a case with rapid clinical progression. Open Orthop J 2011;5(1):13–6.

72. Kalil RK, Unni KK. Malignancy in pigmented villonodular synovitis. Skeletal Radiol 1998;27(7): 392–5.

73. Narváez JA, Narváez J, Aguilera C, et al. MR imaging of synovial tumors and tumor-like lesions. Eur Radiol 2001;11(12):2549–60.

74. Murphey MD, Vidal JA, Fanburg-Smith JC, et al. Imaging of synovial chondromatosis with radiologic-pathologic correlation. Radiographics 2007;27(5):1465–88.

75. Wittkop B, Davies AM, Mangham DC. Primary synovial chondromatosis and synovial chondrosarcoma: a pictorial review. Eur Radiol 2002;12(8): 2112–9.

76. Lawrence RC, Helmick CG, Arnett FC, et al. Estimates of the prevalence of arthritis and selected musculoskeletal disorders in the United States. Arthritis Rheum 1998;41(5):778–99.

77. Sacks JJ, Luo YH, Helmick CG. Prevalence of specific types of arthritis and other rheumatic conditions in the ambulatory health care system in the United States, 2001-2005. Arthritis Care Res (Hoboken) 2010;62(4):460–4.

78. Duivenvoorden T, Vissers MM, Verhaar JA, et al. Anxiety and depressive symptoms before and after total hip and knee arthroplasty: a prospective multicentre study. Osteoarthr Cartil 2013;21(12): 1834–40.

79. Oliveria SA, Felson DT, Reed JI, et al. Incidence of symptomatic hand, hip, and knee osteoarthritis among patients in a health maintenance organization. Arthritis Rheum 1995; 38(8):1134–41.

80. Dillon CF, Rasch EK, Gu Q, et al. Prevalence of knee osteoarthritis in the United States: arthritis data from the Third National Health and Nutrition Examination Survey 1991-94. J Rheumatol 2006; 33(11):2271–9.

81. Losina E, Weinstein AM, Reichmann WM, et al. Lifetime risk and age at diagnosis of symptomatic knee osteoarthritis in the US. Arthritis Care Res (Hoboken) 2013;65(5):703–11.

82. Felson DT. Risk factors for osteoarthritis: understanding joint vulnerability. Clin Orthop Relat Res 2004;(Suppl 427):S16–21.

83. Srikanth VK, Fryer JL, Zhai G, et al. A meta-analysis of sex differences prevalence, incidence and severity of osteoarthritis. Osteoarthr Cartil 2005; 13(9):769–81.

84. Berenbaum F. Osteoarthritis as an inflammatory disease (osteoarthritis is not osteoarthrosis!). Osteoarthritis Cartilage 2013;21(1):16–21. Elsevier Ltd.

85. Scanzello CR, Goldring SR. The role of synovitis in osteoarthritis pathogenesis. Bone 2012;51(2): 249–57.

86. Crema MD, Felson DT, Roemer FW, et al. Peripatellar synovitis: comparison between non-contrast-enhanced and contrast-enhanced MRI and association with pain. The MOST study. Osteoarthritis Cartilage 2013;21(3):413–8.

87. Baker K, Grainger A, Niu J, et al. Relation of synovitis to knee pain using contrast-enhanced MRIs. Ann Rheum Dis 2010;69(10):1779–83.

88. Zanetti M, Bruder E, Romero J, et al. Bone marrow edema pattern in osteoarthritic knees: correlation between MR imaging and histologic findings. Radiology 2000;215(3):835–40.

89. Carrino JA, Blum J, Parellada JA, et al. MRI of bone marrow edema-like signal in the pathogenesis of subchondral cysts. Osteoarthr Cartil 2006;14(10): 1081–5.

90. Glass TA, Dyer R, Fisher L, et al. Expansile subchondral bone cyst. AJR Am J Roentgenol 1982; 139(6):1210–1.

91. Kleemann RU, Krocker D, Cedraro A, et al. Altered cartilage mechanics and histology in knee osteoarthritis: relation to clinical assessment (ICRS Grade). Osteoarthritis Cartilage 2005;13(11):958–63.

MR Imaging of Extrasynovial Inflammation and Impingement About the Knee

Higor Grando, MD[a,b,*], Eric Y. Chang, MD[a,c],
Karen C. Chen, MD[a,c], Christine B. Chung, MD[a,c]

KEYWORDS

- Knee fat pad impingement • Hoffa disease • Patellofemoral friction syndrome • Quadriceps fat pad
- Prefemoral fat pad • Pericruciate fat pad • Adhesive capsulitis knee • Iliotibial band syndrome

KEY POINTS

- The knee has unique anatomy regarding the relationship between the synovial and capsular layers, with interposed fat pads at certain locations.
- The extrasynovial impingement and inflammation syndromes about the knee are underdiagnosed and should be included in the differential diagnosis of anterior knee pain.
- MR imaging is the best imaging modality for evaluation of the anatomy and disorders of these extrasynovial compartments.

INTRODUCTION

The knee demonstrates unique anatomy with regard to the capsular-synovial relationship and in particular contains several interposed fat pads. The 3 intracapsular fat pads are present within the anterior portion of the knee and include the infrapatellar (Hoffa) fat pad, the anterior suprapatellar (quadriceps) fat pad, and the posterior suprapatellar or prefemoral fat pad (PFP).[1,2] In 1953, MacConaill[3] proposed that fat pads not only occupy dead space in the joint but also help maintain the joint cavity and promote efficient lubrication by helping to distribute synovial fluid. This theory may explain the presence of fat pads in areas of the body exposed to mechanical stresses, such as the knee.

The capsule of the knee is a complex structure with up to 3 different layers. The most internal layer is located just superficial and parallel to the synovial membrane for most of its course. The capsule at the anterior portion of the knee is thinner compared with the capsule at the posterior portion of the knee and the extensor mechanism serves as its anterior and outer margin.[1,2,4] At the inferior aspect of the extensor mechanism, the proximal part of patellar tendon partially replaces the capsule, composed of only a thin expansion attached to the patellar margins and patellar tendon.[5] The boundaries of the synovial

E.Y. Chang, MD, gratefully acknowledges grant support from the VA (Clinical Science Research and Development Career Development Award: 1IK2CX000749).

Conflicts of Interest: None.

[a] Department of Radiology, San Diego Medical Center, University of California, 200 West Arbor Drive, San Diego, CA 92126, USA; [b] Department of Radiology, Hospital do Coração (HCor) and Teleimagem, Desembargador Eliseu Guilherme, 147, Paraíso, São Paulo 04004-030, Brazil; [c] Department of Radiology, VA San Diego Healthcare System, 3350 La Jolla Village Drive, MC 114, San Diego, CA 92161, USA

* Corresponding author. Department of Radiology, Mail Code 0868, 8899 University Lane #370, San Diego, CA 92122.

E-mail address: grandohgb@gmail.com

mri.theclinics.com

membrane are more familiar to radiologists and orthopedic surgeons because they are outlined by joint distention during arthrography and arthroscopic surgery. The extrasynovial cruciate ligaments are incompletely surrounded by synovium, however, with the region posterior to the posterior cruciate ligament devoid of synovium.[3,5–7]

Understanding the unique anatomy of the knee is essential toward the goal of understanding extrasynovial disorders and impingement syndromes (**Fig. 1**). Anterior knee disease includes many conditions whose nosologic framework is still not fully standardized. Extrasynovial inflammation and impingement syndromes about the knee are certainly underdiagnosed and should be in the differential diagnosis for patients presenting with anterior knee pain. This article reviews the inflammation and impingement syndromes affecting the superior fat pad, inferior fat pad, pericruciate fat pad, and PFP in the knee, including Hoffa disease, iliotibial band (ITB) syndrome, and adhesive capsulitis (AC).

HOFFA DISEASE
Introduction

The infrapatellar fat pad (IFP), or Hoffa fat pad, composed of large conglomerates of adipose tissue with a surrounding net of fibrous connective tissue and vascularization, is the site of Hoffa disease.

First described in 1904, acute or repetitive trauma to the fat pad causes internal hemorrhage leading to an inflammatory cascade with edema and hypertrophy of the fat pad. This morphologic change in the fat pad results in mechanical impingement between the femur and the tibia. A vicious cycle of inflammation and pain ensues with subsequent deposition of fibrin and hemosiderin, with fibrous tissue, leukocytes, perivascular cells, and fibrin-occluded blood vessels seen on histologic examination.[8] At the end stage of disease, scarring, fibrosis, and calcification may occur.[8–14] Ogilvie-Harris and Giddens[13] found Hoffa disease present in 1% of patients undergoing knee

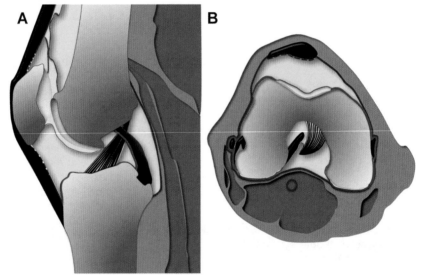

Fig. 1. (*A*) Schematic of midsagittal nondistended knee image. The thick blue line, posterior, represents the posterior capsule. At the anterior portion of the knee, the capsule is thin (*thin blue line*) abutting the quadriceps and patellar tendons (*black*); no synovial layer is seen. Close to the patella, the capsule is quite thin (*dashed blue lines*). A distinct layer of synovium (*red line*) covers the bone (*patchy gray*), the cruciate ligaments (*black*), and the fat pads (*yellow*) except at the posterior-most fat pad interposed between the posterior capsule and posterior cruciate ligament and the parts that have contact with the extensor mechanism. Note a single synovial layer (*red line*) covering the posterior part of the IFP separate from the trochlear cartilage by the intra-articular fluid (*light blue*). (*B*) Schematic of axial image just below the patella. The knee capsule is represented by a thick blue line but is quite thin (*dashed blue line*) behind the patellar tendon (*black*). The synovial layer is represented by the red lines covering most of the knee joint. In this nondistended joint, dual layers of apposed synovium are represented with a thicker red line whereas a single layer of synovium is represented with a thinner red line, such as that surrounding the cruciate ligaments (*black*). Note the same single synovial layer (*red line*) covering the posterior part of the IFP (*yellow*) separated from the trochlear cartilage (*light gray*) by the intra-articular fluid (*light blue*).

arthroscopy, suggesting that this entity may be underdiagnosed by imaging.

Several mechanical abnormalities can occur in the IFP, including acute injury or microtrauma due to blunt impact, shear injury with anterior cruciate ligament tearing, patellar dislocation, torsion, or impingement,[15] each showing different MR imaging patterns.

Similar imaging findings have been reported in patients with HIV (**Fig. 2**), characterized by global homogeneous increase in signal intensity throughout the IFP on fluid-sensitive sequences. In this subset of patients, the quadriceps and PFPs may also be involved and show signal alteration.[16] Structures adjacent to the IFP can be affected by synovial processes and mimic symptoms of IFP impingement. The deep infrapatellar bursa is located immediately posterior to the distal portion of the patellar tendon and can be affected by inflammatory bursitis with or without an associated Hoffitis or other disorders.[17–19]

Clinical

Clinical features consist of pain around the patellar tendon, close to the femorotibial joint line with loss of normal hyperextension.[20] Hoffa[8] reported that affected patients feel pain when pressure was applied to both sides of the patellar tendon during passive extension of the knee.

Most IFP pathologies are successfully managed with the combination of antiinflammatory drugs, physical therapy, taping, muscle training, gait training, and injections of local anesthetic and corticosteroids to decrease pain and inflammation.[15] For patients who fail conservative therapy, arthroscopic resection of the impinging fat pad produces sustained relief of symptoms with low rates of morbidity and complications.[20]

Imaging

Sagittal and axial images on T1-weighted and T2-weighted fat-suppressed sequences provide optimal evaluation of the IFP. The acute phase of the disease demonstrates high T2 and low T1 signal in the IFP (**Fig. 3**). The IFP may be enlarged with accompanying mass effect on the patellar tendon. Enhancement may be present in the fat pad after intravenous gadolinium administration. Chronic cases can demonstrate fibrosis, hemorrhagic deposition, and rarely calcification, characterized by hypointense signal on T1- and T2-weighted images.[8,9,21,22]

Deep infrapatellar bursitis is another cause of anterior knee pain and has a different pathophysiology from Hoffa disease but may result in reactive changes in the IFP given its contiguity with the anterior surface of the fat pad. The imaging findings include a focal collection of high signal

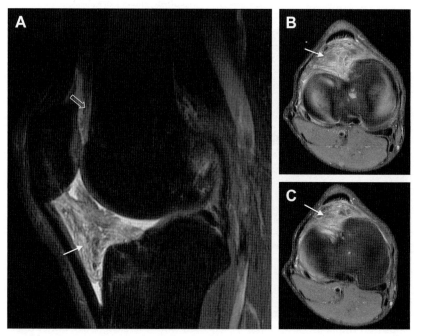

Fig. 2. A 49-year-old man, HIV positive. Sagittal short tau inversion recovery (A) and axial PD fat-suppressed (B, C) images show marked, diffuse edema of Hoffa fat pad (*arrows*) with mild edema of the PFP (*white open arrow*).

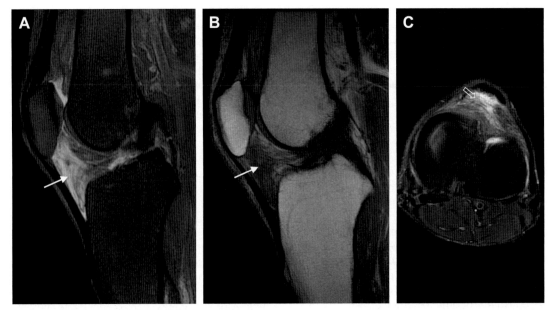

Fig. 3. A 41-year-old man with anterior knee pain and no history of HIV or systemic disease. Sagittal PD fat-suppressed (*A*) and sagittal T1 (*B*) images demonstrate increased and decreased signal intensity (*white arrows*), respectively, of the IFP. Axial PD fat-suppressed image (*C*) confirming that the signal alteration is more at the anterior part of the fat pad (*white open arrow*). (*Courtesy of* Diego Lessa Garcia, MD, Hospital Beneficiência Portuguesa, MedImagem, Sao Paulo, Brazil.)

intensity on T2-weighted sequences confined between the distal portion of the patellar tendon and the anterior aspect of the IFP.[17] The adjacent fat pad can show signs of inflammation with signal abnormality (**Fig. 4**).

PATELLOFEMORAL FRICTION SYNDROME
Introduction

Patellofemoral pain and patellar instability are the 2 main symptoms in patellofemoral disease that includes many conditions.[23]

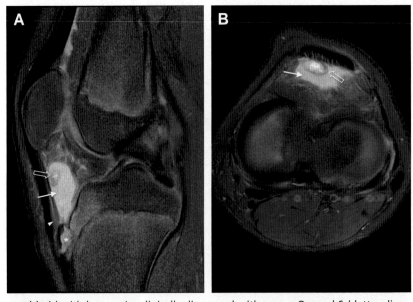

Fig. 4. A 12-year-old girl with knee pain, clinically diagnosed with severe Osgood-Schlatter disease. Sagittal (*A*) and axial PD fat-suppressed (*B*) images show bone marrow edema in the TT (*asterisk*), patellar tendinosis (*arrowhead*), deep infrapatellar bursitis (*white arrow*), and focal edema involving the fat pad apron,[17] (*white open arrow*), which extends inferiorly from Hoffa fat pad.

The Lyon School of Knee Surgery classified patellofemoral disease into 3 distinct entities[24,25]:

1. Objective patellar instability (OPI), which is defined by the presence of at least 1 episode of true patellar dislocation or radiologic sequelae and at least 1 anatomic abnormality confirmed by imaging: trochlear dysplasia, patella alta, patellar tilt, or tibial tuberosity (TT)–trochlear groove (TG) distance abnormality
2. Potential patellar instability (PPI), which is characterized by the presence of subjective patellar pain and/or instability (reflex) with no history of true patellar dislocation and the same anatomic abnormalities as in OPI
3. Patellar pain syndrome (PPS) without a major morphologic abnormality on radiographs.

The symptoms include a combination of patellar pain, reflex buckling, and occasional pseudolocking. The 2 first topics (OPI and PPI) are necessarily related with anatomic abnormalities. Patients presenting with anterior knee pain in the infrapatellar region related to a friction syndrome often fall into the spectrum of PPS but eventually can also have patellofemoral malalignment and fall into the spectrum of PPI or OPI.

Brukner and colleagues[26] first used the term, *infrapatellar fat pad impingement*, in 1999 and Chung and colleagues[27] introduced the term, *patellofemoral friction syndrome*, in a study of 42 patients. These patients with chronic anterior and lateral knee pain showed edema within the anterolateral fat of the anterior compartment of the knee (**Fig. 5**).[26,27] The edema described may be the result of impingement between the lateral femoral condyle and the posterior aspect of the patellar tendon.[22,27,28]

The IFP contains adipocytes, macrophages, lymphocytes, and granulocytes as well as nociceptive nerve fibers that could in part be responsible for anterior pain.[15,29] It plays a role in stabilizing the patella in extremes of flexion and extension.[30]

Clinical

Clinically, the patellafemoral friction syndrome is characterized by anterior pain and tenderness, typically at the lower lateral pole of the patella.[27] This is more common in young patients who engage in routine physical activities.[23,27,31] Similar to a majority of other fat pad impingement syndromes, this friction syndrome occurs with flexion, extension, and mechanical maltracking of the patella. These movements result in remodeling of the morphology of the fat pad, adjusting its shape to the space between the joint (**Fig. 6**). Knee pain can be exacerbated by hyperextension, and physical examination can demonstrate focal point tenderness at the inferior pole of the patella.[28] IFP pathology, including friction syndrome, is

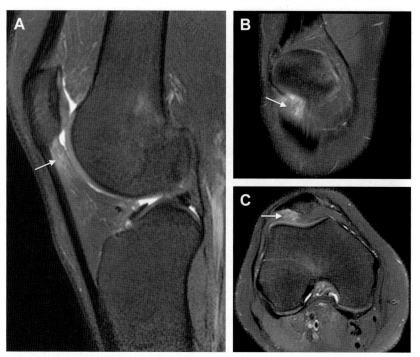

Fig. 5. A 20-year-old man with anterior knee pain. Sagittal (*A*), coronal (*B*), and axial (*C*) PD fat-suppressed images of the knee showing edema (*arrows*) in the superolateral aspect of Hoffa fat pad.

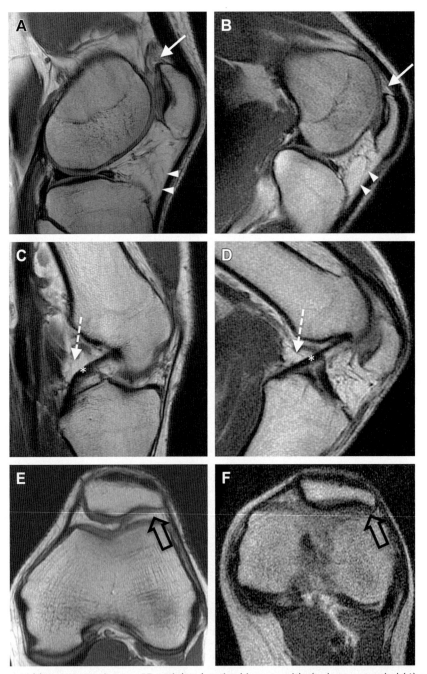

Fig. 6. A 33-year-old asymptomatic man. PD-weighted sagittal images with the knee extended (*A*) and with 90° flexion (*B*) demonstrate deformation of the suprapatellar (*white arrows*) and quadriceps fat pad (*arrowheads*) during knee flexion. PD-weighted sagittal images, knee extended (*C*) and with 90° flexion (*D*), demonstrate deformation of the pericruciate fat pad during knee flexion (*dashed arrows*) with the PCL (*asterisk*) full extended (*D*). Axial PD-weighted images, with the knee extended (*E*) and with 90° flexion (*F*), demonstrate deformation of the superolateral aspect of Hoffa fat pad during knee flexion (*black open arrows*).

usually successfully managed with conservative therapy, including physical therapy targeted at restoring the biomechanics of patellar tracking and taping with the attempt to unload the inferior fat pad.[15]

Imaging

Sagittal and axial imaging planes best demonstrate the patellar tendon and its relationship with the lateral femoral condyle.[27]

Focal increased signal intensity on fluid-sensitive MR images of the superolateral portion of the IFP between the patellar tendon and the lateral femoral condyle has been described as edema related to the friction syndrome (**Fig. 7**).[22,27,31] Enhancement can be seen after intravenous contrast administration.[27]

Anatomic abnormalities of the extensor mechanism, including patellofemoral malalignment,[31] may be related to patellar tendon lateral femoral condyle friction syndrome. Patella alta[23,27] and an increased TT-TG distance are 2 associated findings observed in patients with edema of the superolateral portion of the IFP.[28,31]

Values for patella alta and patella baja were described for radiographs; however, minor adjustments for CT and MR imaging show excellent reproducibility for the 3 classic methods described.[32] The Insall-Salvati (ISI) index uses the ratio of patellar tendon length divided by patellar length (TL/PL). Prior investigators have defined patella alta as TL/PL greater than 1.2 and patella baja as TL/PL less than 0.8.[33,34] The modified ISI ratio is based on the distance between the distal end of the articular surface of the patella and the patellar tendon insertion on the tibia (PT) and the length of the articular surface of the patella (P). The original publication only defined the patela alta value with a PT/P ratio greater than 2.[35] The

Caton-Deschamps method measures the distance between the distal point of the patellar articular surface and the anterior-superior border of the tibia divided by P. The values determined by Caton were greater than or equal to 1.2 and less than or equal to 0.6 for patella alta and patella baja, respectively.[36]

The TT-TG distance was first described for CT[37] but has been shown to be reproducible for MR imaging.[38] Measurements are made on axial images. The TG point represents the deepest cartilaginous point of the most superior image that depicts the complete cartilaginous trochlea. The TT point represents the center of the patellar tendon insertion onto the TT. To obtain the TT-TG measurement, a tangent line to the cartilaginous border of the posterior condyles is drawn with a perpendicular line to the previously determined TG point. These 2 lines are transferred to the level of the TT point, where a perpendicular line is also drawn to the epicondylar tangent. The distance between the TG line and the TT line is the TT-TG value. Pandit and colleagues[39] suggested a value of 10 ± 1 mm in the normal control group, using the MR imaging technique. In one of the most cited articles regarding TT-TG, using CT, Dejour and colleagues[40] found that the TT-TG was 12.7 ± 3.4 mm in their control group and that a value of greater than 20 mm was pathologic.

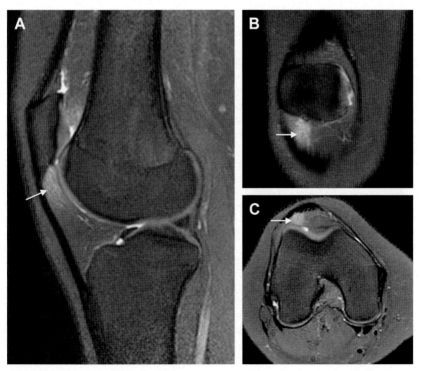

Fig. 7. A 35-year-old woman runner with anterior knee pain. Sagittal (*A*), coronal (*B*), and axial (*C*) PD fat-suppressed of the knee showing edema (*white arrows*) on the superolateral aspect of Hoffa fat pad.

Patella alta may allow the patellar tendon to lie in front of the lateral trochlear facet. The increased TT-TG distance in patients with edema of the superolateral IFP could lead to a lateral displacement of the patellar tendon such that it is opposed to the lateral femoral condyle, facilitating an impingement between these 2 structures.[28] A reduced distance of the patellar ligament to the lateral trochlear facet is directly related to the presence of edema at the lateral portion of the IPFP.[27,28] Patellar tendon abnormalities are also associated with this friction syndrome.[26–28]

QUADRICEPS FAT PAD IMPINGEMENT
Introduction

The anterior suprapatellar fat pad (ASPFP) or quadriceps fat pad is the smallest of the 3 fat pads in the anterior knee with a triangular shape and an average of 7 ± 2 mm in women to 8 ± 2 mm in men.[41] It fills the gap between posterior part of the quadriceps tendon insertion, the posterosuperior aspect of the patella, and the superior part of the retropatellar articular cartilage. It is lined with a synovial surface at the posterior portion that improves the patellofemoral engagement of the extensor mechanism.[41] Posteriorly, the suprapatellar joint recess separates the suprapatellar fat pad from the PFP.[21] The quadriceps tendon is continuous with the ASPFP and is the tendon that contains the most adipose tissue between its fibers at the entheses. This fat is believed to promote stress dissipation or act as a mechanosensory organ.[42]

In contrast with edema of the IFP that is richly innervated and demonstrates a directly relationship with knee pain, the ASPFP has a controversial clinical relationship with knee pain. Roth and colleagues[43] found that there was a relationship between anterior knee pain and imaging findings of edema and enlargement of the superior fat pad. In a recent retrospective study of 879 knee MR imaging examinations, Tsavalas and Karantanas[21] reported that imaging findings of edema and enlargement of the superior fat pad are not related with anterior knee pain.

Clinical

Although the pathogenesis of quadriceps fat pad inflammation is not clearly understood, there may be an association with anterior knee pain.[43] ASPFP edema may be similar to Hoffa disease.[9] Shabshin and colleagues[14] described the histologic appearance in a patient with quadriceps fat pad edema and revealed vasculitis with an inflammatory response similar to the histologic changes described in Hoffa disease. Alternatively, it has been shown that the ASPFP articulates with the femoral trochlea at high angle knee flexion,[44] which may be the mechanism[43] for the fat pad inflammation.

Imaging

When evaluating the quadriceps fat pad, radiologists should note its size, morphology, and signal intensity. Sagittal midline imaging planes on T2-weighted fat-saturated MR images best demonstrate signal alterations and mass effect of the quadriceps fat pad (Fig. 8). Abnormal fat pad signal on fluid-sensitive MR images is defined as present if signal is greater than muscle and less than fluid.[14] As ASPFP signal approaches fluid signal on fluid sensitive sequences, mass effect with a posterior convex border is more likely to be present.[43] The involvement of the intratendinous fat of the adjacent quadriceps tendon (entheseal fat) is observed in some cases (Fig. 9). This secondary involvement may be more symptomatic because of the innervation of fat enthesis.[42]

PREFEMORAL FAT PAD IMPINGEMENT
Introduction

The posterior suprapatellar fat pad, or PFP, is anterior to the femur and is separated from the quadriceps fat pad by the suprapatellar bursa.[9] There is a limited amount of literature on PFP abnormalities, and pathology of this structure is likely underestimated due to underdiagnosis.[45]

PFP impingement may result from alterations in joint mechanics or the presence of superior patella osteophytes associated with repeated microtrauma between the patella and the anterior surface of the distal femur, especially on the lateral side of the fat pat. It may follow a similar pathophysiology of Hoffa disease and quadriceps fat pad.[8,46–48]

Investigators have found a statistically significant association between the presence of superolateral Hoffa fat pad edema and PFP edema.[31] Fat pad edema can be used as an indirect sign of synovial proliferation in patients with joint effusions. In particular, edema within the PFP has highest sensitivity, specificity, and accuracy among the fat pads.[1]

Clinical

The main symptom is chronic anterior knee pain proximal to the superior pole of the patella. In some cases it is debilitating.[45,46] Intermittent mechanical symptoms can occur if the fat pad snaps over the femoral condyles causing a catching sensation during motion.[46,47] Subhawong and

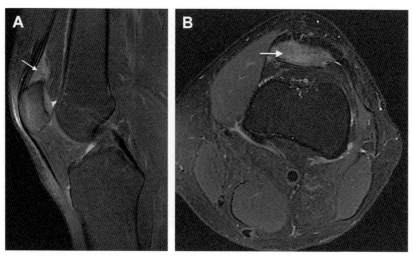

Fig. 8. A 35-year-old woman with knee pain related to running. Sagittal (*A*) and axial (*B*) PD fat-suppressed images showing high signal intensity and mass effect of the quadriceps fat pad (*arrows*).

colleagues[31] show PFP edema in 68% of patients with knee pain and superolateral Hoffa fat pad edema.

The management of PFP impingement is initially conservative, with analgesia, antiinflammatory medications, and physiotherapy, consisting of stretching the quadriceps and flexor muscles to decrease the downward pressure of the patella on the fat pad.[45,47] Arthroscopy can be considered in refractory cases. Kim and colleagues[46] resected a partially fibrosed PFP in a patient with PFP impingement with complete resolution of symptoms and no recurrence at 1-year follow-up.

Imaging

Because of the variety of pathologies, MR imaging is critical in patients with chronic knee pain.[49] The imaging findings of PFP impingement include edema and enlargement of the PFP characterized by high signal intensity on fluid-sensitive images and low signal intensity on T1-weighted images, better appreciated on sagittal and axial planes (**Fig. 10**).

Zakhary and colleagues,[48] in a retrospective study of 478 knee MR imaging examinations, described 2 patterns of PFP edema, one at the

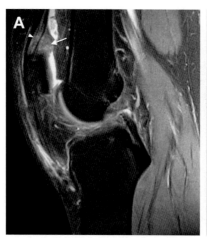
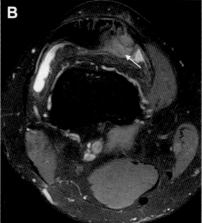

Fig. 9. A 45-year-old man with anterior knee pain. Sagittal PD fat-suppressed image (*A*) demonstrates marked edema at the anterior Suprapatellar (quadriceps) fat pad (*arrow*) and enthesis fat in the distal quadriceps tendon (*arrowhead*). Axial PD fat-suppressed image (*B*) confirms the enlargement of the lateral part of the suprapatellar fat pad (*arrow*).

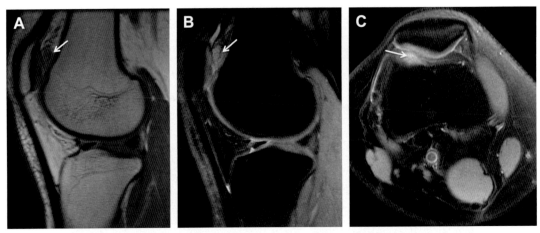

Fig. 10. A 20-year-old woman with anterior knee pain. Sagittal PD (*A*), sagittal PD fat-suppressed (*B*), and axial PD fat-suppressed (*C*) images show PFP edema and mass effect (*arrows*). Patient symptoms resolved after physical therapy.

superior central part of the fat pad, believed related to a prominent superior patella osteophyte causing impingement, and a second at the infero-lateral part of the fat pad, believed related to prior shear injury or impingement. The latter pattern had a high association with lateral patellofemoral friction syndrome.

PERICRUCIATE FAT PAD IMPINGEMENT
Introduction

As discussed previously, several studies have outlined the anatomy and shown the importance of the 3 anterior fat pads with regard to impingement and anterior knee pain. More recently, the pericruciate fat pad has been described in the radiologic literature as a potential location for impingement. Affected patients have been described as participating in intense sports activities, such as soccer, and present with posterior knee pain.[50]

The pericruciate fat pad fills the gap between the anterior and posterior cruciate ligaments and is intimate with both. Similar to the anterior fat pads about the knee, the pericruciate fat pad is intracapsular and extrasynovial.[50] The synovial membrane surrounds the anterior, medial, and lateral portions of the cruciate ligaments but is reflected posteriorly from the PCL to adjoining parts of the joint capsule.[51]

Clinical

In their report, Skaf and colleagues[50] described all the patients with pericruciate fat pad edema as extremely active and presenting with debilitating posterior knee pain, limiting their participation in sports activities. One patient had follow-up

imaging showing improvement of the symptoms and resolution of the signal abnormalities after conservative therapy with rest and nonsteroidal antiinflammatory medication.

Imaging

In the sagittal plane, the PFP appears as a triangular-shaped structure located above the posterior cruciate ligament and posterior to the fibers of the anterior cruciate ligament. In the axial plane, the relation with the cruciate ligaments can be observed within the ACL located more laterally and superiorly, and the PCL formed the inferior limit of the fat pad (**Fig. 11**).[50]

Signal abnormality within the PFP can be seen on all 3 planes but is best appreciated on the sagittal plane as low signal intensity on T1-weighted and high signal intensity on fluid-sensitive images (**Fig. 12**). Diffuse enhancement of the fat pad is observed after the intravenous administration of gadolinium contrast agent. The imaging appearance is similar to that of the IFP in Hoffa disease and the quadriceps fat pad in quadriceps fat pad impingement.[9,22,43]

ADHESIVE CAPSULITIS OF THE KNEE
Introduction

AC was first described in the shoulder as a "periarthritis scapulahumerale" by Duplay[52] in 1896. Neviaser[53] coined the term, *adhesive capsulitis*, in 1945 to describe the findings of chronic inflammation and fibrosis of the joint. It has become evident that AC is not unique to the glenohumeral joint because it has also been reported in the wrist,[4] hip,[5] and most recently knee.[3] Clinical and

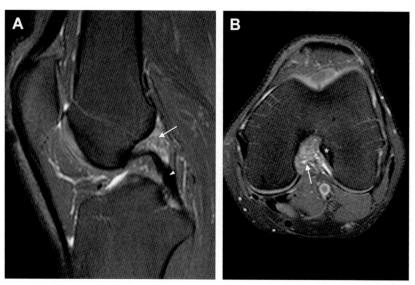

Fig. 11. A 28-year-old professional soccer player with knee pain during training for 2 months. Sagittal (*A*) and axial (*B*) T2 fat-suppressed images show high signal intensity in the pericruciate fat pad (*arrows*). The edematous fat pad is medial to the ACL (*asterisk*) and proximal to the PCL (*arrowhead*). (*Courtesy of* Guinel Hernandez Filho, MD, Tele-imagem, Hospital do Coração e Santa Casa de Misericórdia de São Paulo, Sao Paulo, Brazil.)

histologic findings seem similar regardless of the affected joint. Due to the far greater amount of data and literature available as well as likely identical pathoetiology, this discussion begins with the glenohumeral joint.

In the glenohumeral joint, AC is a common condition that is often reported in many studies as affecting approximately 2% to 5% of the general population. It most typically affects women between 40 and 60 years of age[54–56] and has an association with diabetes[54] and Dupuytren disease.[57] The American Shoulder and Elbow Surgeons have defined AC as "a condition of uncertain etiology characterized by significant restriction of both

active and passive shoulder motion that occurs in the absence of a known intrinsic shoulder disorder."[58]

The disease is thought to be a combination of synovial inflammation and capsular fibrosis,[56] beginning in the synovium and progressing to fibroblastic infiltration and further adhesion and retraction of the capsule.[53,57,59]

Clinical

In the classic description of AC, pain presents first, followed by progressive loss of motion; the pain then subsides and motion may or may not be

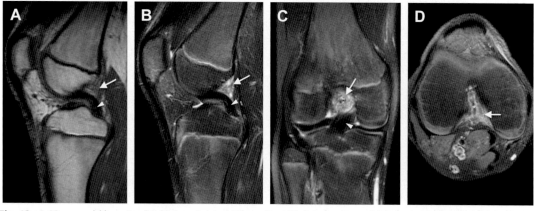

Fig. 12. A 12-year-old boy. Sagittal PD-weighted (*A*), sagittal PD fat-suppressed (*B*), and coronal PD fat-suppressed (*C*) images show edema of the pericruciate fat pad (*arrows*) proximal to the superior aspect of the PCL (*arrowheads*). Axial PD fat-suppressed image (*D*) confirms the edema (*arrow*) of the pericricuate fat pad, located medial and posterior to the femoral foot print of the ACL (*asterisk*).

slowly restored. In the literature, AC of the knee has been described in a 42-year-old woman who presented with knee pain with limitations of both flexion and extension. There was no identifiable joint effusion, and no meniscus, cartilage, or ligament injuries were found. The patient demonstrated complete resolution over a course of 24 months.[60]

Imaging

Imaging findings include high signal intensity on fluid-sensitive images and contrast enhancement of the pericapsular tissues, such as around the anterior cruciate ligament, the popliteal tendon insertion into the lateral condyle, and at the posteromedial and lateral capsule (**Fig. 13**).[60] de Abreu and colleagues[60] additionally described the involvement of the quadriceps fat pad with the presence of signal abnormality most likely representing edema (**Fig. 14**). The overlap of this finding between suprapatellar fat pad impingement and the AC of the knee raises the possibility that isolated suprapatellar fat pad signal alteration may represent a forme fruste of AC of the knee.[60] Additionally, it is possible that the suprapatellar fat pad and other fat pads are a window to synovial abnormalities, with fat pad edema an intermediate step

during migration of the inflammatory reaction as it makes its way from the synovium to the capsule.[1] This particular manifestation is unique to the knee because of the fat pad interposition between the synovium and the capsule at these locations. Although current knowledge of this entity is incomplete, there is evidence that there are certain molecules,[61] beyond the generalized histologic inflammation, that might be used as markers for AC, at least of the shoulder. Further studies are needed to better characterize and understand this disorder.

ILIOTIBIAL BAND SYNDROME
Introduction

The iliotibial tract (ITT) or ITB is a sheet of connective tissue[62] originating at the iliac crest and includes fascial components from the gluteus maximus, gluteus medius, and tensor fasciae latae, which extend distally toward the tibia.[63] On the distal femur, a fibrous band connects the ITT immediately above and on the lateral femoral epicondyle (LFE) and the intermuscular septum, and this is continuous with the patellar retinacula.[64] The main distal insertion is onto Gerdy tubercle at the anterolateral aspect of the tibia.[63,65] The lateral synovial recess and highly vascularized

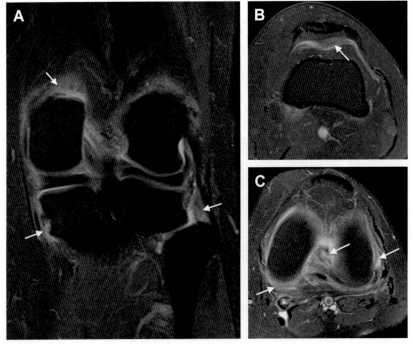

Fig. 13. A 63-year-old woman without history of systemic disease presents with 3 months of knee pain and restricted flexion and extension. Coronal (*A*) and axial (*B, C*) T1 fat-suppressed images after intravenous contrast show marked capsular and synovial enhancement (*arrows*) through the knee. (*Courtesy of* Luis Pecci Neto, MD, Teleimagem, Hospital do Coração, e Universidade Federal de São Paulo, Sao Paulo, Brazil.)

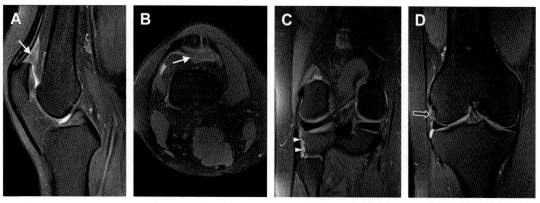

Fig. 14. A 40-year-old woman with 1 month of diffuse knee pain and movement restriction. Sagittal (*A*) and axial (*B*) PD-weighted fat-suppressed shows signal abnormality most likely representing edema of the quadriceps fat pad (*white arrows*). Coronal (*C, D*) PD-weighted fat-suppressed images reveal edema of the pericapsule tissues of the posterolateral capsule (*arrowheads*) and around the popliteal tendon insertion (*open white arrow*). (*Courtesy of* Marcelo Rodrigues de Abreu, MD, Hospital Mãe de Deus, RS, Brasil.)

adipose tissue fill the space between the femur and the ITT that extends proximally to the vastus lateralis muscle.[63,64] The ITT acts as a lateral hip stabilizer resisting hip adduction[62] and it has different functions depending on the position of the knee. With the knee in full extension up to 20° to 30° of flexion, the ITT lies anterior to the LFE and serves as an active knee extensor.[66,67] At 30° of flexion, the ITT assumes a posterior position relative to the LFE and becomes an active knee flexor.[66,67]

The ITB friction syndrome (ITBFS) was first specifically described by Renne (1975) as "a painful, disabling condition in the region lateral to the knee and was initially reported in a group of men undergoing vigorous military physical training."[68] ITBFS is the most common running injury in the lateral knee in runners, accounting for up to 12% of all injuries,[69] especially in downhill and long-distance running. Among cyclists, it is believed to account for 15% to 24% of overuse injuries.[70]

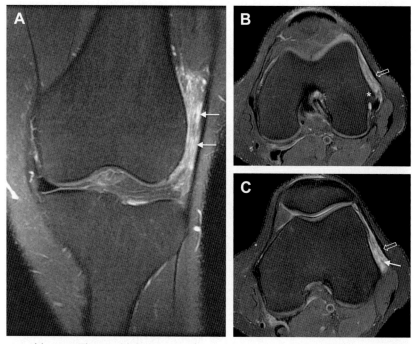

Fig. 15. A 24-year-old soccer player with knee pain. Coronal (*A*) and axial (*B, C*) PD fat-suppressed images of the knee show extensive edema (*arrows*) in the fat between the lateral femoral condyle (LFC) and the ITB (*open arrow*) anterior to the lateral epicondyle (*asterisk*).

Different theories regarding etiology have been proposed for the ITBS. The most cited is the friction-type syndrome. Repetitive knee internal rotation, flexion, and extension, combined with femoral adduction, increase the strain and friction of the ITB fibers as they slide over the LFE causing the ITBS.[71,72] The impingement zone occurs near foot strike or the early stance phase of running when the knee flexion is at or slightly below 30°.[73] In a functional anatomy and radiology study in specimens and patients, Fairclough and colleagues[64] proposed that the injury may not be the consequence of friction of the ITT over the epicondyle but of compression against a layer of highly innervated fat that intervenes between the ITT and the epicondyle. Another hypothesis that has been proposed is the presence of an inflamed bursa[74] but anatomic studies have not supported this theory because no bursa has been identified.[63,64]

Clinical

The diagnosis of ITBFS is based on clinical examination. A complete knee examination and provocative test are performed for the assessment of this pathology. Patients localize the pain over the distal ITB at the level of the LFE, a few centimeters proximal to the knee joint. In the early stages, symptoms occur with exercises involving repetitive flexion and extension, including running and cycling. As the condition worsens, pain is often experienced earlier in the athletic activity and may begin to be present at rest.[66]

The treatment of ITBS is normally conservative and focused on rest, ice application, and physiotherapy as well as analgesic and nonsteroidal antiinflammatory drugs. Refractory cases may eventually require a local corticosteroid injection to relieve the symptoms. Most patients have symptomatic relief within 6 to 8 weeks.[75] In a study by Federicson and colleagues,[76] runners with ITBS may exhibit decreased hip abductor strength with resolution of symptoms after a 6-week program of hip abductor strengthening.

Imaging

The lateral corner of the knee has a complex anatomic interrelationship between several structures, and knowledge of the main structures is important for the location and characterization of the ITT. The LFE is an important landmark for the ITT (**Fig. 15**). Some posterior fibers of the ITT normally insert on the LFE at the level of the insertion of the lateral collateral ligament. The main fibers of the ITT are located anterior and lateral to the biceps femoris tendon, lateral to the fibular collateral ligament and popliteus tendon with knee extension. With knee flexion, the ITT moves posteriorly and comes in contact with the LFE.[63] The lateral recess of the knee contains fatty tissue and is located anterior to the LFE.[63,64] The best sequences to detect ITBS are proton density (PD) and T2-weighted images with fat suppression in the coronal and axial plans. Normally, the ITT demonstrates low signal intensity with a fibrillar pattern.

On MR imaging, ITBS is characterized by poorly defined signal intensity abnormalities between the ITB and the femur with obliteration of the normal fatty tissue (**Fig. 16**). A circumscribed fluid collection deep and medial to the ITB and a thickened ITT can also be associated with ITBS.[63,74]

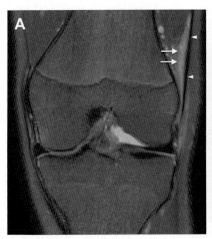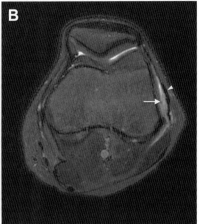

Fig. 16. A 17-year-old athlete with pain while running. Coronal (*A*) and axial (*B*) PD fat-suppressed images reveal high signal intensity in the fat (*white arrow*) deep to the ITB (*arrowhead*).

SUMMARY

The fat pads of the knee are of great importance and are the main structures of the extrasynovial compartment. They have been underappreciated in the literature. The fat pads should be recognized as more than passive, space-occupying structures: they serve to protect the knee by remodeling their shape to adapt to the various degrees of flexion and assist in preserving the compartments of the knee joint by modulating direct contact.[6] Fat pads are richly vascularized and innervated, functioning like a window between the synovium and the capsular layers, and may provide indirect evidence for synovial pathology. The extrasynovial impingement and inflammation syndromes about the knee should be in the differential diagnosis for patients presenting with knee pain.

REFERENCES

1. Schweitzer ME, Falk A, Pathria M, et al. MR imaging of the knee: can changes in the intracapsular fat pads be used as a sign of synovial proliferation in the presence of an effusion? AJR Am J Roentgenol 1993;160(4):823–6.

2. Warren LF, Marshall JL. The supporting structures and layers on the medial side of the knee: an anatomical analysis. J Bone Joint Surg Am 1979; 61(1):56–62.

3. MacConaill MA. The movements of bones and joints. V. The significance of shape. J Bone Joint Surg Br 1953;35B(2):290–7.

4. Seebacher JR, Inglis AE, Marshall JL, et al. The structure of the posterolateral aspect of the knee. J Bone Joint Surg Am 1982;64(4):536–41.

5. Standring S. Gray's anatomy. 40th edition. London: Churchill Livingstone Elsevier; 2008.

6. Davies DV, White JE. The structure and weight of synovial fat pads. J Anat 1961;95:30–7.

7. Gallagher J, Tierney P, Murray P, et al. The infrapatellar fat pad: anatomy and clinical correlations. Knee Surg Sports Traumatol Arthrosc 2005;13(4):268–72.

8. Hoffa A. Influence of adipose tissue with regard to the pathology of the knee joint. JAMA 1904;43: 795–6.

9. Jacobson JA, Lenchik L, Ruhoy MK, et al. MR imaging of the infrapatellar fat pad of Hoffa. Radiographics 1997;17(3):675–91.

10. Maurel B, Le Corroller T, Cohen M, et al. Le corps adipeux infra-patellaire: carrefour anterieur du genou. [Infrapatellar fat pad: anterior crossroads of the knee]. J Radiol 2010;91(9 Pt 1):841–55.

11. Abreu MR, Chung CB, Trudell D, et al. Hoffa's fat pad injuries and their relationship with anterior cruciate ligament tears: new observations based on MR imaging in patients and MR imaging and anatomic correlation in cadavers. Skeletal Radiol 2008;37(4):301–6.

12. Skiadas V, Perdikakis E, Plotas A, et al. MR imaging of anterior knee pain: a pictorial essay. Knee Surg Sports Traumatol Arthrosc 2013;21(2):294–304.

13. Ogilvie-Harris DJ, Giddens J. Hoffa's disease: arthroscopic resection of the infrapatellar fat pad. Arthroscopy 1994;10(2):184–7.

14. Shabshin N, Schweitzer ME, Morrison WB. Quadriceps fat pad edema: significance on magnetic resonance images of the knee. Skeletal Radiol 2006;35(5):269–74.

15. Dragoo JL, Johnson C, McConnell J. Evaluation and treatment of disorders of the infrapatellar fat pad. Sports Med 2012;42(1):51–67.

16. Torshizy H, Pathria MN, Chung CB. Inflammation of Hoffa's fat pad in the setting of HIV: magnetic resonance imaging findings in six patients. Skeletal Radiol 2007;36(1):35–40.

17. LaPrade RF. The anatomy of the deep infrapatellar bursa of the knee. Am J Sports Med 1998;26(1): 129–32.

18. Paulos LE, Wnorowski DC, Greenwald AE. Infrapatellar contracture syndrome. Diagnosis, treatment, and long-term followup. Am J Sports Med 1994; 22(4):440–9.

19. Lagier R, Albert J. Bilateral deep infrapatellar bursitis associated with tibial tuberosity enthesopathy in a case of juvenile ankylosing spondylitis. Rheumatol Int 1985;5(4):187–90.

20. Kumar D, Alvand A, Beacon JP. Impingement of infrapatellar fat pad (Hoffa's disease): results of high-portal arthroscopic resection. Arthroscopy 2007;23(11):1180–6.e1.

21. Tsavalas N, Karantanas AH. Suprapatellar fat-pad mass effect: MRI findings and correlation with anterior knee pain. AJR Am J Roentgenol 2013;200(3): W291–6.

22. Saddik D, McNally EG, Richardson M. MRI of Hoffa's fat pad. Skeletal Radiol 2004;33(8):433–44.

23. Barbier-Brion B, Lerais JM, Aubry S, et al. Magnetic resonance imaging in patellar lateral femoral friction syndrome (PLFFS): prospective case-control study. Diagn Interv Imaging 2012;93(3):e171–82.

24. Dejour H. Instabilités de la rotule. Traité d'Appareil locomotur. France: Encyclopedia Medico-Chirugicale; 1996.

25. Dejour DH. The patellofemoral joint and its historical roots: the Lyon School of Knee Surgery. Knee Surg Sports Traumatol Arthrosc 2013;21(7):1482–94.

26. Brukner JM, Bergman A, Bealieu C, et al. Infrapatellar fat pad impingement: correlation between clinical and MR findings. Med Sci Sports Exerc 1999;31(Suppl 5):1.

27. Chung CB, Skaf A, Roger B, et al. Patellar tendon-lateral femoral condyle friction syndrome: MR imaging in 42 patients. Skeletal Radiol 2001;30(12):694–7.

28. Campagna R, Pessis E, Biau DJ, et al. Is superolateral Hoffa fat pad edema a consequence of impingement between lateral femoral condyle and patellar ligament? Radiology 2012;263(2):469–74.

29. Clockaerts S, Bastiaansen-Jenniskens YM, Runhaar J, et al. The infrapatellar fat pad should be considered as an active osteoarthritic joint tissue: a narrative review. Osteoarthritis Cartilage 2010;18(7):876–82.

30. Bohnsack M, Hurschler C, Demirtas T, et al. Infrapatellar fat pad pressure and volume changes of the anterior compartment during knee motion: possible clinical consequences to the anterior knee pain syndrome. Knee Surg Sports Traumatol Arthrosc 2005;13(2):135–41.

31. Subhawong TK, Eng J, Carrino JA, et al. Superolateral Hoffa's fat pad edema: association with patellofemoral maltracking and impingement. AJR Am J Roentgenol 2010;195(6):1367–73.

32. Lee PP, Chalian M, Carrino JA, et al. Multimodality correlations of patellar height measurement on X-ray, CT, and MRI. Skeletal Radiol 2012;41(10):1309–14.

33. Insall J, Salvati E. Patella position in the normal knee joint. Radiology 1971;101(1):101–4.

34. Shabshin N, Schweitzer ME, Morrison WB, et al. MRI criteria for patella alta and baja. Skeletal Radiol 2004;33(8):445–50.

35. Grelsamer RP, Meadows S. The modified Insall-Salvati ratio for assessment of patellar height. Clin Orthop Relat Res 1992;(282):170–6.

36. Caton J. Methode de mesure de la hauteur de la rotule. [Method of measuring the height of the patella]. Acta Orthop Belg 1989;55(3):385–6.

37. Goutallier D, Bernageau J, Lecudonnec B. Mesure de l'ecart tuberosite tibiale anterieure - gorge de la trochlee (T.A.-G.T.). Technique. Resultats. Interet. [The measurement of the tibial tuberosity. Patella groove distanced technique and results (author's transl)]. Rev Chir Orthop Reparatrice Appar Mot 1978;64(5):423–8.

38. Schoettle PB, Zanetti M, Seifert B, et al. The tibial tuberosity-trochlear groove distance; a comparative study between CT and MRI scanning. Knee 2006;13(1):26–31.

39. Pandit S, Frampton C, Stoddart J, et al. Magnetic resonance imaging assessment of tibial tuberosity-trochlear groove distance: normal values for males and females. Int Orthop 2011;35(12):1799–803.

40. Dejour H, Walch G, Nove-Josserand L, et al. Factors of patellar instability: an anatomic radiographic study. Knee Surg Sports Traumatol Arthrosc 1994; 2(1):19–26.

41. Staeubli HU, Bollmann C, Kreutz R, et al. Quantification of intact quadriceps tendon, quadriceps tendon insertion, and suprapatellar fat pad: MR arthrography, anatomy, and cryosections in the sagittal plane. AJR Am J Roentgenol 1999;173(3): 691–8.

42. Benjamin M, Redman S, Milz S, et al. Adipose tissue at entheses: the rheumatological implications of its distribution. A potential site of pain and stress dissipation? Ann Rheum Dis 2004; 63(12):1549–55.

43. Roth C, Jacobson J, Jamadar D, et al. Quadriceps fat pad signal intensity and enlargement on MRI: prevalence and associated findings. AJR Am J Roentgenol 2004;182(6):1383–7.

44. Huberti HH, Hayes WC, Stone JL, et al. Force ratios in the quadriceps tendon and ligamentum patellae. J Orthop Res 1984;2(1):49–54.

45. Brukner P, Karim K. Clinical sports medicine. 3rd edition. Sydney: McGraw-Hill; 2006.

46. Kim YM, Shin HD, Yang JY, et al. Prefemoral fat pad: impingement and a mass-like protrusion on the lateral femoral condyle causing mechanical symptoms. A case report. Knee Surg Sports Traumatol Arthrosc 2007;15(6):786–9.

47. Borja MJ, Jose J, Vecchione D, et al. Prefemoral fat pad impingement syndrome: identification and diagnosis. Am J Orthop 2013;42(1):E9–11.

48. Zakhary M, Slattery TR, Thein R, et al. Prefemoral fat pad edema in the knee. MRI findings in 44 patients along with clinical correlation and assessment of prevalence. Chicago: RSNA; 2012.

49. Faletti C, De Stefano N, Giudice G, et al. Knee impingement syndromes. Eur J Radiol 1998; 27(Suppl 1):S60–9.

50. Skaf AY, Hernandez Filho G, Dirim B, et al. Pericruciate fat pad of the knee: anatomy and pericruciate fat pad inflammation: cadaveric and clinical study emphasizing MR imaging. Skeletal Radiol 2012; 41(12):1591–6.

51. de Abreu MR, Kim HJ, Chung CB, et al. Posterior cruciate ligament recess and normal posterior capsular insertional anatomy: MR imaging of cadaveric knees. Radiology 2005;236(3):968–73.

52. Duplay S. De la periarthrite scapulohumerale. Rev Frat D Trav De Med 1896;53:226.

53. Neviaser J. Adhesive capsulitis of the shoulder: a study of the pathological findings in periarthritis of the shoulder. J Bone Joint Surg Am 1945;27: 211–22.

54. Bridgman JF. Periarthritis of the shoulder and diabetes mellitus. Ann Rheum Dis 1972;31(1):69–71.

55. Hand C, Clipsham K, Rees JL, et al. Long-term outcome of frozen shoulder. J Shoulder Elbow Surg 2008;17(2):231–6.

56. Hsu JE, Anakwenze OA, Warrender WJ, et al. Current review of adhesive capsulitis. J Shoulder Elbow Surg 2011;20(3):502–14.

57. Bunker TD, Anthony PP. The pathology of frozen shoulder. A Dupuytren-like disease. J Bone Joint Surg Br 1995;77(5):677–83.

58. Matsen FA, Fu FH, Hawkins RJ. The shoulder: a balance of mobility and stability. Rosemont (IL): American Academy of Orthopaedic Surgeons; 1993.

59. Rodeo SA, Hannafin JA, Tom J, et al. Immunolocalization of cytokines and their receptors in adhesive capsulitis of the shoulder. J Orthop Res 1997;15(3): 427–36.

60. de Abreu MR, Falcao M, Sprinz C, et al. Skeletal Radiol 2013;42(5):741–6.

61. Kim YS, Kim JM, Lee YG, et al. Intercellular adhesion molecule-1 (ICAM-1, CD54) is increased in adhesive capsulitis. J Bone Joint Surg Am 2013; 95(4):e181–8.

62. Hamill J, Miller R, Noehren B, et al. A prospective study of iliotibial band strain in runners. Clin Biomech 2008;23(8):1018–25.

63. Muhle C, Ahn JM, Yeh L, et al. Iliotibial band friction syndrome: MR imaging findings in 16 patients and MR arthrographic study of six cadaveric knees. Radiology 1999;212(1):103–10.

64. Fairclough J, Hayashi K, Toumi H, et al. The functional anatomy of the iliotibial band during flexion and extension of the knee: implications for understanding iliotibial band syndrome. J Anat 2006; 208(3):309–16.

65. Terry GC, Hughston JC, Norwood LA. The anatomy of the iliopatellar band and iliotibial tract. Am J Sports Med 1986;14(1):39–45.

66. Strauss EJ, Kim S, Calcei JG, et al. Iliotibial band syndrome: evaluation and management. J Am Acad Orthop Surg 2011;19(12):728–36.

67. Choi L. Orthopaedic sports medicine. 3rd edition. Philadelphia: Saunders Elsevier; 2010.

68. Renne JW. The iliotibial band friction syndrome. J Bone Joint Surg Am 1975;57(8):1110–1.

69. Taunton JE, Ryan MB, Clement DB, et al. A retrospective case-control analysis of 2002 running injuries. Br J Sports Med 2002;36(2): 95–101.

70. Holmes JC, Pruitt AL, Whalen NJ. Iliotibial band syndrome in cyclists. Am J Sports Med 1993; 21(3):419–24.

71. Orava S. Iliotibial tract friction syndrome in athletes–an uncommon exertion syndrome on the lateral side of the knee. Br J Sports Med 1978; 12(2):69–73.

72. Noehren B, Davis I, Hamill J. ASB clinical biomechanics award winner 2006 prospective study of the biomechanical factors associated with iliotibial band syndrome. Clin Biomech 2007;22(9): 951–6.

73. Orchard JW, Fricker PA, Abud AT, et al. Biomechanics of iliotibial band friction syndrome in runners. Am J Sports Med 1996;24(3):375–9.

74. Ekman EF, Pope T, Martin DF, et al. Magnetic resonance imaging of iliotibial band syndrome. Am J Sports Med 1994;22(6):851–4.

75. Lavine R. Iliotibial band friction syndrome. Curr Rev Musculoskelet Med 2010;3(1–4):18–22.

76. Fredericson M, Cookingham CL, Chaudhari AM, et al. Hip abductor weakness in distance runners with iliotibial band syndrome. Clin J Sport Med 2000;10(3):169–75.

Magnetic Resonance Imaging of the Pediatric Knee

Kara G. Gill, MD[a],*, Blaise A. Nemeth, MD, MS[b],
Kirkland W. Davis, MD[c]

KEYWORDS

- Knee • Pediatric • Normal • Trauma • Developmental • Arthritis • Neoplasm

KEY POINTS

- Marrow conversion begins in the epiphyses 6 months after the radiographic appearance of the secondary ossification center. Transition to fatty marrow then continues from the mid-diaphysis toward the metaphyses.
- Irregular ossification involving the posterior femoral condyle epiphysis should be considered normal variation rather than an osteochondral lesion (OCD) in the absence of overlying cartilage abnormality and underlying bone marrow edema.
- Unlike adults who are more likely to suffer from ligamentous and meniscal injuries, trauma in pediatric patients characteristically involves the physis and adjacent bones.
- In contrast to adult OCDs, the hyperintense signal between the osteochondral fragment and native bone must mirror joint fluid to suggest instability in children.
- Synovial sarcoma is the most underrecognized malignant tumor that commonly occurs about the knee; lack of recognition is due to its seemingly benign magnetic resonance imaging characteristics.

INTRODUCTION

In pediatric patients, the knee is the most common joint to be assessed with magnetic resonance (MR) imaging. MR imaging of the knee is performed in children and adolescents to evaluate various traumatic, inflammatory, developmental, and neoplastic conditions. Its high resolution and excellent soft-tissue contrast allow for complete evaluation of both osseous and soft-tissue structures around the knee joint, and its lack of ionizing radiation makes it a preferred modality for advanced imaging in children. At younger ages, sedation is often necessary to obtain diagnostic images, presenting risks that must be taken into account when deciding on the necessity of the study. Furthermore, one must have a solid understanding of the normal skeletal development and variations in development of the distal femur, proximal tibia, and proximal fibula to avoid misdiagnoses.

Older children and adolescents are most commonly imaged to evaluate athletic and traumatic injuries. From infancy through school age,

No disclosures.

[a] Division of Pediatric Radiology, Department of Radiology, University of Wisconsin School of Medicine and Public Health, 600 Highland Avenue, CSC E3/366, Madison, WI 53792-3252, USA; [b] Department of Orthopedics and Rehabilitation, University of Wisconsin School of Medicine and Public Health, UW Medical Foundation Centennial Building, 1652 Highland Avenue, Room 6170-11D, Madison, WI 53705-2281, USA; [c] Musculoskeletal Radiology, University of Wisconsin School of Medicine and Public Health, E3/366, 600 Highland Avenue, Madison, WI 53792-3252, USA
* Corresponding author.
E-mail address: kgill@uwhealth.org

mri.theclinics.com

however, MR imaging is more often performed to evaluate developmental conditions such as Blount disease or to assess for causes of atraumatic pain such as infection or inflammatory arthritis. Neoplasms, both benign and malignant, commonly occur about the knee throughout childhood. Only the most common benign tumors and the most underdiagnosed malignancy are discussed in this article.

NORMAL SKELETAL MATURATION

To appropriately interpret pediatric musculoskeletal images, one must be aware of normal changes that occur with skeletal maturation. The epiphyses at both ends of tubular bones are positioned between the primary physis (growth plate) and the joint. Initially, the epiphysis is entirely cartilaginous. The secondary ossification center forms through endochondral ossification, beginning at the center of the epiphysis. Whereas the primary physis is responsible for longitudinal growth of the bone at each metaphysis, the secondary physis surrounding the secondary ossification center is responsible for spherical growth.[1]

The normal sequence of marrow conversion in pediatric patients must be understood, so as not to delay the diagnosis of infiltrative malignancy, such as leukemia, when imaging children who present with vague joint pain, swelling, or even pathologic fracture. At birth the marrow is entirely hematopoietic, resulting in relatively low signal intensity that is similar to or slightly higher than that of skeletal muscle on T1-weighted images. Normal marrow is usually higher in signal intensity than marrow infiltrated by disease. On T2-weighted images, hematopoietic marrow shows high signal intensity which is less than that of simple fluid and similar to that of muscle. Therefore, very low signal intensity marrow on T1-weighted images and increased signal intensity on water-sensitive sequences is concerning for malignancy.

During the first year of life, conversion from hematopoietic to fatty marrow begins. This marrow conversion progresses from the periphery to the center of each bone in the appendicular skeleton. Epiphyseal conversion occurs first, within 6 months of the radiologic appearance of the secondary ossification center. Transition to fatty marrow then continues, beginning at the mid-diaphysis and progressing toward the metaphyses. Hematopoietic marrow can be seen into early adulthood within the proximal metaphyses of the femora and humeri, as these are the last sites to convert. The transition back to red marrow in patients with anemia or who are receiving growth factors occurs in the reverse order, extending from

the metaphyses centrally to the diaphysis before conversion in the epiphyses occurs. Residual hematopoietic marrow about the knee will appear flame-shaped, with a base adjacent to the physis.[1]

The periosteum is a thin, linear, hypointense structure paralleling the bone. It is tightly bound at the level of the physis but loosely attached along the shaft of the bone. Blood, pus, or tumor easily elevates the periosteum. In children, a layer of fibrovascular tissue separates the periosteum, resolving after physeal closure. This feature is most evident in long bones at the level of the metaphysis, and is best seen along the posterior distal femoral metaphysis as high signal intensity on water-sensitive sequences with intense contrast enhancement (**Fig. 1**). This "metaphyseal stripe" should not be mistaken for a subperiosteal fluid collection.[1]

Normal signal characteristics of the physeal structures on T2-weighted images vary. From distal to proximal, the cartilage of the primary physis (growth plate) is hyperintense, with the adjacent zone of provisional calcification appearing as a thin hypointense line. Immediately proximal resides the primary spongiosa of the metaphysis, which is hyperintense because of its vascularity.[1] The hyaline cartilage of the unossified epiphysis appears hypointense compared with the overlying articular cartilage.[1,2] During early

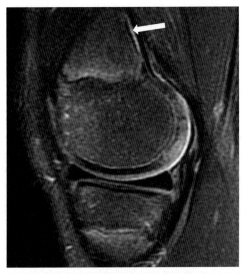

Fig. 1. Parasagittal T2-weighted, fat-suppressed image of the knee in a 10-year-old boy shows decreased signal intensity of the epiphyseal cartilage along the weight-bearing surface of the medial femoral condyle with the T2 hyperintense overlying articular cartilage. Along the posterior femoral condyle the epiphyseal cartilage is more heterogeneous, with the more focal hyperintense region likely related to early ossification. Note the normal posterior metaphyseal stripe (*arrow*).

ossification, increased signal within the distal femoral epiphyseal cartilage may occur, ranging from patchy to focal. The signal intensity along the weight-bearing surface of the distal femoral epiphyseal cartilage, however, is decreased, presumably because of water loss (see **Fig. 1**).[3] Contrast administration shows vascular channels radiating peripherally through the epiphyseal cartilage, which will appear more prominent in diseases such as inflammatory arthritis in which the synovium is hyperemic.[1]

Focal bone marrow edema centered at the physis can be seen in the central distal femur (**Fig. 2**), proximal tibia, or proximal fibula of adolescents, termed focal periphyseal edema pattern (FOPE). All reported patients with FOPE have unfused but narrowed physes. Because this periphyseal edema pattern is seen in patients presenting with pain and incidentally in asymptomatic patients, it is postulated that this may represent normal signal changes related to physeal fusion. Areas of fused physis have relatively less flexibility, possibly resulting in localized microtrauma, accounting for the pain that some patients experience.[4]

Variation in epiphyseal ossification and signal intensity is most evident along the distal femoral condyles. The development of low signal intensity along the weight-bearing surface of the epiphyseal cartilage begins as soon as the child becomes ambulatory. During the preschool years (ages 3–5 years), increasing signal intensity develops in the posterior condylar cartilage and is initially poorly defined, occurring before radiographically identifiable calcification. This increase in signal intensity becomes more focal as the child grows, and appears radiographically as single or multiple ossification centers that eventually coalesce with the underlying bone.[4] Gebarski and Hernandez[5]

have described 4 different normal variations in ossification of the posterior femoral condyles. The first they describe as a puzzle-piece configuration whereby an osseous defect in the posterior femoral condyle is filled with an ossification that fills the defect. The second is an incomplete puzzle-piece configuration whereby the ossification does not completely fill the defect. The posterior condyle can also have a spiculated appearance (**Fig. 3**) or have many adjacent small ossifications (see **Fig. 3**; **Fig. 4**). Unlike OCD lesions, there is no bone marrow edema seen with any of these variants to suggest abnormality.[5] In addition, these normal variants reside more posteriorly along the non–weight-bearing surface of the femoral condyle. In the absence of adjacent bone marrow edema, these developmental variations should not be mistaken for osteochondritis dissecans.[1,3,5,6]

TRAUMA

Unlike adults who are more likely to suffer from ligamentous and meniscal injuries, trauma in children and adolescents characteristically involves the physis and adjacent bones, which are the weakest link in skeletally immature patients. Thus the pediatric knee is susceptible to multiple types of fractures in addition to chronic repetitive stress injuries. There are various acute and chronic knee injuries unique to the growing pediatric patient. As increasingly more children are involved in competitive sports at a younger age, these injuries are becoming more prevalent. The most common indications for MR imaging of the knee following trauma are refusal to bear weight, persistent pain, or hemarthrosis in the presence of negative radiographs, suggesting internal derangement or occult fracture.[7]

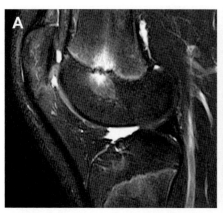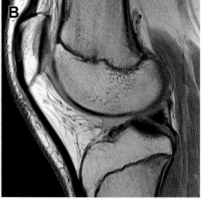

Fig. 2. Sagittal T2-weighted, fat-suppressed (*A*) and proton-density (*B*) images of the knee in a 14-year-old girl with pain show edema on both sides of the narrow mid-femoral physis, consistent with focal periphyseal edema pattern.

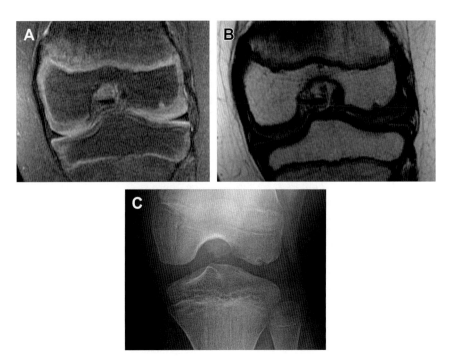

Fig. 3. Coronal fat-suppressed proton-density (*A*), coronal proton-density (*B*), and tunnel radiographic images of the knee (*C*) in a 9-year-old boy with joint pain and swelling shows a focal defect in the posterior lateral femoral condyle that is mildly hyperintense on fat-suppressed images. The adjacent epiphyseal cartilage is slightly hypointense to the overlying articular cartilage, both of which are intact. There is no underlying bone marrow edema, consistent with normal developmental variation.

Acute

Ligamentous injuries are overall less common in pediatric patients than in adults, owing to ligamentous laxity in combination with relative weakness of the physis; as such, osseous injuries are more common. The most common ligament injured in the pediatric population is the anterior cruciate ligament (ACL). ACL tears are more common in girls, likely related to a combination of hormonal influence, valgus alignment, and increased joint laxity.[6–8] MR criteria for the diagnosis of ACL tear is the same as that in adults, with loss of parallelism with the Blumensaat line being a more sensitive finding than fiber discontinuity in this age group.[9] Unlike adults, the classic pattern of bone marrow edema involving the lateral femoral condyle and posterolateral tibial plateau ("kissing

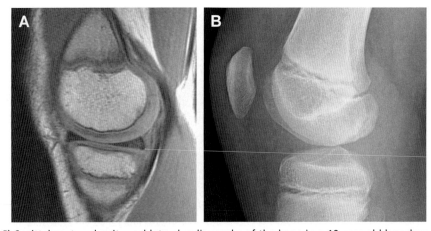

Fig. 4. (*A*, *B*) Sagittal proton-density and lateral radiographs of the knee in a 10-year-old boy show mild undulation along the posterior lateral femoral condyle.

contusions") is not always associated with an ACL tear in pediatric patients, owing to normal ligamentous laxity.[6,9,10]

In even younger patients, the same mechanism of injury produces tibial spine avulsion fractures rather than ACL tears,[7,8] especially if the intercondylar notch is wide.[11] Type I tibial spine avulsion fractures are, at most, minimally displaced and are managed conservatively.[7,10] The remaining types require surgical intervention. Type II fractures show anterior elevation from the parent bone. Type III and IV fractures show progressive separation of the fragment (**Fig. 5**). Type V fractures are displaced and have a rotational component.[10] Hinged or displaced avulsion fractures require surgery.[7] Posterior cruciate and collateral ligament injuries are uncommon, as severe valgus or varus stress on the knee joint more likely result in physeal fracture.[7]

Before physeal fusion occurs, meniscal injury is uncommon. Meniscal tears in pediatric patients appear similar to those in adults: linear increased signal within the meniscus extending to the articular surface, abnormal morphology, or displaced meniscal fragments.[9] Longitudinal tears and peripheral detachments are the most common, with the posterior horns more often injured.[7] Normal vascular tissue can produce increased signal within the meniscus, but differs from a tear in that the increased signal intensity does not extend to the articular surface. Most meniscal injuries in children younger than 10 years are due to discoid meniscus (see later discussion).[7,8]

Fractures involving the distal femoral or proximal tibial physes are considered high risk for causing abnormal growth (**Figs. 6–9**).[7] These Salter-Harris fractures can be subtle on radiographs, and often require subsequent MR imaging to further define the extent of the fracture and associated soft-tissue injuries.[7,12] Metaphyseal fractures in the distal femur or proximal tibia appear as linear foci of high signal intensity with surrounding marrow edema on fluid-sensitive sequences. The injured portion of the adjacent physis shows high signal intensity and widening. Periosteal elevation and disruption are commonly seen adjacent to the injured physis. Periosteum may even become trapped within the fracture.[7,8] Associated effusions, predominantly suprapatellar, are common.[12] Salter-Harris type II fractures of the distal femur are the most common type diagnosed on MR imaging. Follow-up imaging may be indicated to evaluate for premature physeal fusion, either with radiographs, computed tomography, or MR imaging.[7]

Acute extensor mechanism injuries include transient patellar dislocation (TPD), patellar sleeve fractures, and tibial tubercle avulsion fractures. TPD usually occurs between the ages of 14 and 16 years during a twisting injury of the mildly flexed knee with the foot planted, resulting in the quadriceps muscle pulling the patella laterally.[13] During lateral dislocation, the inferomedial patellar facet impacts the trochlear articular surface, resulting in osteochondral defects in both the inferomedial patella and lateral trochlea.[14] Of note, the patellar lesion should be seen on at least 2 consecutive images.[15] As the patella relocates during leg extension, it impacts the anterolateral femoral condyle, resulting in the characteristic bone contusions of the medial patella and anterolateral femoral condyle. The femoral contusion is located just anterior to the trochlear osteochondral lesion,[14] more anterior and superior to those seen in older adolescents and adults with ACL injury.[15]

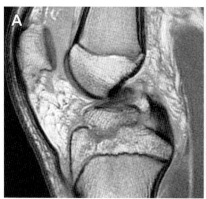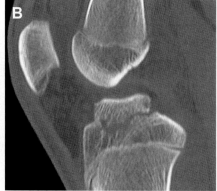

Fig. 5. Sagittal proton-density (*A*) and sagittal computed tomography (CT) (*B*) images of the knee in a 16-year-old boy who fell while skateboarding show a type III tibial spine avulsion; the tibial spine is diffusely displaced from the plateau without rotation.

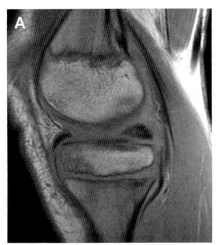
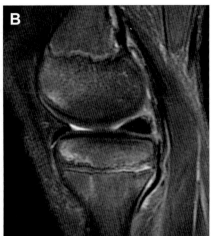

Fig. 6. Sagittal proton-density (*A*) and T2-weighted fat-suppressed (*B*) images of the knee in a 10-year-old boy with pain after a hyperextension injury show widening and increased signal intensity within the posterior proximal tibial physis, consistent with a Salter-Harris type I fracture. Note contusions in the anterior tibial epiphysis and anterior femoral condyle.

It is also imperative to evaluate the images for evidence of medial patellar restraint injury. Both the medial patellar retinaculum (MPR) and the medial patellofemoral ligament (MPFL) require

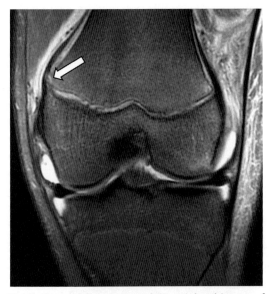

Fig. 7. Coronal fat-suppressed T2-weighted image of the left knee in a 15-year-old boy with pain following a soccer injury shows cortical discontinuity of the very distal medial femoral metaphysis with widening and increased signal intensity of the medial physis, consistent with a Salter-Harris type II fracture (*arrow*). This subtle cortical fracture was not visible radiographically. Note the adjacent thin subperiosteal hematoma, which is wider and more heterogeneous in signal intensity than the normal metaphyseal stripe seen along the lateral distal femoral metaphysis. Significant soft-tissue edema is also present.

scrutiny. Previously, disruption of the MPR at its patellar insertion was thought to be of greatest importance. More recent studies, however, have demonstrated that the MPFL is the major ligament limiting lateral patellar movement. The vastus medialis obliquus muscle (VMO) also plays an important role, as it acts as a dynamic stabilizer, counteracting the pull of the vastus lateralis muscle.[15] The MPFL provides 50% to 80% of the medial restraint of the patella[14]; therefore, injury to this structure often results in persistent instability. The MPFL travels anteriorly from the region of the adductor tubercle on the medial femoral condyle deep to the VMO to attach to the superomedial patella. MPFL tears are common after TPD and usually occur at its femoral attachment. As this structure is difficult to discretely identify, the secondary signs of substantial edema at its origin near the adductor tubercle and elevation of the VMO by edema are used to diagnose a tear.[14–16] Edema may also be seen on occasion in the adductor tubercle itself.[16] The medial retinaculum is seen as a low signal intensity band extending posteriorly from the medial patella and becoming continuous with the fascia of the VMO. The medial retinaculum may be torn at its patellar attachment, possibly with an associated cortical avulsion fragment, or along its mid-substance.[15] T2 hyperintense edema adjacent the medial patellar pole indicates retinacular injury. Wrinkling of the MPR indicates a tear.[14] Additional MR findings in patients with TPD include joint effusion, hemarthrosis, lateral patellar subluxation or tilt, patella alta, and trochlear dysplasia.[16]

Predisposing factors for TPD include genu valgum, ligamentous laxity, trochlear dysplasia,

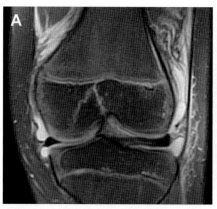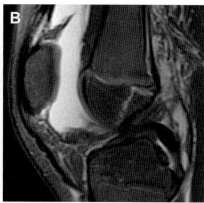

Fig. 8. Coronal fat-suppressed proton-density (A) and sagittal fat-suppressed T2-weighted (B) images of the knee in a 7-year-old boy who fell 3 stories show a comminuted distal femoral epiphysis fracture extending to the physis. There is a large associated joint effusion in addition to soft-tissue edema. This Salter-Harris type III fracture was not visible on radiographs.

patellar tilt, patella alta, and a dysplastic, flattened patella.[7,8,17] Trochlear dysplasia can be diagnosed when the trochlear line lies anterior to the lateral femoral condyle on a well-positioned lateral radiograph (the trochlear crossover sign). On a midsagittal MR image, a sharp, step-like transition from the anterior femoral cortex to the trochlear articular surface is seen rather than a smooth one. Trochlear depth can be evaluated on an axial image 3 cm above the weight-bearing surface of the condyles. If the depth measures 3 to 5 mm or less, the trochlea can be called shallow and is associated with patellar instability.[14]

Patellar sleeve avulsion fractures are osteocartilaginous injuries at the inferior patellar pole[9] (**Fig. 10**) and occur most commonly between the ages of 8 and 12 years.[17] Cartilage surrounding the ossifying patella blends directly with patellar tendon fibers rather than by distinct Sharpey fibers that are found in adults. For this reason, patellar tendon injury in children occurs at the proximal or distal ends of the tendon, rather than at the mid-substance.[18] MR imaging helps distinguish between this entity and Sinding-Larsen-Johansson (SLJ) syndrome following episodes of trauma, as radiographs will show bone fragments adjacent to the inferior patellar pole in both entities. With patellar sleeve avulsion fracture, the fragment includes both bone and apophyseal cartilage.[10] The extent of the cartilaginous injury is often significantly underestimated on radiographs.[17] This aspect has clinical implications, as SLJ is managed symptomatically, whereas patellar sleeve avulsion fractures require open reduction and internal fixation for displaced fractures or at least immobilization and non–weight-bearing if nondisplaced.

The tibial tubercle is an anterior extension of the proximal tibial epiphysis. The proximal tibial physis closes between the ages of 13 and 15 years in girls and between the ages of 15 and 19 years in boys. The tubercle apophysis differs from the physis in that it is composed of fibrocartilage rather than columnar cartilage. Fibrocartilage has greater tensile strength, allowing the tubercle to tolerate the strong forces exerted during quadriceps contraction. During skeletal maturation the cartilage gradually converts to columnar cartilage, resulting in greater risk of physeal fracture as the patient grows.[17] The Odgen classification is used to categorize tibial tubercle avulsion fractures into 3 types, each with 2 subtypes. Type I fractures involve only the distal tubercle, without (A) or with (B) displacement (**Fig. 11**). Type II fractures involve the entire ossification center. Type II-A fractures are separated from the metaphysis; type II-B fractures are comminuted. Type III fractures extend through the proximal tibial epiphysis to the joint space without (A) or with (B) displacement.[17] This final type can also be classified as a Salter-Harris type III fracture. The risk of compartment syndrome is high, and most avulsions require surgical intervention.

Unlike adults in whom Baker cysts are typically associated with internal derangement, popliteal cysts in children are more frequently idiopathic or posttraumatic, although they can be associated with septic or inflammatory arthritis. As in adults, MR imaging shows well-defined fluid-filled structures in the posteromedial knee, extending between the gastrocnemius and semimembranosus tendons. Fine septations may be present within Baker cysts.[7,19] Rupture of popliteal cysts in children is rare[7,8]; spontaneous involution generally occurs.

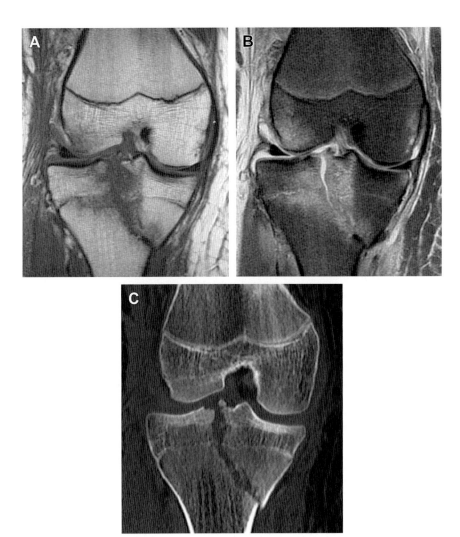

Fig. 9. Coronal T1-weighted (*A*) and fat-suppressed proton-density (*B*) images of the knee in a 14-year-old girl with pain after a fall down stairs show a mildly displaced fracture extending from the tibial plateau through the metaphysis with surrounding edema, consistent with a Salter-Harris type IV fracture. Note also the contusion of the lateral condyle. A noncontrast enhanced CT image (*C*) at the same level also shows the fracture, and a tibial spine fracture fragment.

Chronic

In order of decreasing frequency, osteochondritis dissecans (OCD) most commonly affects the posterolateral aspect of the medial femoral condyle (**Fig. 12**), the lateral femoral condyle, the femoral trochlea, and the patella (**Fig. 13**).[20] When the patella is involved the lower pole is affected, differentiating this entity from the normal variant dorsal patellar defect, which occurs in the superior pole (see later discussion).[9] Repetitive microtrauma is thought to be the primary mechanism of injury, resulting in delamination and sequestration of a fragment of subchondral bone and its overlying cartilage.[9] OCD occurs bilaterally in one-third of patients but with asymmetric severity.

Peak incidence is around 12 to 13 years of age.[7] Affected patients present with activity-related pain. Locking or effusion may occur with unstable or loose fragments. MR imaging confirms the diagnosis and evaluates lesion stability, the most important prognostic indicator.[8,20] Larger fragment size (>1 cm), cystic change at the donor site, and T2 hyperintensity between the fragment and the donor bone indicate instability in adults.[7,20] Kijowski and colleagues[20] demonstrated that adult MR criteria for stability resulted in 100% sensitivity but only 11% specificity for unstable juvenile OCD lesions. If the hyperintense signal between the fragment and the native bone mirrored joint fluid and if there was a second outer

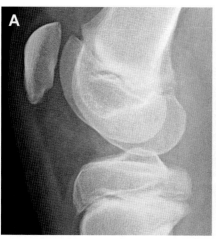 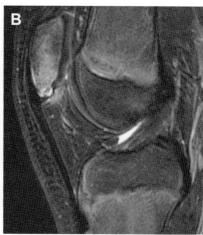

Fig. 10. (*A*) Lateral radiograph of an 8-year-old boy with pain and swelling after a fall shows a subtle, minimally displaced fracture at the inferior patellar pole without adjacent thickening of the patellar tendon, consistent with a patellar sleeve fracture. (*B*) Sagittal T2-weighted fat-suppressed image shows the minimally displaced fracture fragment with edema throughout much of the patella in addition to adjacent fat.

rim of low T2 signal or multiple breaks in the subchondral bone, specificity increased to 100%. The presence of multiple cysts or a single cyst greater than 5 mm in diameter also had high specificity for unstable lesions in juvenile OCD. Pediatric patients have better clinical outcomes than adults, although this may be overestimated as misdiagnosis of normal variation in femoral condyle ossification, as OCD is common. As stated previously, the absence of associated bone marrow signal abnormalities and cartilage injury suggests normal variation.

Chronic repetitive stress injuries to the distal femoral and proximal tibial physes may be identified on MR imaging in some patients with insidious onset of knee pain.[7] Focal widening of the physis results from disruption in endochondral ossification. Periphyseal edema and discontinuity in the zone of provisional calcification is also an indication of physeal injury (**Fig. 14**).[1]

Chronic extensor mechanism injuries include Osgood-Schlatter disease (OSD) and SLJ disease. Clinical diagnosis is possible in most cases, but MR imaging assists in differentiation from acute

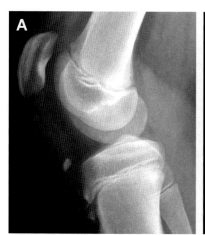 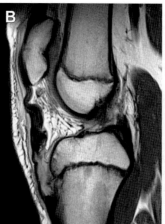 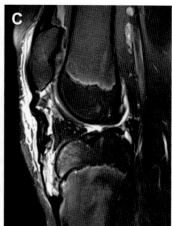

Fig. 11. Lateral radiograph (*A*) of a 13-year-old boy with pain and swelling after a fall while skateboarding shows partial avulsion of the tibial tubercle with displacement and significant soft-tissue swelling (type I-B fracture). Calcification inferior to the patella was presumably related to prior trauma. Sagittal proton-density (*B*) and fat-suppressed T2-weighted (*C*) images show the displaced fracture fragment attached to undulating patellar tendon. The most superficial portion of the tendon remains attached to the inferior tubercle. There is significant surrounding soft-tissue edema.

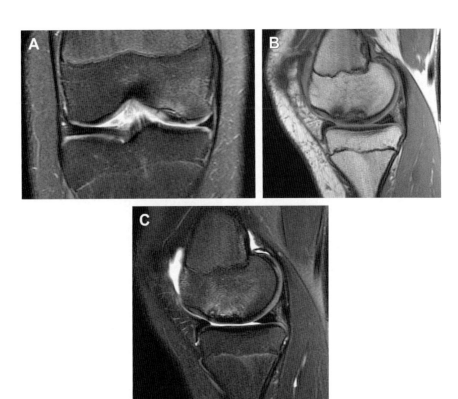

Fig. 12. Coronal fat-suppressed proton-density (*A*), sagittal proton-density (*B*), and sagittal fat-suppressed T2-weighted (*C*) images of the medial femoral condyle of a 15-year-old girl show an unstable osteochondral lesion along the weight-bearing surface. The underlying cartilage shows abnormal signal intensity. The lesion is larger than 1 cm with underlying bone marrow edema and cystic change. The coronal image best shows the fluid signal intensity rim between the fragment and the donor site, suggesting instability.

injury in the presence of radiographic findings and a recent traumatic event. OSD is a traction apophysitis occurring after repetitive trauma at the patellar tendon insertion onto the tibial tuberosity.[7,9,10] Typical presentation is an adolescent male with anterior knee pain and soft-tissue swelling over the tibial tubercle. The abnormality is present bilaterally in up to 50% of cases.[10] In the early stage, abnormal high signal intensity will be seen in the tibial tubercle ossification center. In progressive disease, high signal abnormality also occurs in the adjacent physeal cartilage. A hypointense linear tear can be seen in the ossification center, the anterior part of which appears to be displaced proximally. The patellar tendon now appears edematous and thickened at its insertion onto the tuberosity (**Fig. 15**). In the terminal stage, separate T1 and T2 hypointense ossicles, representing avulsed pieces of the tubercle, have been displaced superiorly from the tubercle and are surrounded by edema. The patellar tendon continues to be thickened and edematous.[21] The tubercle can appear enlarged or fragmented; however, in the absence of inflammatory change this is considered a normal variant. Infrapatellar bursitis may be seen.[7,9,10]

SLJ disease is a similar traction apophysitis involving the origin of the patellar tendon at the inferior patella pole. These patients present with inferior patellar pain often associated with running, climbing, or kneeling. MR imaging shows fragmentation at the inferior patellar pole in addition to thickening and edema of the proximal patellar tendon, which may or may not contain ossification.[7,8] T2 high signal is also seen within Hoffa's fat pad (**Fig. 16**).[14] In the absence of edema, irregularity of the inferior patellar pole is considered a normal variant of ossification. MR imaging is helpful in differentiating SLJ disease from patellar sleeve avulsion. In the former, only bone is avulsed from the inferior patellar pole. With the latter, both bone and its associated cartilage are avulsed.[10]

DEVELOPMENTAL
Discoid Meniscus

Discoid menisci are large and dysplastic, lacking the normal semilunar shape, and most often involve the lateral meniscus. Affected children and adolescents present with pain, clicking, snapping, or locking. On coronal MR imaging, the

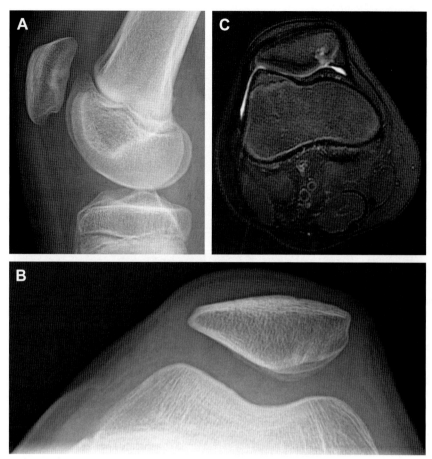

Fig. 13. Lateral (*A*) and Laurin (*B*) view radiographs of the knee in a 12-year-old boy with knee pain show irregularity of the medial patella facet with marginal sclerosis. The presence of a stable patellar osteochondral lesion was confirmed on subsequent axial fat-suppressed T2-weighted image (*C*) as a T2 hyperintense subchondral lesion with overlying cartilage signal abnormality. The lesion measures 7 mm in greatest dimension and has no underlying fluid-intensity rim.

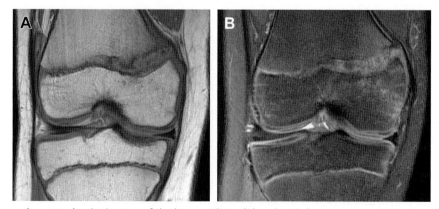

Fig. 14. Coronal proton-density images of the knee without (*A*) and with fat suppression (*B*) in a 14-year-old boy with medial knee pain show widening and irregularity of the medial distal femoral physis with edema in the adjacent femoral metaphysis, consistent with a chronic repetitive stress injury of the physis.

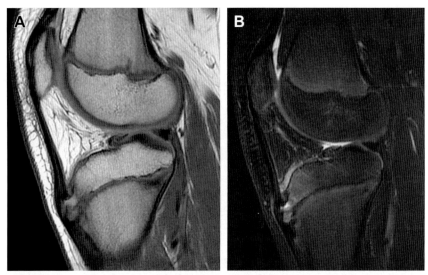

Fig. 15. Sagittal proton-density (*A*) and T2-weighted fat-suppressed (*B*) images of the knee in a 13-year-old boy with anterior knee pain and a palpable lump over the tubercle show thickening and abnormally increased signal intensity of the distal patellar tendon near its insertion. Hypertrophy, early fragmentation, and edema of the tibial tubercle are seen. Findings are consistent with Osgood-Schlatter disease.

discoid meniscus extends farther medially toward the tibial spines (greater than 13 mm in transverse dimension or 2 mm greater than the normal medial meniscus) (**Fig. 17**A). On sagittal images, continuity between the anterior and posterior horns is seen in 3 or more contiguous images 4 to 5 mm thick (see **Fig. 17**B).[22] These images often show diffusely increased T2 signal intensity owing to intrasubstance degeneration, making them prone to tears.[8] Despite the overall abnormal signal characteristics of a discoid meniscus, if high signal intensity contacts the articular surface, a tear should be diagnosed. Cystic degeneration of the meniscus can also be seen.[9]

Congenital Abnormalities of the Cruciate Ligaments

If the ACL is found to be absent at MR imaging, one must question if there is a chronic tear or if it is congenitally absent. Congenital aplasia or hypoplasia of the cruciate ligaments is extremely rare and can be associated with congenital longitudinal limb deficiencies.[23] Either the ACL alone or both of the cruciate ligaments may be affected, though not the posterior cruciate ligament (PCL) in isolation. Manner and colleagues[23] defined 3 patterns of abnormalities. Type 1 deformities are most common, and are characterized by hypoplasia or aplasia of

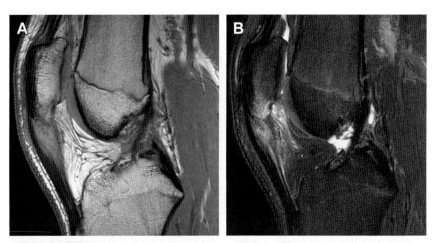

Fig. 16. Sagittal proton-density (*A*) and fat-suppressed T2-weighted (*B*) images of the knee in 16-year-old male basketball player with worsening left knee pain for 1 year show persistent sequelae of Sinding-Larsen-Johansson disease including edema in the inferior patella, thickening and increased signal within the proximal patellar tendon, and edema in Hoffa's fat pad.

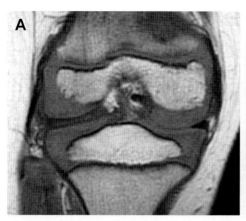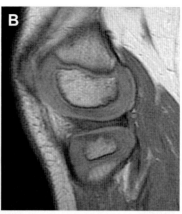

Fig. 17. Coronal T1-weighted (*A*) and sagittal proton-density (*B*) images of the right knee of a 5-year-old girl with knee pain and popping show lateral meniscus that is too wide, extending medially to the intercondylar notch, consistent with a discoid meniscus. The meniscus also shows increased intrasubstance signal, suggesting early degeneration.

the ACL with a normal PCL. As expected, lateral tibial spine hypoplasia or aplasia is seen, with a normal medial tibial spine. The intercondylar notch is also narrowed, with decreased height. Type 2 is characterized by aplasia of the ACL, hypoplasia of the PCL and associated aplasia of the lateral tibial spine, hypoplasia of the medial tibial spine, and a narrowed and shallow intercondylar notch. Type III is characterized by aplasia of both cruciate ligaments, flattening of the tibial eminence, and absence of the femoral intercondylar notch. The distal femoral joint surface is concave and the tibial joint surface is convex, resulting in an abnormal, ball-in-socket knee joint. This final type is the only type shown to have associated discoid meniscus.[23]

When the ACL is absent on MR imaging without evidence of acute rupture and one needs to decide between chronic tear or congenital absence of the ACL, one should assess the osseous structures. If the intercondylar notch and tibial eminence appear abnormally narrowed (hypoplastic), the ligament is congenitally absent. If the bones are normal, the ACL is chronically torn.[9,23]

Bipartite Patella

The patella usually forms from 2 or 3 ossification centers, which begin to develop between 4 and 7 years of age. In a bipartite patella, the secondary ossification center at the superolateral aspect of the patella fails to fuse. It may be a unilateral or bilateral finding.[14] Although bipartite patella is considered a normal variant, it may be painful. The secondary ossification center serves as the insertion of at least part of the vastus lateralis muscle, separated from the remainder of the patella by fibrocartilage. This fibrocartilage can normally exhibit high or low signal depending on the relative

amounts of cartilaginous and fibrous tissue.[14] Acute trauma or chronic abnormal motion between the ossification centers during repetitive stress can cause injury to this synchondrosis. MR imaging assists in determining cases that may benefit from surgical excision of the accessory ossification center based on bone marrow edema on both sides of the synchondrosis (**Fig. 18**).[7,8,14] Degenerative changes such as cysts can also be seen along the margins of the synchondrosis.[9]

Dorsal Defect of the Patella

Dorsal defect of the patella is considered a normal variant, but can be associated with pain. The defect is located at the superolateral aspect of the patella, involving the articular facet, typically measuring 1 to 2 cm. The round lucent region seen on radiographs appears as a T2 hyperintense focus with intact overlying cartilage; however, the cartilage may appear indented or thin. The MR signal of the defect usually is similar to that of the overlying articular cartilage.[7,14] There should be no adjacent bone marrow edema as would be seen in a patellar osteochondral lesion.

Blount Disease

Abnormal endochondral ossification of the medial proximal tibial physis results in Blount disease, formerly called tibia vara. Early or infantile onset and late onset or juvenile versions of Blount disease are differentiated by symptoms occurring before or after 4 years of age, in addition to differences in pathophysiology. Long-term complications of premature degenerative changes resulting from progressive deformity, altered

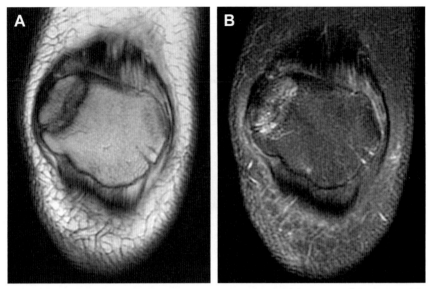

Fig. 18. Coronal proton-density (*A*) and fat-suppressed proton-density (*B*) images of the knee with and without fat saturation in a 15-year-old female basketball player with pain for 5 years show a bipartite patella with edema on both sides of the synchondrosis.

biomechanics, and leg-length discrepancy can occur without appropriate treatment. Radiographs suffice for diagnosis in pediatric patients with genu varum after 2 years of age by identification of medial proximal tibial downsloping and beaking. If surgical correction is indicated, MR imaging may assist in evaluation of physeal bars, meniscal abnormalities, and perichondrial membrane changes. Although the medial compartment is most severely affected, bone marrow signal changes can also be seen in the lateral compartment. The only ligamentous abnormality identified in patients with Blount disease is ACL laxity.[24]

The most well-known abnormalities occur in the proximal tibia. In the coronal plane, the medial tibial epiphysis and metaphysis show abnormal medial downsloping, metaphyseal irregularity, and physeal widening. Posterior downsloping of the proximal tibial is also seen in the sagittal plane. Increased T2 signal within the marrow and transphyseal bony bridging may occur, the latter of which has significant surgical implications. When measured at the mid-femoral condyle on coronal images, the medial tibial epiphyseal cartilage thickness is decreased in comparison with the lateral epiphyseal cartilage. In most cases, this cartilage also shows increased signal intensity on T2-weighted images. The perichondrium along the medial epiphysis is seen as a hypointense linear structure and also becomes deformed (**Fig. 19**).[24]

At the same mid-condylar level on coronal images, the medial joint space is noted to be wider and the meniscus appears thicker than in the lateral compartment. The medial meniscus often shows increased signal intensity, likely related to hypertrophy and intrasubstance degeneration.[24]

Although changes in the lateral femoral condyle are less common, abnormalities may exist. Some patients demonstrate epiphyseal hyperintensity.[24]

Vascular Malformations

Vascular malformations (VMs) may involve the bones, synovium, or extra-articular soft tissues. These malformations are present at birth and grow with the child. Intra-articular lesions may be venous, venolymphatic, lymphatic (LM), or arteriovenous (AVM). These rare lesions present with pain and recurrent swelling, and are most common about the knee.[2] There may or may not be associated overgrowth of the osseous and soft-tissue structures, depending on the degree of limb involvement. VMs are usually isointense to hypointense relative to muscle on T1-weighted images and hyperintense on T2-weighted images. Venous and macrocystic LMs are well circumscribed whereas microcystic LMs and AVMs are more infiltrating. VMs will enhance homogeneously and LMs will enhance peripherally. Phleboliths are seen in VMs because of intralesional clotting. Enlarged draining veins can be seen with both venous and venolymphatic malformations. AVMs will contain numerous flow voids. Synovial VMs are most common in the knee and manifest as recurrent hemarthrosis.[2]

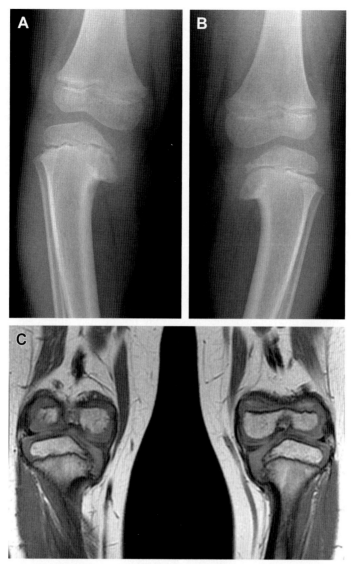

Fig. 19. Anteroposterior radiographs of the right (*A*) and left (*B*) knees and a coronal proton-density image of bilateral knees (*C*) in a 4-year-old boy with Blount disease show medial downsloping and irregularity of the tibial epiphysis and metaphysis. The medial joint space is widened and the medial menisci show abnormal increased signal intensity, especially on the right. The medial perichondrium is deformed.

INFLAMMATORY

Younger children are often imaged to evaluate for possible inflammatory and infectious arthritides in the setting of a history of pain, limp, or swelling. Joint effusions have many possible underlying nontraumatic causes including septic arthritis, juvenile inflammatory arthritis (JIA), hemophilia, and synovial venous malformation.[8,25] Lipoma arborescens and pigmented villonodular synovitis are rare causes of effusions in children.[25]

MR imaging is superior to other modalities in detecting inflammatory changes in joint and cartilage abnormalities, although differentiation among causes often requires clinical correlation. MR imaging also shows the later manifestations of inflammatory arthritides including erosions, joint space loss, and ligamentous involvement.[26]

Normal synovium is low in signal intensity on both T1-weighted and T2-weighted images, and is seen as a smooth rim along the joint capsule and along the cartilage that is no more than 2 mm thick. Synovium homogeneously enhances after contrast administration. When inflamed, the synovium will become similar in signal intensity to joint fluid on both T1-weighted and T2-weighted images. Gadolinium is needed to differentiate the inflamed synovium from the adjacent joint fluid. Rapid enhancement occurs with inflamed synovium, whereas absent, heterogeneous, or poor enhancement is seen in fibrotic synovium.[2,26] It is important to remember that the synovial basement membrane is incomplete, allowing gadolinium to leak into the joint space within as little as 5 minutes of administration. If delayed images are obtained, the degree of synovial thickening may be overestimated,[25,26] thus limiting the evaluation of multiple joints in one setting.

Septic arthritis is a rapidly progressing inflammatory arthritis, most commonly caused by *Staphylococcus aureus*. This disorder is distinguished from nonpyogenic arthritis, which is generally more indolent. Septic arthritis most commonly occurs in young children, with a peak age of 2 to 3 years. The lower extremity joints are more likely to be involved. Patients present with abrupt onset of fever, swelling and warmth over a joint, refusal to bear weight, and limp. When there is clinical concern for septic arthritis, prompt aspiration of the fluid is indicated,[26] followed by surgical irrigation and debridement. Typically imaging is not necessary for diagnosis, but MR imaging aids in identification of associated osteomyelitis and/or subperiosteal abscess. As with sterile inflammatory arthritis, MR imaging will show a joint effusion, synovial thickening, and possibly popliteal lymphadenopathy. The presence of signal abnormalities and enhancement in adjacent bone, however, suggests septic arthritis with associated osteomyelitis.[2]

JIA is defined as a systemic disease affecting patients younger than 16 years with symptoms lasting more than 6 weeks.[7,25,27] The knee is the joint most often affected.[25] Patients present with a nonpainful, warm, swollen joint. In JIA, MR imaging is used to determine disease activity and extent in addition to treatment response. Some studies contend that a negative MR examination at diagnosis predicts a better prognosis, whereas a positive MR exam portends increased risk of disease progression.[2,26] Joint effusion, synovial thickening and nodularity, pannus formation, and inflammation in the infrapatellar fat pad are the most common MR findings.[7,26] Popliteal cysts and popliteal lymphadenopathy are also common secondary findings in JIA.[7,25] If contrast-enhanced images are not performed on initial MR imaging, they should be subsequently obtained because the presence of synovial abnormalities may not be fully appreciated, thus delaying the diagnosis.[26] Mass-like synovial proliferation is called pannus. Both the thickened synovium and pannus show enhancement following gadolinium administration (**Fig. 20**), which may be heterogeneous or homogeneous; necrotic pannus lacks enhancement. Synovium that shows low T1 and T2 signal with heterogeneous enhancement is more severely affected, with the signal characteristics related to fibrin and hemosiderin deposition.

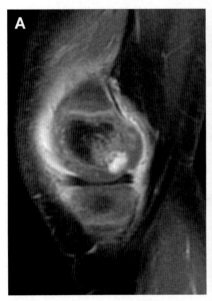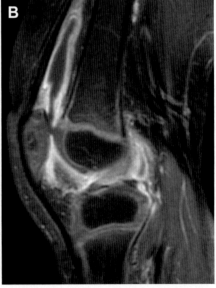

Fig. 20. Sagittal contrast-enhanced T1-weighted images of the knee in a 3-year-old girl with juvenile inflammatory arthritis show enhancing, oval pannus formation within the epiphyseal cartilage of the medial femoral condyle with adjacent bone marrow edema (A). On the more medial sagittal image, a moderate joint effusion is seen with associated synovial thickening. Edema is also seen superiorly in Hoffa's fat pad (B). Findings were confirmed at arthroscopy.

In addition, sloughed synovium produces characteristic low signal intensity foci within the joint fluid, consistent with rice bodies. A moderate to large joint effusion is typical in the suprapatellar bursa.[7,25]

As the disease progresses, bone and cartilage changes can be seen. Narrowing or loss of the joint space will be seen before osseous involvement related to cartilage loss. Subsequent bone changes on MR imaging first manifest as ill-defined areas of marrow edema and enhancement. These early bone changes likely reflect osteitis, and probably predict eventual disease progression to erosions. Erosions can occur anywhere along the joint surface, but are most commonly seen at sites of synovial reflection. These erosions are hypointense on T1-weighted and hyperintense on T2-weighted sequences, and show marked enhancement when active.[2,26] Limb abnormalities may be related to a combination of disease chronicity, steroid therapy, and immobilization. Early on, localized hyperemia results in epiphyseal enlargement and accelerated maturation, resulting in relative increase in length of the affected limb, widening of the intercondylar notch, and squaring of the patella. In long-standing disease the accelerated bone growth promotes premature physeal fusion, resulting in decreased final bone length.[2]

Synovial hypertrophy can cause varying degrees of cruciate ligament atrophy.[2] The menisci become hypoplastic and degenerated owing to surrounding synovial hypertrophy.[2,25] These intra-articular abnormalities are generally not present unless the disease has been poorly controlled for 4 to 5 years.[2,26] In the chronic stage of the disease, the degree of synovial thickening is likely due to a combination of the underlying disease process and the resultant degenerative change.[26]

It is important to remember that enthesitis can also occur in JIA. Enthesitis is diagnosed on MR imaging as increased signal intensity on short-tau inversion recovery or fat-suppressed T2-weighted images, and enhancement at the site of

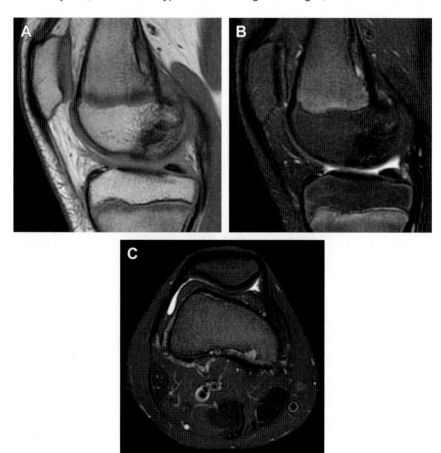

Fig. 21. Sagittal proton-density (A), fat-suppressed T2-weighted (B), and axial fat-suppressed T2-weighted images of the knee (C) in an 8-year-old girl with bilateral knee pain show a cortically based, well-circumscribed heterogeneous hyperintense lesion in the posteromedial femoral metaphysis with no associated bone marrow edema or soft-tissue mass, consistent with a benign, incidental cortical desmoid.

tendon attachments. There may be associated inflammatory changes in adjacent musculature or bursitis. Tendon sheath effusions with synovial thickening and enhancement may also be seen.[2]

Hemophilia is an X-linked recessive disorder affecting boys, resulting in a deficiency of clotting factors. Hemophilia A is due to a deficiency in clotting factor VIII, whereas hemophilia B results from a deficiency in plasma factor IX. Bleeding occurs spontaneously or following minimal trauma. Hemarthrosis accounts for 85% of bleeding episodes, with the knee being the most commonly affected joint followed by the elbow, ankle, hip, and shoulder. Recurrent episodes of bleeding cause synovial hypertrophy and inflammation in addition to cartilaginous and osseous erosions, leading to early degenerative change. Early MR changes include hemarthrosis with or without intra-articular clot and erosions. The synovium shows thickening and decreased T1 and T2 signal intensity caused by hemosiderin deposition, resulting in the characteristic low signal "blooming" on gradient echo imaging. Foci of increased T2 signal within the synovium represent inflammation. The epiphyses appear overgrown and the patella appears squared, as in JIA. The intercondylar notch also widens. Cartilage thinning, subchondral cysts, and osteophytes are seen chronically.[25]

NEOPLASTIC

Incidental benign bone tumors are commonly seen on knee MR imaging. Cortical irregularity along the posteromedial distal femoral metaphysis near the site of medial gastrocnemius muscle origin is commonly seen on radiographs and MR imaging (Fig. 21). Known as cortical desmoids, these are benign and generally incidental findings. These

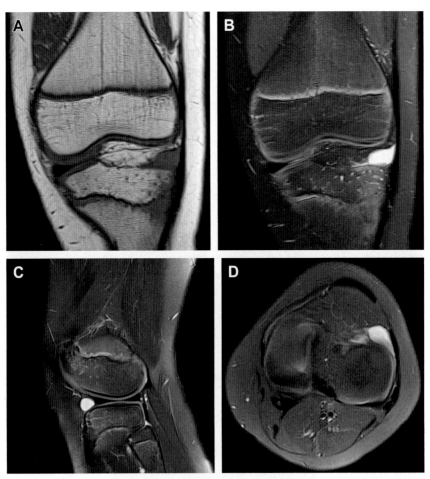

Fig. 22. Non–contrast-enhanced coronal T1-weighted (A), coronal (B) and sagittal (C) fat-suppressed T2-weighted, and axial fat-suppressed proton-density (D) images of the knee in a 10-year-old boy show what appeared to be a parameniscal cyst at the anterolateral aspect of the lateral meniscus. The child underwent arthroscopy for a presumed meniscal tear. No tear was found. The pathologic feature on the resected cystic mass was synovial sarcoma.

are well circumscribed, cortically based lesions without associated soft-tissue mass, which show low signal on T1-weighted images and high signal on T2-weighted images, along with enhancement.[7]

Fibrous cortical defects (<2 cm) and nonossifying fibromas (>2 cm) are other common benign metaphyseal lesions about the knee. The MR characteristics of these lesions correlate well with the radiologic appearance. These defects are well-defined, cortical lesions with MR signal that varies depending on the degree of maturation. On T1-weighted images, the lesions are lower in signal intensity than muscle. Early on these lesions are hyperintense on T2-weighted images, becoming heterogeneous and, finally, low in signal intensity as they mature.[7] This appearance corresponds to the initial lucent appearance on radiographs, which is followed by progressive sclerosis.

Osteochondromas also commonly occur about the knee, and are classified as either pedunculated or sessile. Radiographs typically suffice for diagnosis, but MR imaging may be indicated to assess painful or atypical appearing lesions. Typical osteochondromas show continuity with the marrow cavity of the parent bone; when pedunculated, they project away from the adjacent physis. The cartilage cap exhibits low signal intensity on T1-weighted images and high signal intensity on T2-weighted sequences.[7] Bursae may develop over these tumors at sites of friction.

Although osteosarcoma is the most common malignant primary bone neoplasm about the knee, one of the most underrecognized malignant tumors is synovial sarcoma, the most common soft-tissue sarcoma in pediatric patients following rhabdomyosarcoma.[2,28] Ninety percent of synovial sarcomas in children occur in the extremities, with the lower

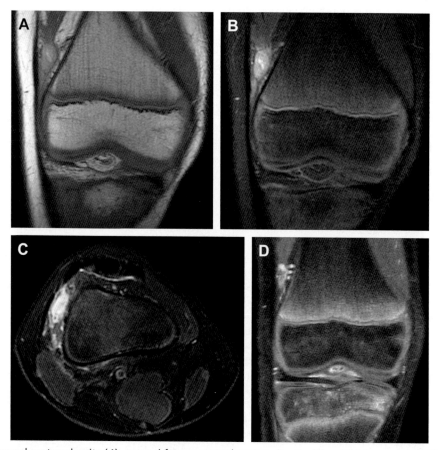

Fig. 23. Coronal proton-density (A), coronal fat-suppressed proton-density (B), axial fat-suppressed T2-weighted (C), and contrast-enhanced coronal fat-suppressed T1-weighted (D) images of the knee in a 10-year-old boy with knee pain for 2 years show a solid, heterogeneously T2 hyperintense, heterogeneously enhancing mass with ill-defined margins deep to the iliotibial band, which was thought to represent a hematoma initially. Owing to the chronic pain and lack of interval decrease in size over 8 months, the mass was resected, with pathologic study revealing synovial sarcoma.

extremity being involved 5 times more often than the upper extremity. In pediatric patients, synovial sarcoma paradoxically presents as either a painless mass or an area of tenderness and swelling without obvious mass, appearing as nonaggressive lesions at MR imaging: small in size, well circumscribed, and noninvasive. Most are T2 hyperintense, but can be heterogeneous and contain septations, appearing cystic (**Fig. 22**), solid (**Fig. 23**), or mixed with heterogeneous enhancement. If calcifications are present, they will appear as foci of low signal intensity on both T1-weighted and T2-weighted images. Though typically localized to the deep soft tissues, synovial sarcoma can occur within joints, occasionally mistaken for a parameniscal cyst. More proximal lesions, those with local invasive characteristics, and tumors larger than 5 cm portend a worse prognosis.[2,28]

SUMMARY

MR imaging of the knee is performed in pediatric patients to evaluate traumatic injuries, developmental abnormalities, inflammatory arthropathies, and neoplasms. Knowledge of normal skeletal maturation and the signal characteristics of normal structures about the knee helps in understanding the pathophysiology of various MR imaging findings, and limits misdiagnoses.

REFERENCES

1. Laor T, Jaramillo D. MR imaging insights into skeletal maturation: what is normal? Radiology 2009; 250:28–38.
2. Kim HK, Zbojniewicz AM, Merrow AC, et al. MR findings of synovial disease in children and young adults: part 2. Pediatr Radiol 2011;41:512–24.
3. Varich LJ, Laor T, Jaramillo D. Normal maturation of the distal femoral epiphyseal cartilage: age-related changes at MR imaging. Radiology 2000;214:705–9.
4. Zbojniewicz AM, Laor T. Focal periphyseal edema (FOPE) zone on MRI of the adolescent knee: a potentially painful manifestation of physiologic physeal fusion? AJR Am J Roentgenol 2011;197:998–1004.
5. Gebarski K, Hernandez RJ. Stage-1 osteochondritis dissecans versus normal variants of ossification in the knee in children. Pediatr Radiol 2005;35:880–6.
6. Jans LB, Jaremko JL, Ditchfield M, et al. Evolution of femoral condylar ossification at MR imaging: frequency and patient age distribution. Radiology 2011;258:880–8.
7. Sanchez R, Strouse PJ. The knee: MR imaging of uniquely pediatric disorders. Radiol Clin North Am 2009;47:1009–25.
8. Strouse PJ. MRI of the knee: key points in the pediatric population. Pediatr Radiol 2010;40:447–52.
9. Davis KW. Imaging pediatric sports injuries: lower extremity. Radiol Clin North Am 2010;48:1213–35.
10. Gottsegen CJ, Eyer BA, White EA, et al. Avulsion fractures of the knee: imaging findings and clinical significance. Radiographics 2008;28:1755–70.
11. Kocher MS, Mandiga R, Klingele K, et al. Anterior cruciate ligament injury versus tibial spine fracture in the skeletally immature knee: a comparison of skeletal maturation and notch width index. J Pediatr Orthop 2004;24(2):185–8.
12. Close BJ, Strouse PJ. MR of physeal fractures of the adolescent knee. Pediatr Radiol 2000;30:756–62.
13. Beasley LS, Vidal AF. Traumatic patellar dislocation in children and adolescents; treatment update and review. Curr Opin Pediatr 2004;16:29–36.
14. Dwek JR, Chung CB. The patellar extensor apparatus of the knee. Pediatr Radiol 2008;38:925–35.
15. Elias DA, White LM, Fithian DC. Acute lateral patellar dislocation at MR imaging: injury patterns of medial patellar soft-tissue restraints and osteochondral injuries of the inferomedial patella. Radiology 2002; 225:736–43.
16. Zaidi A, Babyn P, Astori I, et al. MRI of traumatic patellar dislocation in children. Pediatr Radiol 2006;36:1163–70.
17. Dupuis CS, Westra SJ, Makris J, et al. Injuries and conditions of the extensor mechanism of the pediatric knee. Radiographics 2009;29:877–86.
18. Hunt DM, Somashekar N. A review of sleeve fractures of the patella in children. Knee 2005;12:3–7.
19. De Maeseneer M, Debaere C, Desprechins B, et al. Popliteal cysts in children: prevalence, appearance and associated findings at MR imaging. Pediatr Radiol 1999;29:605–9.
20. Kijowski R, Blankenbaker DG, Shinki K, et al. Juvenile versus adult osteochondritis dissecans of the knee: appropriate MR imaging criteria for instability. Radiology 2008;248:571–8.
21. Hirano A, Fukubayashi T, Ishii T, et al. Magnetic resonance imaging of Osgood-Schlatter disease: the course of the disease. Skeletal Radiol 2002;31:334–42.
22. Silverman JM, Mink JH, Deutsch AL. Discoid menisci of the knee: MR imaging appearance. Radiology 1989;173(2):351–4.
23. Manner HM, Radler C, Ganger R, et al. Dysplasia of the cruciate ligaments: radiographic assessment and classification. J Bone Joint Surg Am 2006;88: 130–7.
24. Ho-fung V, Jaimes C, Delgado J, et al. MRI evaluation of the knee in children with infantile Blount disease: tibial and extra-tibial findings. Pediatr Radiol 2013;43:1316–26.
25. Kim HK, Zbojniewicz AM, Merrow AC, et al. MR findings of synovial disease in children and young adults: part 1. Pediatr Radiol 2011;41:495–511.
26. Johnson K. Imaging of juvenile idiopathic arthritis. Pediatr Radiol 2006;36:743–58.

27. Eich GF, Halle F, Hodler J, et al. Juvenile chronic arthritis: imaging of the knees and hips before and after intraarticular steroid injection. Pediatr Radiol 1994;24:558–63.

28. Bixby SD, Hettmer S, Taylor GA, et al. Synovial sarcoma in children: imaging features and common benign mimics. AJR Am J Roentgenol 2010;195: 1026–32.

Imaging the Knee in the Setting of Metal Hardware

Eric Y. Chang, MD[a,b,*], Won C. Bae, PhD[b],
Christine B. Chung, MD[a,b]

KEYWORDS

- Metal artifact reduction sequences • Metal imaging • Metal hardware • View angle tilting
- Slice encoding for metal artifact correction • Multiacquisition variable-resonance image combination
- Ultrashort echo time-MAVRIC • Knee

KEY POINTS

- Magnetic resonance (MR) imaging will be increasingly used to evaluate the knee in the setting of metal hardware as techniques continue to improve.
- Protocols that are optimized for the evaluation of the painful knee without hardware are suboptimal in the presence of metal.
- Knowledge of the basic principles behind MR imaging metal artifact reduction sequences will allow the radiologist to tailor examinations to match the degree of metal artifact.
- MR imaging metal artifact reduction sequences can show diseases that are occult on other imaging modalities.

INTRODUCTION

Magnetic resonance (MR) imaging is an established modality for the evaluation of musculoskeletal structures, including the knee. This situation is because of the superior soft tissue contrast of MR imaging compared with radiography or computed tomography (CT). In addition, MR imaging can frequently detect osseous abnormalities that may not be visible with other imaging modalities.[1,2] Over the past several years, clinical guidelines for the use of knee MR imaging have broadened.[3,4] Furthermore, metallic implants are increasingly used, particularly for total knee replacement (TKR).[5–7] In part because of prosthetic device wear over time, the number of revision surgeries has also increased.[8] Coupled with continuing improvements in techniques designed to minimize artifacts, it is not uncommon for the radiologist to encounter a patient presenting for MR imaging of the knee in the setting of metal hardware. This article reviews the general principles behind the effects of metal on MR imaging, various MR techniques that are available or have been recently described in the literature, and diseases that can be encountered on MR imaging of patients related to knee arthroplasty, hardware after internal fixation, or hardware used for soft tissue fixation.

Conflicts of interest: none.
[a] Radiology Service, VA San Diego Healthcare System, 3350 La Jolla Village Drive, San Diego, CA 92161, USA;
[b] Department of Radiology, University of California San Diego Medical Center, 200 West Arbor Drive, San Diego, CA 92103, USA
* Corresponding author. Radiology Service, VA San Diego Healthcare System, 3350 La Jolla Village Drive, MC 114, San Diego, CA 92161.
E-mail address: ericchangmd@gmail.com

Magn Reson Imaging Clin N Am 22 (2014) 765–786
http://dx.doi.org/10.1016/j.mric.2014.07.009
1064-9689/14/$ – see front matter Published by Elsevier Inc.

GENERAL PRINCIPLES
Magnetic Susceptibility

Magnetic susceptibility, expressed in parts per million (ppm), is a measure of the tendency of a material to interact with and distort the main magnetic field (B_0).[9] Negative susceptibility values indicate magnetism that opposes B_0, or diamagnetism, and positive susceptibility values indicate the tendency to increase B_0, including paramagnetism or ferromagnetism. In clinical MR imaging, the material of interest is typically water, and therefore, the scanner hardware is tuned to the resonance frequency of protons attached to water molecules, which is 64 MHz at 1.5 T (termed the on-resonance frequency).[10] Water has a magnetic susceptibly value of −9 ppm[9] and materials of different magnetic properties than water create perturbations in the local field, causing precession frequency to increase or decrease (off-resonance frequencies). Susceptibility differences can be small and in the order of a few ppm, such as the differences between biological tissues (water, bone, and fat).[9,11] In contrast, implanted metals show marked susceptibility differences to human tissue in the order of hundreds to thousands of ppm. Implants containing ferromagnetic materials such as nonmagnetic (MR-safe) stainless steel alloys can show a positive shift of 6700 ppm, and cobalt-chromium alloys can show a shift of 1370 ppm.[12,13] Paramagnetic materials show lower susceptibility, such as titanium (182 ppm) and zirconium (109 ppm).[9] **Table 1** provides a list of approximate magnetic susceptibilities of materials commonly encountered during imaging of orthopedic implants about the knee. The susceptibility is heavily dependent on the composition of the implant, and this information is often not easily ascertained. Radiographically similar appearing prostheses can have vastly different composition and susceptibility, such as cobalt-chromium alloys and oxidized zirconium femoral components.[14] In addition, the terms cobalt-chromium alloy, cobalt-chromium-molybdenum alloy, and titanium alloy do not specify the precise composition of a prosthesis. For instance, cobalt-based and cobalt-chromium have both been used to describe implants containing various amounts of cobalt, chromium, manganese, nickel, molybdenum, iron, carbon, and silicon.[13,15] Minute differences in implant composition beyond what is typically controllable through the manufacturing process can cause differences in measurable magnetic susceptibility.[9]

Imaging Artifacts in the Setting of Metal Hardware

When a clinical magnet is appropriately shimmed, the B_0 field is typically homogeneous over a 45-cm

Table 1
Comparison of magnetic susceptibilities

Material	Approximate Magnetic Susceptibility (ppm)	Reference
Zirconium oxide	−8.3	9
Water	−9.1	9,126
Bone (cortical)	−8.9 to −12.8	9,126,127
Fat	−7.8 to −12	9,128
Polyethylene	~0.0[a]	129
Air	0.4	9
Titanium alloys	14.6	130
Zirconium	109	9
Tantalum	178	9
Titanium	182	9
Cobalt-chromium alloys	900 to 1370	12,13
Stainless steel alloys (nonmagnetic, MR-safe)	3520 to 6700	9

Values represent a guide because susceptibilities differ depending on the precise composition of metal alloys.
[a] Value converted from originally reported value of mass susceptibility.

diameter to at least 1.5 ppm.[12,16] In the setting of orthopedic implants, the static magnetic field becomes inhomogeneous, typically because of magnetic susceptibility but also influenced by implant size, shape, and orientation. These inhomogeneities cause 3 main types of artifacts on conventional, clinical MR images: T2* dephasing, displacement artifacts, and failure of fat suppression (**Fig. 1**A).[17] These artifacts are described in further detail later, and conventional techniques used to decrease these artifacts are summarized in **Table 2**.

T2* dephasing
T2* dephasing occurs because of varying rates of precession inside a voxel (see **Fig. 1**B). Dephasing effects can be minimized through the use of refocusing pulses, such as those used with spin-echo or fast spin-echo (FSE) imaging. T2* dephasing can also be minimized with decreasing effective echo time (TE),[18] such as with ultrashort TE (UTE) techniques (**Fig. 2**).

Displacement artifacts
Displacement artifacts arise because of frequency variations in both the slice selection (through-plane, z-axis) and readout (in-plane, x-y–axis) directions. In clinical MR imaging, spatial variation

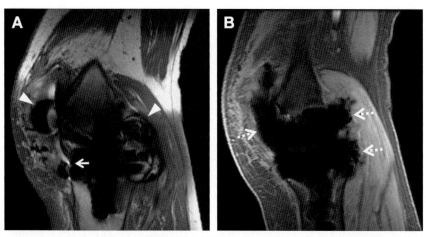

Fig. 1. A 65-year-old woman status post TKR with oxidized zirconium femoral component and titanium alloy tibial component, imaged at 3 T. Sagittal two-dimensional fast spin-echo image (*A*) with chemical fat suppression shows marked artifact including signal pile-up (*arrow*), distortion (*arrowheads*), and poor fat suppression. Sagittal three-dimensional fast spoiled gradient-echo (FSPGR) image (*B*) with iterative decomposition of water and fat with echo asymmetry and least squares estimation fat suppression (water image) shows increased signal loss caused by T2* dephasing (*dashed arrows*), but homogeneous fat suppression, including near the prosthesis and at edges of field of view.

of frequency is tightly controlled through the use of gradients. Alterations of this frequency because of susceptibility cause mismapping of signal with mild cases showing geometric distortion and severe cases showing signal loss in 1 region and pile-up artifact in another.[17]

Displacement artifacts can be reduced by using stronger imaging gradients. This factor allows for

Table 2
Conventional techniques used to decreased metal artifact

Technique	Trade-off
Use a lower field strength magnet	Higher tesla magnets may have more powerful gradients Lower SNR
Avoid conventional gradient sequences	Gradient sequences are often faster than other sequences and allow a lower echo time
Decrease slick thickness	Lower SNR Increased time to cover same volume
Increase matrix	Lower SNR Increased time
Increase receiver bandwidth	Lower SNR
Decrease TE	Alters contrast, may decrease visualization of fluid/edema
Increasing echo train length	T2 blurring
Swap phase-frequency directions to improve visualization of an obscured area	May result in increased imaging time to avoid wrap Vascular pulsation artifacts along phase direction may obscure anatomy
Use of inversion recovery for fat suppression	Lower SNR
Use of Dixon techniques for fat suppression	Increased time Fat-water swapping artifact
Precontrast and postcontrast subtraction images	Lower SNR Misregistration can cause false-positive enhancement

Abbreviation: SNR, signal-to-noise ratio.

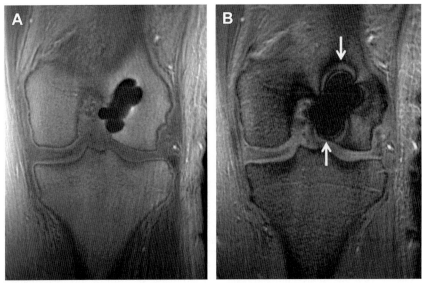

Fig. 2. A 22-year-old woman status post anterior cruciate ligament reconstruction with titanium alloy interference screw in the femoral tunnel. Coronal UTE images with 8 microsecond (*A*) and 4.4 millisecond (*B*) TEs show marked dephasing artifact surrounding the screw at the longer TE (*arrows*).

inclusion of more frequencies within the same voxel, and therefore spreads the metal artifact effects over fewer voxels and a smaller portion of the anatomy. Slice selection gradient strength is increased by selecting a smaller slice thickness. Readout gradient strength is increased by increasing the number of frequencies per pixel (readout bandwidth).[18] Pseudocylindrical structures such as screws often show an arrow (or cloverleaf) artifact pattern, with the direction of the arrow pointing in the frequency encode direction (**Fig. 3A**).[18,19] Generally, swapping the phase-frequency encode directions does not

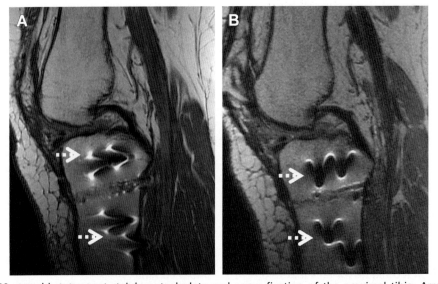

Fig. 3. A 39-year-old status post stainless steel plate and screw fixation of the proximal tibia. Arrow-shaped artifacts from screws (*dashed arrows*) point in the in-plane frequency encode direction, which is anterior-posterior on the sagittal two-dimensional intermediate-weighted FSE image (*A*) and superior-inferior on the three-dimensional (3D) intermediate-weighted CUBE image (*B*). Artifact is approximately the same size on both sequences, despite through-plane phase encode direction on 3D sequence (*B*) caused by thick slab selection.

alter the overall degree of metal artifact,[18,19] but this can allow visualization of otherwise obscured anatomy. However, in some scenarios, empirical evidence suggests that the overall degree of artifact is reduced. For instance, on axial images in patients with TKRs, choosing a left-right frequency encoding direction minimizes artifact surrounding the femoral component.[20]

Alignment of the main magnetic field, long axis of the magnetic object, and frequency encode direction results in optimal reduction of metallic artifacts.[20,21] This situation explains the decreased susceptibility seen with knee arthroplasty pegs/stems and intramedullary rods compared with interlocking screws, which are orthogonal to B_0, or with complex geometric shapes such as the femoral component of a TKR.

Phase encoding, in contrast to frequency encoding, is resistant to displacement artifacts. Conventional two-dimensional (2D) sequences phase encode in 1 direction, whereas three-dimensional (3D) sequences phase encode in 2 directions (through-plane and 1 in-plane direction). However, with most recent 3D FSE sequences including CUBE (GE Medical Systems, Milwaukee, WI), SPACE (Siemens, Erlangen, Germany), and VISTA (Philips, Eindhoven, Netherlands), there is thick slab-selective excitation, and through-plane signal distortion is large, despite phase encoding (see **Fig. 3**B).[17] Displacement artifacts can be minimized with thin slabs at the expense of imaging time. Nonselective 3D imaging would also circumvent these effects, but the entire z-axis direction would have to be imaged to avoid aliasing.[22]

Failure of fat suppression

Failure of fat suppression occurs most dramatically with the use of spectrally selective or chemical fat suppression.[23] Chemical fat suppression relies on the chemical shift difference between the water peak and main fat peak, which is approximately 3.5 ppm ($\sim$220 Hz at 1.5 T and $\sim$440 Hz at 3 T, with fat precessing slower than water).[24] As a preparatory pulse, the fat is selectively excited based on expected precession frequency, and the signal is crushed before application of a standard imaging sequence. In the setting of metal, artifactual frequency shift can easily cause complete failure of fat suppression and in some areas can cause saturation of the water peak (see **Fig. 1**A).

Inversion recovery techniques such as short tau inversion recovery (STIR) are more resistant to B_0 inhomogeneities, because fat is nulled based on the short T1 time relative to water. However, STIR can have several disadvantages. The inversion pulse also affects water with resultant decreased signal-to-noise ratio (SNR) by approximately 40% to 50%.[24] Because of the bandwidth mismatch between the inversion and excitation-refocusing pulses, standard STIR sequences can show distortion artifacts, which obscure surrounding anatomic structures as well as cause inefficient fat suppression. Use of an optimized higher bandwidth inversion pulse has been shown to decrease these artifacts.[25]

In addition, STIR should not be used with exogenous contrast, because enhancing tissue may also be nulled by the inversion pulse. In the setting of contrast administration, subtraction images between non–fat-suppressed T1-weighted precontrast and postcontrast images can be helpful, assuming identical imaging parameters and no patient motion. Even with no appreciable motion between source images, the radiologist should carefully scrutinize edge enhancement on subtraction images, which may be artifactual because of minimal misregistration. Simple subtraction of MR images causes a decrease in SNR,[26] but in our experience, aggressive windowing and leveling can readily show regions of enhancement.

Chemical shift-based fat suppression methods (commonly known as Dixon techniques) rely on phase shifts created by the differences in resonance frequency of fat and water.[24] Many variations of this technique have been used since the initial description. Although Dixon techniques provide for robust fat suppression, they are limited, because of longer scan times. In addition, there is a fundamental ambiguity in distinguishing between fat and water when 1 molecule dominates intravoxel signal. Complex algorithms have been used to resolve this, but most assume a smoothly varying B_0 field, which may not be the case in the presence of metal.[24] Iterative decomposition of water and fat with echo asymmetry and least squares estimation (IDEAL) is a multipoint water–fat separation method, which has been described to be useful in the setting of smaller metal artifact.[27–29] Typically IDEAL should not be used for larger implants, but in some instances, it can be helpful (see **Fig. 1**B).

ADVANCED METAL ARTIFACT REDUCTION TECHNIQUES
View Angle Tilting

View angle tilting (VAT) is a technique used to reduce in-plane displacement artifacts, originally introduced in 1988 by Cho and colleagues.[30] VAT relies on the fact that magnetic susceptibility artifacts cause displacements in both slice selection and readout directions. By viewing the slice from an angle, these displacements can be made to cancel each other (**Fig. 4**). This situation is accomplished by reapplying the slice selection gradient during the readout period. The metal artifact reduction sequence (MARS) has been described as a specific technique that uses the VAT method in conjunction with stronger slice selection gradients and readout bandwidths to further reduce distortions.[31–34] However, with these techniques, through-plane distortions are not corrected, and small blurring artifacts can be seen.[35,36] MARS is now commonly used to refer to all artifact reducing techniques.

Slice Encoding for Metal Artifact Correction

Slice encoding for metal artifact correction (SEMAC) uses the VAT-compensation gradient to suppress in-plane displacements but also adds additional phase encoding steps in the slice selection direction to correct through-plane displacements.[35] An FSE sequence is used to avoid dephasing artifacts. SEMAC is slice selective (2D excitations), but image acquisition is 3D. Early versions of SEMAC used 16 through-plane phase encode steps, which could register off-resonance contributions of up to ±16 kHz (**Fig. 5**).[35,37] The number of through-plane phase encoding steps is limited to save time and encodes subvolumes centered on the excited slice volumes. Phase encoding rather than slice selection resolves the

position in the slice direction, and slice selection thickness does not affect the final through-slice resolution.[37,38] Largely because of the extra phase encode steps, SEMAC can be time consuming, and multiple acceleration techniques have been used, including parallel imaging and partial Fourier reconstruction.[38,39] In addition, to achieve 5-minute to 6-minute scan times per sequence, the number of through-plane phase encode steps has been reduced to 8 to 12 when imaging after TKR.[39] Significant residual artifacts are seen with the decrease in number of phase encode steps, particularly adjacent to implants with higher susceptibility such as cobalt-chromium-molybdenum alloys (>80 kHz off-resonance at 1.5 T) or steel (>192 kHz at 1.5 T) (**Fig. 6**). On the Siemens platform, SEMAC combined with increased readout and radiofrequency pulse bandwidths is termed WARP-Turbo Spin Echo (Siemens, Erlangen, Germany).[40,41] On the Philips platform (Philips, Eindhoven, Netherlands), SEMAC with decreased phase encode steps has been combined with off-resonance suppression (different radiofrequency bandwidths for excitation and refocusing pulses) to achieve faster imaging times.[42,43]

Multiacquisition Variable-Resonance Image Combination

Multiacquisition variable-resonance image combination (MAVRIC) is a technique described by Koch and colleagues in 2009.[44] MAVRIC uses

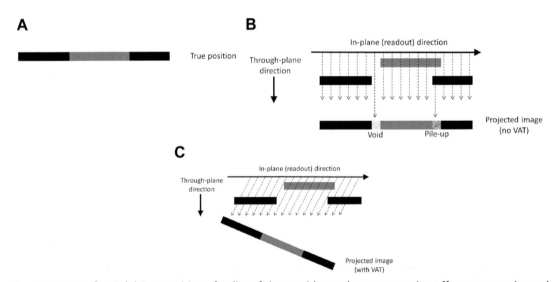

Fig. 4. Concept of VAT. (*A*) True position of a slice of tissue, with gray bars representing off-resonance spins and black bars representing on-resonance spins. (*B*) Conventional 2D techniques show susceptibility-induced shift in 2 directions (through-plane and in-plane directions), which after readout results in a projected image containing displacement artifacts including signal void and signal pile-up. (*C*) VAT applies a slice encoding gradient during the readout, which results in a projected image, in which the shifts in 2 orthogonal directions are transformed into a shift in just 1 oblique direction.

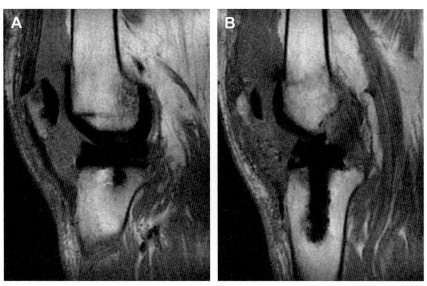

Fig. 5. Artifact correction with SEMAC at 1.5 T in patient with *Staphylococcus aureus* septic arthritis after TKR using oxidized zirconium femoral component and titanium alloy tibial component. Two sagittal T1-weighted SEMAC images (*A, B*) using 16 through-plane phase encoding steps show near perfect correction of through-plane and in-plane artifacts.

limited bandwidth frequency selective excitation to suppress in-plane displacements.[17,44] Narrow spectral bandwidth imaging is performed for the on-resonance frequency and repeated for multiple partially overlapping offset frequencies, each regarded as individual spectral bins (**Fig. 7**).[37] Spectral bins closer to the on-resonance frequency image farther away from the implant, whereas off-resonance bins image closer to the implant. After excitation, a standard 3D-FSE sequence is used for acquisition. Phase encoding is used to resolve displacements in the through-plane direction, and the refocusing pulse avoids dephasing artifacts (**Fig. 8**). Similar to SEMAC

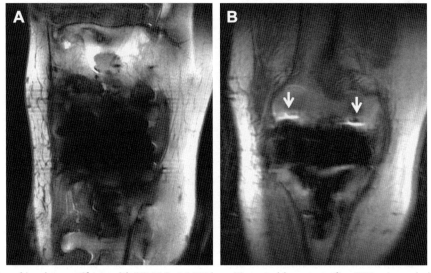

Fig. 6. Reduced in-plane artifacts with SEMAC at 1.5 T in a 47-year-old woman after TKR using cobalt-chromium alloy femoral component and titanium alloy tibial component. Conventional 2D FSE T1-weighted image (*A*) shows marked in-plane and through-plane artifacts. SEMAC T1-weighted image (*B*) with sparse phase encodes to minimize time shows marked improvement in image quality; however, through-plane pile-up artifacts (*arrows*) remain because of limited phase encoding steps.

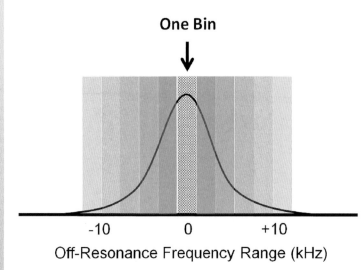

One Bin

-10   0   +10

Off-Resonance Frequency Range (kHz)

Fig. 7. Concept of MAVRIC. Gaussian distribution of spin frequency range is shown in the setting of metal (*black curve*). Each narrow rectangular spectral bin independently excites and images a 3D FSE dataset. After all 3D datasets are acquired (11 total in this figure), images are combined for a single final dataset. Checkered bin in the figure represents the on-resonance condition, which images protons not affected and farther away from the implant. For illustrative purposes, multiple radiofrequency pulses with rectangular profiles are shown, although in practice Gaussian pulse profiles are used with partial overlap between adjacent bins.

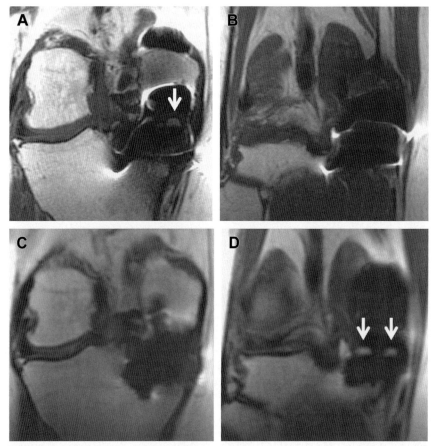

Fig. 8. A 54-year-old woman status post medial unicompartmental knee arthroplasty using cobalt-chromium alloy components, imaged at 1.5 T. Optimized conventional 2D T1-weighted FSE images (*A, B*) show significant artifacts, including distortion, which are markedly improved on T1-weighted MAVRIC images (*C, D*). On MAVRIC image at the posterior portion of the joint (*D*), 2 intra-articular bodies are evident (*arrows*). Because of through-plane distortions, these bodies were mismapped into the central portion of the joint on conventional images (*A, arrow*) and not recognized prospectively.

data, MAVRIC spectral bin subimages are combined through quadrature summation (sum of squares) to form a composite image.[37] The total number of spectral bins affects imaging time, and typically, bins with 2.25 kHz full width at half maximum and 1 kHz bin separation are used. Coverage of a range of ±12 kHz off-resonance has been described for use with clinically compatible imaging times.[37] However, by limiting the number of off-resonance spectral bins to save time, tissue immediately adjacent to higher susceptibility implants is not excited or imaged and is represented by regions of signal void. Another potential limitation of MAVRIC is aliasing in the through-plane direction because of nonselective volume excitation, although this is generally more problematic in hip or shoulder imaging and less so when imaging the knee.[17]

Current Generation Hybrid Techniques

More recently, the similarities between the multi-spectral imaging approaches of SEMAC and MAVRIC were highlighted by Koch and colleagues,[37] who introduced the MAVRIC-SEMAC hybrid technique. This technique adds a through-plane gradient to the multiple spectral acquisitions of MAVRIC. This gradient is applied during excitation, thereby adding slice selectivity, and during readout, thereby adding VAT. Additional phase encoding steps in the through-plane direction are also performed, similar to SEMAC. This hybrid approach was originally termed volume-selective 3D multispectral imaging (VS-3D-MSI), but has now been productized as MAVRIC SeLective on the GE platform. Similar approaches have been described on other vendor platforms, such as multiple slab acquisition with VAT based on a SPACE sequence (MSVAT-SPACE) on the Siemens platform.[22,45] Advances to the techniques listed earlier are rapidly progressing, in particular in combination with acceleration methods, such as parallel imaging and compressed sensing.[38,45–48]

UTE-MAVRIC

UTE techniques use TEs in the order of microseconds, which allow for rapid encoding of the signal before decay. Compared with conventional TEs, in which short T2/T2* structures are hypointense, musculoskeletal tissues such as ligaments, tendons, and cortical bone are directly visible with UTE. In addition, use of UTE sequences can allow direct visualization of solid polymers such as the polyethylene spacer of implants.[49]

UTE-MAVRIC combines UTEs with the multi-spectral approach of the MAVRIC sequence to minimize intravoxel dephasing and excite/image spins closer to the implant, which would have otherwise been excluded (**Fig. 9**).[50] Unlike other imaging techniques, UTE-MAVRIC generates 3D images with isotropic voxels, which allows reconstruction into any imaging plane after acquisition. Imaging time with UTE-MAVRIC is optimized through undersampling of the off-resonance bins.[50] If the composition of the particular metal implant is known, the examination can be further tailored by increasing or decreasing the number of off-resonance bins. For instance, more bins should be used with higher susceptibility implants such as cobalt-chrome (see **Fig. 9A**) compared with titanium (see **Fig. 9C**).

CLINICAL APPLICATION
MR Imaging After Knee Arthroplasty

Knee arthroplasty has increased at a staggering rate over the last decade and is now more common than hip arthroplasty.[5–7] Although implant survival rates for TKR are approximately 93% at 15 years and 83% at 20 years,[51,52] failures still occur, and imaging is integral for diagnosis and management decisions. Although there are more than 150 different knee implant designs in use,[53,54] the most common femoral component consists of a cobalt-chromium-molybdenum alloy.[55] Another commonly used femoral component consists of a ceramic-surfaced oxidized zirconium (Oxinium, Smith and Nephew, Memphis, TN).[56] Compared with cobalt-chromium alloys, oxidized zirconium may have decreased wear[57] and be hypoallergenic.[58] The most common tibial component consists of a titanium alloy (titanium-aluminum-vanadium or titanium-aluminum-niobium).[53,55,59] More recently, porous tantalum has been used for orthopedic products, including a tibial component (Trabecular Metal, Zimmer, Warsaw, IN), with encouraging early and mid-term results.[60,61] As shown in **Table 1**, cobalt-chromium alloys generally show more artifacts than zirconium, titanium, or tantalum, although as described earlier, the susceptibility of a metal alloy is heavily dependent on the precise composition.

Complications after knee arthroplasty can be grouped into 2 broad categories: extra-articular and intra-articular causes.[62] Extra-articular abnormalities include bursitis, tendonitis, or peri-prosthetic fracture. Intra-articular abnormalities include infection, instability, malalignment, aseptic loosening, prosthesis fracture, polyethylene wear, osteolysis, focal scar tissue formation, soft tissue impingement, and extensor mechanism problems. Some abnormalities can be readily diagnosed with

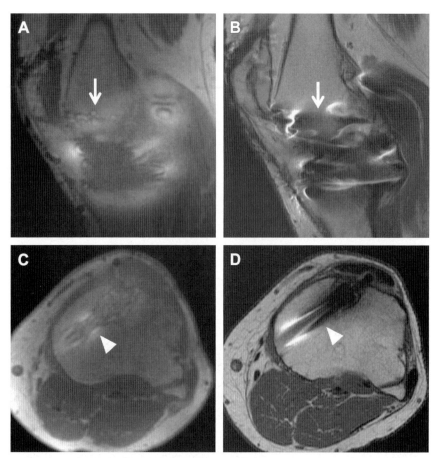

Fig. 9. Improved periprosthetic visualization with UTE-MAVRIC compared with T1-weighted FSE. Patient status after medial unicompartmental knee arthroplasty several years previously using cobalt-chromium alloy components (*A, B*). Sagittal UTE-MAVRIC image (*A*) allows visualization of a pin tract used for the distal femoral cutting block (*arrows*), which was not evident on the conventional sequence (*B*). Different patient with titanium screw in the proximal tibia (*C, D*) shows decreased susceptibility artifact around the screw (*arrowheads*) on axial UTE-MAVRIC (*C*) compared with FSE image (*D*).

radiographs or fluoroscopy, such as periprosthetic fractures or instability.[63] However, many complications can be best visualized with cross-sectional imaging, and MR imaging offers superior contrast as well as having the benefit of being noninvasive, reproducible, and lacking ionizing radiation. Complications that can be readily detected on MR imaging include aseptic loosening, osteolysis, and infection.

Aseptic loosening

Aseptic loosening was initially used to describe a linear radiolucency around a previously well-fixed cemented component, which was often slowly progressive.[64,65] In contrast, osteolysis often refers to a rapidly expanding periprosthetic lucency.[66] Although many investigators often use these terms interchangeably when describing bone loss after

arthroplasty,[67] for this review, aseptic loosening is used according to the classic radiographic description. Other investigators use linear osteolysis[68] and interfacial bone resorption[69] to describe this same process. For the interested reader, there are several articles[70–73] reviewing the cellular and pathogenetic mechanisms behind osteolysis and aseptic loosening.

Studies have shown that one of the most common causes of late TKR failure is aseptic loosening.[74,75] Historically, radiography is the standard imaging modality for detection of loosening. Radiographic signs of loosening include fractures of the prosthesis, cement, or periprosthetic bone,[76] as well as widened or progressively enlarging radiolucency at the cement-bone, metal-cement, or metal-bone interface.[54,77] Radiography has limited sensitivity and specificity for detecting loosening compared with surgery, with sensitivity as low as 77% for detecting loosening of the femoral component and specificity as low as 72% for detecting loosening of the tibial component.[78] Loosening of the tibial component is more common than the femoral component.[79] MR imaging can detect component loosening (**Fig. 10**), and studies have shown that optimized conventional sequences tailored to reduce susceptibility artifacts can be helpful in evaluating the implant-bone interface.[80]

Osteolysis

Osteolysis refers to an expansile periprosthetic lucency, which is often rapidly progressive.[66] This disease has also been termed focal osteolysis,[68] particle disease,[81] and aggressive granulomatosis.[82] Particles from the prosthesis (including cement, polyethylene, metal, or ceramic) can induce a foreign body and chronic inflammatory reaction, which accelerates bone destruction and inhibits bone formation.[73]

Patients with periprosthetic osteolysis can remain asymptomatic despite extensive bone loss.[83] In addition, studies with long-term follow-up have shown that osteolysis may not necessarily progress and may not necessarily lead to revision.[84] However, once an osteolytic lesion is identified, annual follow-up to determine lesion progression may be indicated. Small lesions that are nonprogressive and asymptomatic usually require no treatment (**Fig. 11**).[85]

MR imaging has the potential to detect intracapsular synovial deposits before the osteoclastic resorption of bone.[81] If osteolysis is suspected, optimized conventional MR imaging has been shown to be superior to radiographs for detecting the true extent of osteolysis and for showing

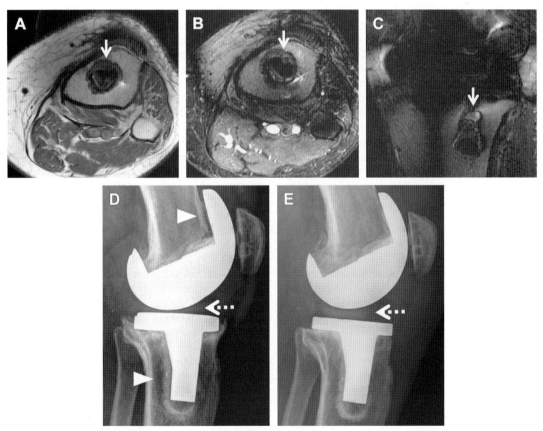

Fig. 10. A 61-year-old woman with knee pain 2 years after TKR using cobalt-chromium alloy femoral and tibial components. Axial T1-weighted (*A*), axial STIR (*B*), and coronal STIR (*C*) images show interfacial bone resorption around the tibial component (*arrows*). Findings of periprosthetic lucency (*arrowheads*) and polyethylene wear (*dashed arrows*) are confirmed on radiographs at presentation (*D*) compared with those obtained 2 years previously (*E*), consistent with aseptic loosening. Fat suppression with STIR (*B, C*) can fail when susceptibility is sufficient to dramatically alter T1.

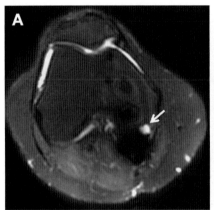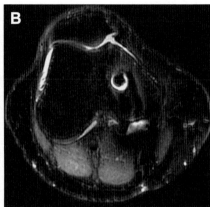

Fig. 11. Patient status post medial unicompartmental knee arthroplasty 4 years previously using cobalt-chromium alloy femoral and tibial components presenting with pain at the lateral aspect of the knee. Axial MAVRIC STIR image (*A*) shows 7 mm hyperintense focus adjacent to the femoral component (*arrow*), which was obscured by artifact on the conventional STIR image (*B*). This lesion was not present on preoperative MR imaging and is consistent with small focal osteolysis, but is not likely to be clinically significant. The patient had a lateral meniscus tear, which was suspected on clinical history and examination.

additional, radiographically occult lesions.[86] Although osteolysis and stress shielding may also appear similar on radiographs,[87] MR imaging may be useful for distinguishing between these 2 entities. A study using a 128-slice CT scanner and 1.5-T magnet with conventional artifact reduction techniques (including maximum receiver bandwidth and reduction of interecho spacing) reported similar accuracies in volume measurements of osteolytic defects.[88] More recent studies have shown that techniques such as SEMAC are superior to conventional MR sequences for the detection of osteolytic foci,[39] and as advanced MR imaging techniques continue to improve, it is likely that MR may become the cross-sectional imaging modality of choice for evaluation of osteolysis.

Signal characteristics of periprosthetic osteolysis are variable. Relative to skeletal muscle, they may appear similar or slightly hyperintense on T1-weighted sequences and similar or hyperintense on fluid-sensitive sequences.[86,89–93] Contrast can be helpful to distinguish the osteolytic mass from other lesions, because there should be relatively little enhancement compared with neoplasm. Post-contrast appearances that have been described include peripheral rim enhancement, irregular internal enhancement, and lack of central intralesional enhancement.[91,94] In some cases, no discernable enhancement is seen (**Fig. 12**).

Infection

Infection after knee arthroplasty can occur early or late.[74,95] Infection is a serious complication,

and the clinical diagnosis may not be obvious. Patients typically present with pain, but fever, chills, erythema, and swelling may be absent in a chronically infected knee (**Fig. 13**).[76] In addition, positive laboratory findings are often nonspecific.[96,97] However, when both erythrocyte sedimentation rate (ESR) and C-reactive protein (CRP) are negative, the diagnosis of infection is highly unlikely.[98]

Although aspiration is the gold standard for diagnosis,[98–101] imaging may be performed because of a confusing clinical picture. Several entities can mimic infection, including aseptic loosening, hemarthrosis, crystal arthritis, and metastases (**Fig. 14**).[102–105] Although not always present, patients often present with a joint effusion.[106,107] Other nonspecific findings include edema of the adjacent soft tissues and bone marrow. Osseous erosions, sinus tracts, and extracapsular soft tissue or fluid collections are more specific signs of infection on MR imaging.[105,107] The presence of lamellated hyperintense synovitis on intermediate-weighted MR images has been shown to be a reliable sign for infection, with sensitivity of 0.86 to 0.92 and specificity of 0.85 to 0.87.[81,108]

Painful Hardware After Internal Fixation

Internal fixation is commonly used for fractures about the knee. In the setting of painful hardware, imaging can be helpful for the orthopedic surgeon. Certain complications such as implant failure, periprosthetic fractures, and osseous nonunion may

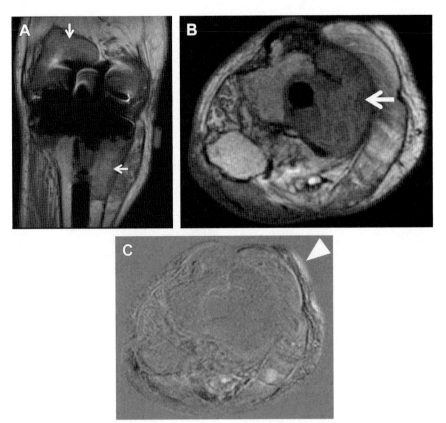

Fig. 12. A 77-year-old man status post TKR 14 years previously with a cobalt-chromium alloy femoral component and titanium alloy tibial component. The patient had a history of malignancy and presented with knee pain and 6.8-kg (15-lb) weight loss. Conventional coronal T1-weighted precontrast image (*A*) and axial T1-weighted postcontrast image (*B*) show aggressive osteolytic masses surrounding the femoral and tibial components (*arrows*). Regions of T1 shortening were present on precontrast (*A*) and postcontrast images (*B*), precluding accurate qualitative evaluation of enhancement. Subtraction images of axial precontrast and postcontrast T1-weighted images were performed (*C*), which did not show any significant enhancement, suggesting osteolysis, which was confirmed on biopsy. Note pseudoenhancement at edges caused by minor misregistration (*arrowhead*).

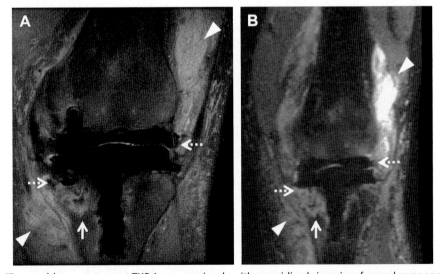

Fig. 13. A 47-year-old man status post TKR 1 year previously with an oxidized zirconium femoral component and titanium alloy tibial component, presenting with worsening pain. Clinical presentation was atypical, because the patient was afebrile, ESR/CRP were only mildly positive, and patient had 2 negative aspirations. Coronal 2D FSE image with IDEAL fat suppression (*A*) and SEMAC STIR image (*B*) show osseous erosions (*arrows*) and extracapsular soft tissue collections (*arrowheads*), most consistent with infection, which was confirmed on a subsequent aspiration. Note improved visualization of periprosthetic tissue with SEMAC acquisition compared with FSE acquisition (*dashed arrows*).

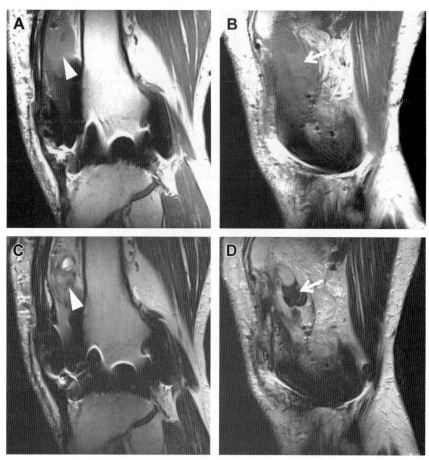

Fig. 14. A 64-year-old man status post TKR with cobalt-chromium femoral and titanium alloy tibial components, presenting with acute onset knee pain and weakness. Clinical concern was for either possible extensor mechanism disruption or infection. Conventional T1-weighted (*A, B*) and T2-weighted (*C, D*) FSE images in the sagittal plane show masses in the suprapatellar (*arrowheads*) and lateral recesses (*arrows*), with heterogeneous signal most consistent with spontaneous hemarthrosis and blood clots. Aspiration yielded 40 mL of blood, and additional history and laboratory examinations showed the patient was supratherapeutic on Coumadin.

be readily seen on radiographs or CT. However, other complications, such as infection or soft tissue compromise, may be best evaluated with MR imaging.

Hardware used for internal fixation includes intramedullary nails with interlocking screws as well as extramedullary plates and screws. Traditionally, stainless steel was the most widely used material, although titanium alloys have become increasingly favored because of their superior clinical performance,[109] improved biocompatibility,[110,111] increased strength,[112] and decreased susceptibility effects. Cobalt-chromium alloys are not frequently used for trauma implants.[15] Broken hardware is typically encountered in the presence of nonunion or delayed union of the fracture.[113]

Because of a more narrow diameter, interlocking screws are more prone to failure than intramedullary nails or plates.[114] In some cases of broken screws, overlapping hardware may obscure visualization on radiographs. Patients may present with pain,[114,115] and a bone marrow edema pattern may be seen (**Fig. 15**).

Iatrogenic soft tissue injury can also be seen after fracture fixation, including injury to the common peroneal nerve during placement of the proximal tibial interlocking screws.[116,117] Injury to a branch of the profunda femoris artery with resultant pseudoaneurysm has also been reported 4 weeks[118] to 4 years[119] after placement of a femoral intramedullary nail with a distal interlocking screw (**Fig. 16**).

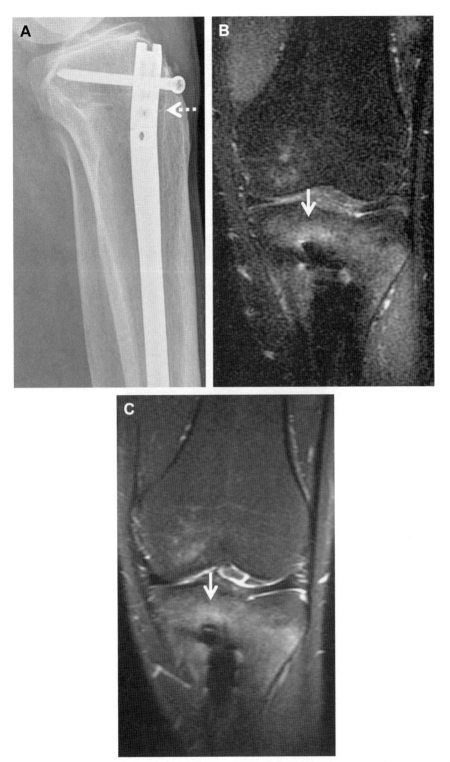

Fig. 15. A 25-year-old man status post internal fixation for a distal tibial shaft fracture with a titanium alloy intramedullary nail and screw. One of the 2 proximal interlocking screws was previously removed; however, the patient complained of persistent proximal knee pain. Radiograph (*A*) shows lucency anterior to the proximal aspect of the nail, suggesting loosening (*dashed arrow*). On conventional STIR image with high receiver bandwidth (*B*) and MAVRIC STIR image (*C*), abundant bone marrow edema pattern is present (*arrows*). There were no clinical signs of infection; edema suggested that hardware was the source of pain. A radiographically occult fractured screw was surgically retrieved, and the patient's pain resolved. Note the decreased periprosthetic artifact and improved SNR on MAVRIC image compared with conventional image.

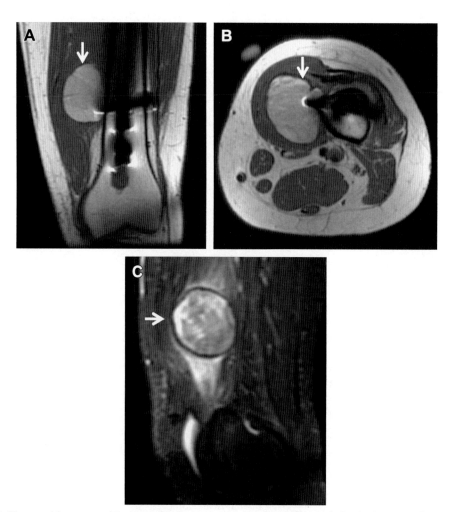

Fig. 16. A 22-year-old woman with metastatic breast cancer treated with prophylactic titanium alloy intramedullary rod and distal interlocking screw 2 years previously, presenting with new onset mass. Conventional coronal T1-weighted (*A*), axial T1-weighted (*B*), and sagittal STIR (*C*) images show a circumscribed mass adjacent to the medial tip of the distal interlocking screw (*arrows*). Mass shows intrinsic T1 shortening and a T2-hypointense rim with mild surrounding edema, consistent with a thrombosed pseudoaneurysm.

Soft Tissue Fixation

Fixation of soft tissue, such as ligaments and tendons, to bone is common in orthopedic surgery. This fixation includes intra-articular procedures such as anterior cruciate ligament (ACL) reconstruction and extra-articular tendon/ligament repair or reconstruction. One of the most common knee injuries is an ACL tear, and current ACL reconstruction techniques use biological tissue grafts, typically either a bone-patellar tendon-bone or hamstring tendon graft. There are several types of fixation,[120] but generally, these can be divided into aperture fixation with interference screws or suspensory fixation with cortical buttons, staples, screws, spiked washers, or cross-pins.[121] For extra-articular soft tissue repair, suture anchors and staples are commonly used. Most currently available metallic implants used for soft tissue fixation are composed of titanium alloy or stainless steel,[122] although aluminum and cobalt-chromium alloys have been used in the past.[15,122] Interference screws, suture anchors, and cross-pins are also available in polymer or composite form,[120,122] and these have fewer susceptibility effects compared with their metallic counterparts. MR imaging is the preferred modality for evaluation of complications related to soft tissue fixation,[123] including broken[124] or displaced hardware (**Figs. 17 and 18**).[125]

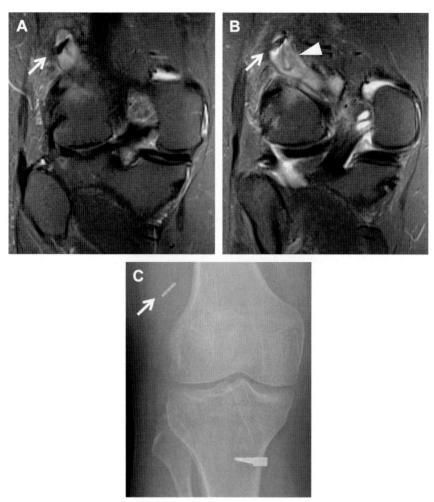

Fig. 17. A 31-year-old man status post ACL reconstruction with suspensory femoral fixation using an EndoButton (Smith & Nephew, Andover, MA) made of titanium alloy. Two coronal STIR images (*A, B*) show a displaced EndoButton (*arrows*), which is disconnected from the graft, but still attached to the preloaded continuous loop of suture (*arrowhead*). A displaced EndoButton is confirmed on radiographs (*C, arrow*).

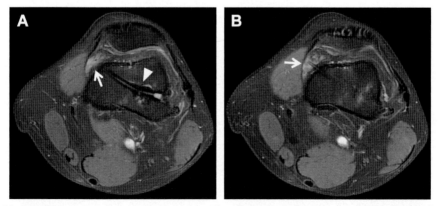

Fig. 18. A 41-year-old man status post ACL reconstruction 3 years previously using bioabsorbable (poly-L-lactic-acid) femoral cross-pin fixation presents with pain and catching at the medial aspect of the knee. Axial intermediate-weighted images with chemical fat suppression (*A, B*) show a fractured cross-pin (*arrowhead*) with distal end protruding through the anteromedial femoral cortex and irritating the prefemoral fat pad (*arrows*). Magnetic susceptibility of cross-pin is well matched to tissue and does not cause any appreciable artifact.

SUMMARY

As techniques continue to improve, MR imaging will be increasingly used to evaluate the knee in the setting of metal hardware. Pulse sequences and protocols that are optimized for the evaluation of the painful knee without hardware are suboptimal in the presence of metal. Radiologists should eschew the 1-protocol-fits all approach in the setting of metal because of the widely variant magnetic susceptibilities of implants. Knowledge of the basic principles behind MR MARS allows the radiologist to tailor examinations to match the degree of metal artifact as well as properly interpret images generated from these sequences. Optimization of MR imaging in this setting is clearly necessary in the era of personalized medicine. Hybrid techniques in combination with acceleration may be the most successful in the near future, and these techniques will allow optimal anatomic visualization and diagnosis of postoperative disease.

ACKNOWLEDGMENTS

E.Y. Chang, MD, gratefully acknowledges grant support from the VA (Clinical Science Research and Development Career Development Award 1IK2CX000749).

REFERENCES

1. Yao L, Lee JK. Occult intraosseous fracture: detection with MR imaging. Radiology 1988;167(3):749–51.
2. Berquist TH. Osseous and myotendinous injuries about the knee. Radiol Clin North Am 2007;45(6):955–68, vi.
3. Espeland A, Natvig NL, Loge I, et al. Magnetic resonance imaging of the knee in Norway 2002-2004 (national survey): rapid increase, older patients, large geographic differences. BMC Health Serv Res 2007;7:115.
4. Solomon DH, Katz JN, Carrino JA, et al. Trends in knee magnetic resonance imaging. Med Care 2003;41(5):687–92.
5. Weinstein AM, Rome BN, Reichmann WM, et al. Estimating the burden of total knee replacement in the United States. J Bone Joint Surg Am 2013;95(5):385–92.
6. Losina E, Thornhill TS, Rome BN, et al. The dramatic increase in total knee replacement utilization rates in the United States cannot be fully explained by growth in population size and the obesity epidemic. J Bone Joint Surg Am 2012;94(3):201–7.
7. Kurtz SM, Lau E, Ong K, et al. Future young patient demand for primary and revision joint replacement: national projections from 2010 to 2030. Clin Orthop Relat Res 2009;467(10):2606–12.
8. Cram P, Lu X, Kates SL, et al. Total knee arthroplasty volume, utilization, and outcomes among Medicare beneficiaries, 1991-2010. JAMA 2012;308(12):1227–36.
9. Schenck JF. The role of magnetic susceptibility in magnetic resonance imaging: MRI magnetic compatibility of the first and second kinds. Med Phys 1996;23(6):815–50.
10. Brown MA, Semelka RC. MRI: basic principles and applications. 4th edition. Hoboken (NJ): Wiley-Blackwell/John Wiley; 2010.
11. Young IR, Bydder GM, Fullerton GD. MRI of tissues with short T2s or T2*s. Chichester (West Sussex): John Wiley; 2012.
12. Koch KM, Hargreaves BA, Pauly KB, et al. Magnetic resonance imaging near metal implants. J Magn Reson Imaging 2010;32(4):773–87.
13. Bartusek K, Dokoupil Z, Gescheidtova E. Magnetic field mapping around metal implants using an asymmetric spin-echo MRI sequence. Meas Sci Technol 2006;17(12):3293–300.
14. Kim YH, Park JW, Kim JS. Comparison of the Genesis II total knee replacement with oxidised zirconium and cobalt-chromium femoral components in the same patients: a prospective, double-blind, randomised controlled study. J Bone Joint Surg Br 2012;94(9):1221–7.
15. Leung KS, Taglang G, Schnettler R. Practice of intramedullary locked nails new developments in techniques and applications. Berlin (London): Springer; 2006. Available at: http://dx.doi.org/10.1007/3-540-32345-7.
16. Analoui M, Bronzino JD, Peterson DR. Medical imaging: principles and practices. Boca Raton (FL): Taylor & Francis/CRC Press; 2013.
17. Hargreaves BA, Worters PW, Pauly KB, et al. Metal-induced artifacts in MRI. AJR Am J Roentgenol 2011;197(3):547–55.
18. Vandevenne JE, Vanhoenacker FM, Parizel PM, et al. Reduction of metal artefacts in musculoskeletal MR imaging. JBR-BTR 2007;90(5):345–9.
19. Suh JS, Jeong EK, Shin KH, et al. Minimizing artifacts caused by metallic implants at MR imaging: experimental and clinical studies. AJR Am J Roentgenol 1998;171(5):1207–13.
20. Lee KY, Slavinsky JP, Ries MD, et al. Magnetic resonance imaging of in vivo kinematics after total knee arthroplasty. J Magn Reson Imaging 2005;21(2):172–8.
21. Guermazi A, Miaux Y, Zaim S, et al. Metallic artefacts in MR imaging: effects of main field orientation and strength. Clin Radiol 2003;58(4):322–8.
22. Ai T, Padua A, Goerner F, et al. SEMAC-VAT and MSVAT-SPACE sequence strategies for metal

artifact reduction in 1.5T magnetic resonance imaging. Invest Radiol 2012;47(5):267–76.

23. Keller PJ, Hunter WW Jr, Schmalbrock P. Multisection fat-water imaging with chemical shift selective presaturation. Radiology 1987;164(2):539–41.

24. Bley TA, Wieben O, Francois CJ, et al. Fat and water magnetic resonance imaging. J Magn Reson Imaging 2010;31(1):4–18.

25. Ulbrich EJ, Sutter R, Aguiar RF, et al. STIR sequence with increased receiver bandwidth of the inversion pulse for reduction of metallic artifacts. AJR Am J Roentgenol 2012;199(6): W735–42.

26. Martel AL, Fraser D, Delay GS, et al. Separating arterial and venous components from 3D dynamic contrast-enhanced MRI studies using factor analysis. Magn Reson Med 2003;49(5):928–33.

27. Cha JG, Hong HS, Park JS, et al. Practical application of iterative decomposition of water and fat with echo asymmetry and least-squares estimation (IDEAL) imaging in minimizing metallic artifacts. Korean J Radiol 2012;13(3):332–41.

28. Cha JG, Jin W, Lee MH, et al. Reducing metallic artifacts in postoperative spinal imaging: usefulness of IDEAL contrast-enhanced T1- and T2-weighted MR imaging–phantom and clinical studies. Radiology 2011;259(3):885–93.

29. Lee JB, Cha JG, Lee MH, et al. Usefulness of IDEAL T2-weighted FSE and SPGR imaging in reducing metallic artifacts in the postoperative ankles with metallic hardware. Skeletal Radiol 2013; 42(2):239–47.

30. Cho ZH, Kim DJ, Kim YK. Total inhomogeneity correction including chemical shifts and susceptibility by view angle tilting. Med Phys 1988;15(1): 7–11.

31. Chang SD, Lee MJ, Munk PL, et al. MRI of spinal hardware: comparison of conventional T1-weighted sequence with a new metal artifact reduction sequence. Skeletal Radiol 2001;30(4): 213–8.

32. Olsen RV, Munk PL, Lee MJ, et al. Metal artifact reduction sequence: early clinical applications. Radiographics 2000;20(3):699–712.

33. Kolind SH, MacKay AL, Munk PL, et al. Quantitative evaluation of metal artifact reduction techniques. J Magn Reson Imaging 2004;20(3):487–95.

34. Toms AP, Smith-Bateman C, Malcolm PN, et al. Optimization of metal artefact reduction (MAR) sequences for MRI of total hip prostheses. Clin Radiol 2010;65(6):447–52.

35. Lu W, Pauly KB, Gold GE, et al. SEMAC: slice encoding for metal artifact correction in MRI. Magn Reson Med 2009;62(1):66–76.

36. Butts K, Pauly JM, Gold GE. Reduction of blurring in view angle tilting MRI. Magn Reson Med 2005; 53(2):418–24.

37. Koch KM, Brau AC, Chen W, et al. Imaging near metal with a MAVRIC-SEMAC hybrid. Magn Reson Med 2011;65(1):71–82.

38. Hargreaves BA, Chen W, Lu W, et al. Accelerated slice encoding for metal artifact correction. J Magn Reson Imaging 2010;31(4):987–96.

39. Sutter R, Hodek R, Fucentese SF, et al. Total knee arthroplasty MRI featuring slice-encoding for metal artifact correction: reduction of artifacts for STIR and proton density-weighted sequences. AJR Am J Roentgenol 2013;201(6):1315–24.

40. Griffin JF, Archambault NS, Mankin JM, et al. Magnetic resonance imaging in cadaver dogs with metallic vertebral implants at 3 Tesla: evaluation of the WARP-turbo spin echo sequence. Spine 2013;38(24):E1548–53.

41. Sutter R, Ulbrich EJ, Jellus V, et al. Reduction of metal artifacts in patients with total hip arthroplasty with slice-encoding metal artifact correction and view-angle tilting MR imaging. Radiology 2012; 265(1):204–14.

42. Bos C, den Harder CJ, Yperen G. MR imaging near orthopedic implants with artifact reduction using view-angle tilting and off-resonance suppression. Presented at: ISMRM 18th Annual Meeting. Stockholm, Sweden, May 1–7, 2010.

43. Den Harder CJ, Blume UA, Bos C. MR imaging near orthopedic implants using slice-encoding for metal artifact correction and off-resonance suppression. Presented at: ISMRM 19th Annual Meeting. Montréal, Québec, Canada, May 7–13, 2011.

44. Koch KM, Lorbiecki JE, Hinks RS, et al. A multispectral three-dimensional acquisition technique for imaging near metal implants. Magn Reson Med 2009;61(2):381–90.

45. Li G, Nittka M, Paul D, et al. MSVAT-SPACE for fast metal implants imaging. Presented at: ISMRM 19th Annual Meeting. Montréal, Québec, Canada, May 7–13, 2011.

46. Koch KM, King KF. Combined parallel imaging and compressed sensing on 3D multi-spectral imaging near metal implants. Presented at: ISMRM 19th Annual Meeting. Montréal, Québec, Canada, May 7–13, 2011.

47. Nittka M, Otazo R, Rybak LD, et al. Highly accelerated SEMAC metal implant imaging using joint compressed sensing and parallel imaging. Presented at: ISMRM 21st Annual Meeting. Salt Lake City, Utah, April 20–26, 2013.

48. Worters PW, Sung K, Stevens KJ, et al. Compressed-sensing multispectral imaging of the postoperative spine. J Magn Reson Imaging 2013; 37(1):243–8.

49. Springer F, Martirosian P, Schwenzer NF, et al. Three-dimensional ultrashort echo time imaging of solid polymers on a 3-Tesla whole-body MRI scanner. Invest Radiol 2008;43(11):802–8.

50. Carl M, Koch K, Du J. MR imaging near metal with undersampled 3D radial UTE-MAVRIC sequences. Magn Reson Med 2013;69(1):27–36.

51. Dixon MC, Brown RR, Parsch D, et al. Modular fixed-bearing total knee arthroplasty with retention of the posterior cruciate ligament. A study of patients followed for a minimum of fifteen years. J Bone Joint Surg Am 2005;87(3):598–603.

52. Ma HM, Lu YC, Ho FY, et al. Long-term results of total condylar knee arthroplasty. J Arthroplasty 2005;20(5):580–4.

53. Mulcahy H, Chew FS. Current concepts in knee replacement: features and imaging assessment. AJR Am J Roentgenol 2013;201(6):W828–42.

54. Math KR, Zaidi SF, Petchprapa C, et al. Imaging of total knee arthroplasty. Semin Musculoskelet Radiol 2006;10(1):47–63.

55. Raphael B, Haims AH, Wu JS, et al. MRI comparison of periprosthetic structures around zirconium knee prostheses and cobalt chrome prostheses. AJR Am J Roentgenol 2006;186(6):1771–7.

56. Laskin RS. An oxidized Zr ceramic surfaced femoral component for total knee arthroplasty. Clin Orthop Relat Res 2003;(416):191–6.

57. Heyse TJ, Elpers ME, Nawabi DH, et al. Oxidized zirconium versus cobalt-chromium in TKA: profilometry of retrieved femoral components. Clin Orthop Relat Res 2014;472(1):277–83.

58. Nasser S. Orthopedic metal immune hypersensitivity. Orthopedics 2007;30(8 Suppl):89–91.

59. Munzinger UK, Boldt JG, Keblish PA. Primary knee arthroplasty. Berlin (NY): Springer; 2004.

60. Wilson DA, Richardson G, Hennigar AW, et al. Continued stabilization of trabecular metal tibial monoblock total knee arthroplasty components at 5 years measured with radiostereometric analysis. Acta Orthop 2012;83(1):36–40.

61. Unger AS, Duggan JP. Midterm results of a porous tantalum monoblock tibia component clinical and radiographic results of 108 knees. J Arthroplasty 2011;26(6):855–60.

62. Brown EC 3rd, Clarke HD, Scuderi GR. The painful total knee arthroplasty: diagnosis and management. Orthopedics 2006;29(2):129–36 [quiz: 137–8].

63. Mulcahy H, Chew FS. Current concepts in knee replacement: complications. Am J Roentgenol 2013;202(1):W76–86.

64. Sinha RK, Shanbhag AS, Maloney WJ, et al. Osteolysis: cause and effect. Instr Course Lect 1998;47:307–20.

65. Gruen TA, McNeice GM, Amstutz HC. "Modes of failure" of cemented stem-type femoral components: a radiographic analysis of loosening. Clin Orthop Relat Res 1979;(141):17–27.

66. Harris WH, Schiller AL, Scholler JM, et al. Extensive localized bone resorption in the femur following total hip replacement. J Bone Joint Surg Am 1976;58(5):612–8.

67. Callaghan JJ, Rosenberg AG, Rubash HE. The adult hip. 2nd edition. Philadelphia: Lippincott Williams & Wilkins; 2007.

68. Yoon TR, Rowe SM, Jung ST, et al. Osteolysis in association with a total hip arthroplasty with ceramic bearing surfaces. J Bone Joint Surg Am 1998; 80(10):1459–68.

69. Schmalzried TP, Callaghan JJ. Wear in total hip and knee replacements. J Bone Joint Surg Am 1999; 81(1):115–36.

70. Gallo J, Goodman SB, Konttinen YT, et al. Osteolysis around total knee arthroplasty: a review of pathogenetic mechanisms. Acta Biomater 2013;9(9): 8046–58.

71. O'Neill SC, Queally JM, Devitt BM, et al. The role of osteoblasts in peri-prosthetic osteolysis. Bone Joint J 2013;95-B(8):1022–6.

72. Jiang Y, Jia T, Wooley PH, et al. Current research in the pathogenesis of aseptic implant loosening associated with particulate wear debris. Acta Orthop Belg 2013;79(1):1–9.

73. Goodman SB, Gibon E, Yao Z. The basic science of periprosthetic osteolysis. Instr Course Lect 2013;62:201–6.

74. Sharkey PF, Hozack WJ, Rothman RH, et al. Insall Award paper. Why are total knee arthroplasties failing today? Clin Orthop Relat Res 2002;(404):7–13.

75. Friedman RJ, Hirst P, Poss R, et al. Results of revision total knee arthroplasty performed for aseptic loosening. Clin Orthop Relat Res 1990;(255): 235–41.

76. Duff GP, Lachiewicz PF, Kelley SS. Aspiration of the knee joint before revision arthroplasty. Clin Orthop Relat Res 1996;(331):132–9.

77. Allen AM, Ward WG, Pope TL Jr. Imaging of the total knee arthroplasty. Radiol Clin North Am 1995; 33(2):289–303.

78. Marx A, Saxler G, Landgraeber S, et al. Comparison of subtraction arthrography, radionuclide arthrography and conventional plain radiography to assess loosening of total knee arthroplasty. Biomed Tech (Berl) 2005;50(5):143–7.

79. Windsor RE, Scuderi GR, Moran MC, et al. Mechanisms of failure of the femoral and tibial components in total knee arthroplasty. Clin Orthop Relat Res 1989;(248):15–9 [discussion: 19–20].

80. Heyse TJ, Chong le R, Davis J, et al. MRI analysis of the component-bone interface after TKA. Knee 2012;19(4):290–4.

81. Potter HG, Foo LF. Magnetic resonance imaging of joint arthroplasty. Orthop Clin North Am 2006;37(3): 361–73, vi–vii.

82. Tigges S, Stiles RG, Roberson JR. Aggressive granulomatosis complicating knee arthroplasty. Can Assoc Radiol J 1994;45(4):310–3.

83. Maloney WJ. Management of osteolysis after total knee replacement. J Bone Joint Surg Br 2010;92-B-(Suppl I):90–1.

84. Colizza WA, Insall JN, Scuderi GR. The posterior stabilized total knee prosthesis. Assessment of polyethylene damage and osteolysis after a ten-year-minimum follow-up. J Bone Joint Surg Am 1995;77(11):1713–20.

85. Scuderi GR. Complications after total knee arthroplasty: how to manage patients with osteolysis. Instr Course Lect 2012;61:397–404.

86. Vessely MB, Frick MA, Oakes D, et al. Magnetic resonance imaging with metal suppression for evaluation of periprosthetic osteolysis after total knee arthroplasty. J Arthroplasty 2006;21(6):826–31.

87. Bono JV, Scott RD. Revision total knee arthroplasty. New York: Springer; 2005.

88. Solomon LB, Stamenkov RB, MacDonald AJ, et al. Imaging periprosthetic osteolysis around total knee arthroplasties using a human cadaver model. J Arthroplasty 2012;27(6):1069–74.

89. Mosher TJ, Davis CM 3rd. Magnetic resonance imaging to evaluate osteolysis around total knee arthroplasty. J Arthroplasty 2006;21(3):460–3.

90. Gupta SK, Chu A, Ranawat AS, et al. Osteolysis after total knee arthroplasty. J Arthroplasty 2007;22(6):787–99.

91. Desai MA, Bancroft LW. The case. Diagnosis: periprosthetic osteolysis. Orthopedics 2008;31(6):518, 615–8.

92. Potter HG, Nestor BJ, Sofka CM, et al. Magnetic resonance imaging after total hip arthroplasty: evaluation of periprosthetic soft tissue. J Bone Joint Surg Am 2004;86-A(9):1947–54.

93. Sofka CM, Potter HG, Figgie M, et al. Magnetic resonance imaging of total knee arthroplasty. Clin Orthop Relat Res 2003;(406):129–35.

94. White LM, Kim JK, Mehta M, et al. Complications of total hip arthroplasty: MR imaging-initial experience. Radiology 2000;215(1):254–62.

95. Fehring TK, Odum S, Griffin WL, et al. Early failures in total knee arthroplasty. Clin Orthop Relat Res 2001;(392):315–8.

96. Magnuson JE, Brown ML, Hauser MF, et al. In-111-labeled leukocyte scintigraphy in suspected orthopedic prosthesis infection: comparison with other imaging modalities. Radiology 1988;168(1):235–9.

97. Virolainen P, Lahteenmaki H, Hiltunen A, et al. The reliability of diagnosis of infection during revision arthroplasties. Scand J Surg 2002;91(2):178–81.

98. Della Valle C, Parvizi J, Bauer TW, et al. American Academy of Orthopaedic Surgeons clinical practice guideline on: the diagnosis of periprosthetic joint infections of the hip and knee. J Bone Joint Surg Am 2011;93(14):1355–7.

99. Bach CM, Sturmer R, Nogler M, et al. Total knee arthroplasty infection: significance of delayed aspiration. J Arthroplasty 2002;17(5):615–8.

100. Leone JM, Hanssen AD. Management of infection at the site of a total knee arthroplasty. Instr Course Lect 2006;55:449–61.

101. Levitsky KA, Hozack WJ, Balderston RA, et al. Evaluation of the painful prosthetic joint. Relative value of bone scan, sedimentation rate, and joint aspiration. J Arthroplasty 1991;6(3):237–44.

102. Karataglis D, Marlow D, Learmonth DJ. Atraumatic haemarthrosis following total knee replacement treated with selective embolisation. Acta Orthop Belg 2006;72(3):375–7.

103. Holt G, Vass C, Kumar CS. Acute crystal arthritis mimicking infection after total knee arthroplasty. BMJ 2005;331(7528):1322–3.

104. Currall VA, Dixon JH. Synovial metastasis: an unusual cause of pain after total knee arthroplasty. J Arthroplasty 2008;23(4):631–6.

105. Bitto DJ, Schweitzer ME, Zoga A. Clinical effectiveness of MRI in diagnosis of infection in patients with total knee arthroplasties. Presented at: ISMRM 11th Annual Meeting. Toronto, Ontario, Canada, July 10–16, 2003.

106. Karchevsky M, Schweitzer ME, Morrison WB, et al. MRI findings of septic arthritis and associated osteomyelitis in adults. AJR Am J Roentgenol 2004;182(1):119–22.

107. Bancroft LW. MR imaging of infectious processes of the knee. Magn Reson Imaging Clin N Am 2007;15(1):1–11.

108. Plodkowski AJ, Hayter CL, Miller TT, et al. Lamellated hyperintense synovitis: potential MR imaging sign of an infected knee arthroplasty. Radiology 2013;266(1):256–60.

109. Riemer BL, DiChristina DG, Cooper A, et al. Nonreamed nailing of tibial diaphyseal fractures in blunt polytrauma patients. J Orthop Trauma 1995;9(1):66–75.

110. Kraft CN, Diedrich O, Burian B, et al. Microvascular response of striated muscle to metal debris. A comparative in vivo study with titanium and stainless steel. J Bone Joint Surg Br 2003;85(1):133–41.

111. Ryhanen J, Kallioinen M, Serlo W, et al. Bone healing and mineralization, implant corrosion, and trace metals after nickel-titanium shape memory metal intramedullary fixation. J Biomed Mater Res 1999;47(4):472–80.

112. Gaebler C, Stanzl-Tschegg S, Heinze G, et al. Fatigue strength of locking screws and prototypes used in small-diameter tibial nails: a biomechanical study. J Trauma 1999;47(2):379–84.

113. Hak DJ, McElvany M. Removal of broken hardware. J Am Acad Orthop Surg 2008;16(2):113–20.

114. Whittle AP, Wester W, Russell TA. Fatigue failure in small diameter tibial nails. Clin Orthop Relat Res 1995;(315):119–28.

115. Mohammed A, Saravanan R, Zammit J, et al. Intramedullary tibial nailing in distal third tibial fractures: distal locking screws and fracture non-union. Int Orthop 2008;32(4):547–9.

116. Drosos GI, Stavropoulos NI, Kazakos KI. Peroneal nerve damage by oblique proximal locking screw in tibial fracture nailing: a new emerging complication? Arch Orthop Trauma Surg 2007;127(6): 449–51.

117. Hems TE, Jones BG. Peroneal nerve damage associated with the proximal locking screws of the AIM tibial nail. Injury 2005;36(5):651–4 [discussion: 655].

118. Rajaesparan K, Amin A, Arora S, et al. Pseudoaneurysm of a branch of the profunda femoris artery following distal locking of an intramedullary hip nail: an unusual anatomical location. Hip Int 2008;18(3): 231–5.

119. Bose D, Hauptfleisch J, McNally M. Delayed pseudoaneurysm caused by distal locking screw of a femoral intramedullary nail: a case report. J Orthop Trauma 2006;20(8):584–6.

120. Harvey A, Thomas NP, Amis AA. Fixation of the graft in reconstruction of the anterior cruciate ligament. J Bone Joint Surg Br 2005;87(5): 593–603.

121. Colvin A, Sharma C, Parides M, et al. What is the best femoral fixation of hamstring autografts in anterior cruciate ligament reconstruction?: a meta-analysis. Clin Orthop Relat Res 2011;469(4):1075–81.

122. Suchenski M, McCarthy MB, Chowaniec D, et al. Material properties and composition of soft-tissue fixation. Arthroscopy 2010;26(6):821–31.

123. Meyers AB, Haims AH, Menn K, et al. Imaging of anterior cruciate ligament repair and its complications. AJR Am J Roentgenol 2010;194(2):476–84.

124. Hasan S, Nayyar S, Onyekwelu I, et al. Complications using bioabsorbable cross-pin femoral fixation: a case report and review of the literature. Case Rep Radiol 2011;2011:6.

125. Hall MP, Hergan DM, Sherman OH. Early fracture of a bioabsorbable tibial interference screw after ACL reconstruction with subsequent chondral injury. Orthopedics 2009;32(3):208.

126. Sumanaweera TS, Glover GH, Binford TO, et al. MR susceptibility misregistration correction. IEEE Trans Med Imaging 1993;12(2):251–9.

127. Ford JC, Wehrli FW, Chung HW. Magnetic field distribution in models of trabecular bone. Magn Reson Med 1993;30(3):373–9.

128. Stroman PW. Essentials of functional MRI. Boca Raton (FL): CRC Press; 2011.

129. Kaye GW, Laby TH. Tables of physical and chemical constants. 16th edition. Essex (England); New York: Longman; 1995.

130. Wichmann W, Von Ammon K, Fink U, et al. Aneurysm clips made of titanium: magnetic characteristics and artifacts in MR. AJNR Am J Neuroradiol 1997;18(5):939–44.

Index

Note: Page numbers of article titles are in **boldface** type.

Magn Reson Imaging Clin N Am 22 (2014) 787–790
http://dx.doi.org/10.1016/S1064-9689(14)00101-9
1064-9689/14/$ – see front matter © 2014 Elsevier Inc. All rights reserved.

mri.theclinics.com

United States Postal Service

Statement of Ownership, Management, and Circulation
(All Periodicals Publications Except Requestor Publications)

1. Publication Title	2. Publication Number	3. Filing Date
Magnetic Resonance Imaging Clinics of North America	0 1 1 - 9 0 0 9	9/14/14

4. Issue Frequency	5. Number of Issues Published Annually	6. Annual Subscription Price
Feb, May, Aug, Nov	4	$375.00

7. Complete Mailing Address of Known Office of Publication (Not printer) (Street, city, county, state, and ZIP+4®)

Elsevier Inc.
360 Park Avenue South
New York, NY 10010-1710

Contact Person
Stephen R. Bushing

Telephone (Include area code)
215-239-3688

8. Complete Mailing Address of Headquarters or General Business Office of Publisher (Not printer)

Elsevier Inc., 360 Park Avenue South, New York, NY 10010-1710

9. Full Names and Complete Mailing Addresses of Publisher, Editor, and Managing Editor (Do not leave blank)

Publisher (Name and complete mailing address)

Linda Belfus, Elsevier Inc., 1600 John F. Kennedy Blvd, Suite 1800, Philadelphia, PA 19103-2899

Editor (Name and complete mailing address)

John Vassallo, Elsevier Inc., 1600 John F. Kennedy Blvd., Suite 1800, Philadelphia, PA 19103-2899

Managing Editor (Name and complete mailing address)

Adrianne Brigido, Elsevier Inc., 1600 John F. Kennedy Blvd., Suite 1800, Philadelphia PA 19103-2899

10. Owner (Do not leave blank. If the publication is owned by a corporation, give the name and address of the corporation immediately followed by the names and addresses of all stockholders owning or holding 1 percent or more of the total amount of stock. If not owned by a corporation, give the names and addresses of the individual owners. If owned by a partnership or other unincorporated firm, give its name and address as well as those of each individual owner. If the publication is published by a nonprofit organization, give its name and address.)

Full Name	Complete Mailing Address
Wholly owned subsidiary of	1600 John F. Kennedy Blvd, Ste. 1800
Reed/Elsevier, US holdings	Philadelphia, PA 19103-2899

11. Known Bondholders, Mortgages, and Other Security Holders Owning or Holding 1 Percent or More of Total Amount of Bonds, Mortgages, or Other Securities. If none, check box ☐ None

Full Name	Complete Mailing Address
N/A	

12. Tax Status (For completion by nonprofit organizations authorized to mail at nonprofit rates) (Check one)
The purpose, function, and nonprofit status of this organization and the exempt status for federal income tax purposes:
☐ Has Not Changed During Preceding 12 Months
☐ Has Changed During Preceding 12 Months (Publisher must submit explanation of change with this statement)

13. Publication Title	14. Issue Date for Circulation Data Below
Magnetic Resonance Imaging Clinics of North America	August 2014

15. Extent and Nature of Circulation		Average No. Copies Each Issue During Preceding 12 Months	No. Copies of Single Issue Published Nearest to Filing Date
a. Total Number of Copies (Net press run)		1,528	1,793
b. Paid Circulation (By Mail and Outside the Mail)	(1) Mailed Outside-County Paid Subscriptions Stated on PS Form 3541. (Include paid distribution above nominal rate, advertiser's proof copies, and exchange copies)	1,050	1,337
	(2) Mailed In-County Paid Subscriptions Stated on PS Form 3541 (Include paid distribution above nominal rate, advertiser's proof copies, and exchange copies)		
	(3) Paid Distribution Outside the Mails Including Sales Through Dealers and Carriers, Street Vendors, Counter Sales, and Other Paid Distribution Outside USPS®	197	195
	(4) Paid Distribution by Other Classes Mailed Through the USPS (e.g. First-Class Mail®)		
c. Total Paid Distribution (Sum of 15b (1), (2), (3), and (4))		1,247	1,532
d. Free or Nominal Rate Distribution (By Mail and Outside the Mail)	(1) Free or Nominal Rate Outside-County Copies Included on PS Form 3541	68	61
	(2) Free or Nominal Rate In-County Copies Included on PS Form 3541		
	(3) Free or Nominal Rate Copies Mailed at Other Classes Through the USPS (e.g. First-Class Mail)		
	(4) Free or Nominal Rate Distribution Outside the Mail (Carriers or other means)		
e. Total Free or Nominal Rate Distribution (Sum of 15d (1), (2), (3) and (4))		68	61
f. Total Distribution (Sum of 15c and 15e)		1,315	1,593
g. Copies not Distributed (See instructions to publishers #4 (page #3))		213	200
h. Total (Sum of 15f and g)		1,528	1,793
i. Percent Paid (15c divided by 15f times 100)		94.83%	96.17%

16. Total circulation includes electronic copies. Report circulation on PS Form 3526-X worksheet.

17. Publication of Statement of Ownership
If the publication is a general publication, publication of this statement is required. Will be printed in the November 2014 issue of this publication.

18. Signature and Title of Editor, Publisher, Business Manager, or Owner

Stephen R. Bushing – Inventory Distribution Coordinator

Date September 14, 2014

I certify that all information furnished on this form is true and complete. I understand that anyone who furnishes false or misleading information on this form or who omits material or information requested on the form may be subject to criminal sanctions (including fines and imprisonment) and/or civil sanctions (including civil penalties).

PS Form 3526, August 2012 (Page 1 of 3 (Instructions Page 3)) PSN 7530-01-000-9931 PRIVACY NOTICE: See our Privacy policy in www.usps.com

PS Form 3526, August 2012 (Page 2 of 3)

Moving?

Make sure your subscription moves with you!

To notify us of your new address, find your **Clinics Account Number** (located on your mailing label above your name), and contact customer service at:

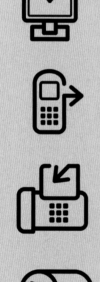

Email: journalscustomerservice-usa@elsevier.com

800-654-2452 (subscribers in the U.S. & Canada)
314-447-8871 (subscribers outside of the U.S. & Canada)

Fax number: 314-447-8029

Elsevier Health Sciences Division
Subscription Customer Service
3251 Riverport Lane
Maryland Heights, MO 63043

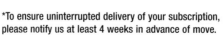